In

e

Reproduction, Obstet

y

Integrated Clinical Science

Reproduction, Obstetrics and Gynaecology

Edited by

M G Elder, MD FRCS (Edin) FRCOG

Professor of Obstetrics and Gynaecology, Institute of Obstetrics and Gynaecology, Royal Postgraduate Medical School, Hammersmith Hospital, London

Heinemann Professional Publishing

Heinemann Medical Books

An imprint of Heinemann Professional Publishing Ltd
Halley Court, Jordan Hill, Oxford OX2 8EJ

OXFORD LONDON MELBOURNE AUCKLAND

First published 1988
© M G Elder 1988

British Library Cataloguing in Publication Data

Elder, M. G.
Reproduction, obstetrics and gynaecology.
1. Gynaecology and obstetrics
I. Title   II. Series
618

ISBN 0 433 16609 6

Photoset by Wilmaset, Birkenhead, Wirral
Printed and bound in Great Britain by
Butler & Tanner Ltd., Frome

Contents

Contributors

M Afnan MBBS MRCOG
Senior Registrar in Obstetrics and Gynaecology
St Helier Hospital
Carshalton

Harold Bourne FRCPsych
Consultant in Child and Family Psychiatry
Charing Cross Hospital, London;
Consultant Psychotherapist
Connolly Unit
Ealing Hospital
London

Ian Burn FRCS (Eng)
Honorary Consulting Surgeon
Charing Cross Hospital
London

Michael Darling MRCOG
Master
Rotunda Hospital
Dublin

D Keith Edmonds MB ChB MRCOG FRACOG
Consultant Obstetrician and Gynaecologist
Queen Charlotte's and Chelsea
Hospital for Women
London

M G Elder MD FRCS (Edin) FRCOG
Professor of Obstetrics and Gynaecology
Institute of Obstetrics and Gynaecology
Royal Postgraduate Medical School
Hammersmith Hospital
London

D Glance BSc PhD
Research Assistant
Institute of Obstetrics and Gynaecology
Royal Postgraduate Medical School
Hammersmith Hospital
London

D F Hawkins DSc FRCOG
Professor of Obstetric Therapeutics
Institute of Obstetrics and Gynaecology
Hammersmith Hospital
London

Stephen G Hillier MSc PhD
Senior Lecturer and Director
Lothian Health Board Reproductive
Endocrinology Laboratory
University of Edinburgh Centre for
Reproductive Biology

Lennox Kane BA MD MRCOG
Consultant Obstetrician and Gynaecologist
St Albans and Hemel Hempstead

Richard J Lilford PhD MRCP MRCOG
Professor of Obstetrics and Gynaecology
St James' University Hospital
Leeds

K B Lim MRCOG
Consultant in Obstetrics and Gynaecology

Norman McWhinney BA FRCS MRCOG
Consultant Obstetrician and Gynaecologist
St Helier Hospital
Carshalton

Norman Morris MD FRCOG
Emeritus Professor of Obstetrics and
Gynaecology
University of London

Philip J Steer BSc MD MRCOG
Senior Lecturer in Obstetrics and Gynaecology
St Mary's Hospital Medical School
London

Beverley Webb FRCS MRCOG LRCP
Consultant Obstetrician and Gynaecologist
Lister Hospital
Stevenage

Andrew G L Whitelaw MD FRCP
Consultant Neonatologist
Hammersmith Hospital
London

Gordon Williams MS FRCS
Consultant Urologist
Hammersmith Hospital;
Honorary Senior Lecturer
Royal Postgraduate Medical School
University of London

Integrated Clinical Science

Series Editor

George P McNicol MD Phd FRCP
(Lond, Edin, Glasg) FRCPath Hon FACP

Principal and Vice Chancellor, University of Aberdeen. Lately Professor of Medicine, The University of Leeds, and Head, The University Department of Medicine, The General Infirmary, Leeds

Advisory Editors

Professor A S Douglas
Department of Medicine, University of Aberdeen

Pathology: Professor C C Bird
Institute of Pathology
University of Leeds

Physiology: Professor P H Fentem
Department of Physiology and
Pharmacology
Nottingham University

Biochemistry: Dr R M Denton
Reader in Biochemistry
University of Bristol

Anatomy: Professor R L Holmes
Department of Anatomy
University of Leeds

Pharmacology: Professor A M Breckenridge
Department of Clinical
Pharmacology
Liverpool University

Other titles:

Cardiovascular Disease*
J R Hampton

Endocrinology
C R W Edwards

Gastroenterology
P Jones, P Brunt,
N A G Mowat

Haematology*
J C Crawley

Musculoskeletal Disease*
V Wright
R Dickson

Nephro-urology
A W Asscher
D B Moffat

Neurology
R W Ross Russell

Psychiatry*
J L Gibbons

Respiratory Disease
G M Sterling

*ELBS low-priced edition also available.

Preface

Within medicine technological innovation has allowed great progress to be made in diagnosis and therapy.

Obstetrics and gynaecology has been no exception, so that within the last decade there have been considerable advances. These include the big improvement in antenatal diagnosis of fetal abnormalities, employing ultrasound and procedures like fetoscopy and chorion villus sampling. This, in turn, allows cytogenetics and molecular biology to make their contributions to the diagnosis and treatment.

The management of high risk pregnancy with a more positive approach to early delivery is producing better survival rates and, in our opinion, lower morbidity rates among low birth weight infants.

The management of gynaecological cancer, particularly ovarian, has become surgically more aggressive, and use of increasing numbers of new cytotoxic drugs has increased survival significantly. The appreciation of the value of colposcopy and laser therapy for cervical intraepithelial disease is coping with the big increase in this condition. The realisation of the need for meticulous surgical techniques for the treatment of tubal disease and the development of in vitro fertilisation has improved the lot of some infertile couples. The latter technique provides an important foundation from which the molecular basis of embryonic development can be determined. These are but a few of the major developments during the last ten years in a specialty which is changing at an increasing rate on all fronts. The next ten years will see bigger increases in our knowledge, and so changes in therapy will evolve as basic science is increasingly applied to the problems of obstetrics and gynaecology.

However, despite such scientific development, the cornerstone of good treatment will always remain clinical acumen based on a sympathetic relationship with the patient, accurate history taking, careful, systematic clinical examination and, very importantly, good communication with the patient and, if necessary, relatives. No amount of science will replace these, and without the foundations of good clinical practice many of the benefits of science will be lost.

The purpose of this book is to provide the reader with an understanding of most of clinical obstetrics and gynaecology, together with some of its underlying scientific basis, with particular emphasis on reproduction.

M G Elder

June, 1988

Introduction

The Practice of Obstetrics and Gynaecology

Obstetrics and gynaecology is concerned with problems of health which are specific to women. Inevitably, many of these problems relate to reproductive issues such as pregnancy, fertility and to sexuality. Obstetrics and gynaecology is, therefore, a rather special and more intimate form of medical practice in which psychosocial as well as physical factors play an important role in the aetiology of ill health.

For this reason, the student of obstetrics and gynaecology needs to have a sound knowledge of women's psychology as well as of anatomy, physiology and biochemistry. At the same time, it is now well established that changes in biochemistry can have a significant influence upon a woman's behaviour and personality. This link between biochemistry and psychology—psychoneuroendrocrinology—illustrates the futility of drawing too fine a distinction between mind and body, since at most times the brain and body are working in an intimate and carefully coordinated relationship. Ill health only arises when psyche or soma are subject to acute or chronic environmental stresses that are beyond their tolerance.

For many years now, traditional medical practice has concentrated its attention upon the physical aspects of male and female ill health. Sadly, the specialty of obstetrics and gynaecology has fallen into the same trap. However, at last there are signs that we are becoming more aware of the psychosocial factors that influence women's health, and it is now increasingly accepted that a holistic approach to the care of women must be adopted.

Students of obstetrics and gynaecology must, therefore, acquaint themselves with the evolution of female psychology during the important phases of childhood, puberty, the reproductive years, the menopause and, finally, old age.

Obtaining a history inevitably involves exploration of sensitive issues related to social status, sexuality, reproduction and sexual experience. It is essential that these matters should be elucidated with tact, patience and understanding. Equally, it must be appreciated that the gynaecological examination is also quite different from other forms of investigation, since in some ways it can be regarded as a form of rape. For this reason, the examination of the vagina needs to be carried out with a special awareness of the embarrassment and the emotional stress that may be involved. This is yet another example of the 'intimate' nature of our specialty.

In particular, obstetrics and gynaecology is concerned with prevention and with very early diagnosis. The steady evolution of antenatal care started with the work of Pinard in France, followed at the very beginning of this century in Scotland by that of Ballantyne. Antenatal care is a classic example of effective and now quite sophisticated preventive medicine.

Pregnancy involves a complex sequence of profound changes throughout a woman's body—every system is involved. Parallel with these physical changes, significant emotional reactions also occur.

Women now receive most careful observation and support throughout their pregnancy. This includes the use of ultrasound, pioneered by Ian Donald in Glasgow, which allows fetal development to be followed throughout the course of pregnancy. As a consequence of effective antenatal care there has been a dramatic fall in maternal and perinatal mortality and morbidity. However, there is still some reluctance to acknowledge the effect that psychosocial stress may have upon the physical course of pregnancy. For example, there remains a very high perinatal mortality in unsupported women in the social class V category. Little, so far, has been done to examine or relieve the environmental stress factors that may be involved in these perinatal deaths.

Inevitably, labour is an experience involving major stress for most women. Modern treatment leads to higher rates of interference which do appear to contribute to lower perinatal death rates. Pain relief is more effective because of the greater use of epidural anaesthesia, but this, in turn, has increased the incidence of forceps delivery.

On the other hand, it is questionable whether the emotional needs of women are met as well as they should be. Labour wards remain tense, noisy, anxious places where intimacy and silence are both very hard to find, and where the constant bustle leaves little opportunity to establish rapport or to provide support and comfort. And yet, effective emotional support is an essential requirement throughout the whole course of labour.

Our policy of prevention and early diagnosis also extends to the field of gynaecology. For example, by regular cervical smears, it is possible to identify precancerous lesions of the cervix which can be treated at an early stage with little or no risk to the woman. In this way, malignant invasion is avoided.

The investigation and relief of infertility constitutes another area where we have a major commitment. The reasons for infertility are various, but the recent introduction of in vitro fertilisation (IVF) and gamete intrafallopian transfer (GIFT) have opened up new areas of hope for the infertile couple.

Finally, we are now much more actively concerned with helping women who have particular problems at, or following, the menopause, which are either physical or emotional, or most often a complex mixture of the two.

In all these areas, powerful emotional reactions are involved, and slowly we are becoming more aware of the psychological support that we need to provide. For example, in several units, specially trained counsellors are now involved with infertility as well as with menopause clinics. It is to be hoped that trained counsellors will eventually be present in all gynaecological departments. Many women who attend gynaecological clinics may have no recognisable physical problem; their symptoms are, in fact, related to recent emotional problems of a domestic or psychosocial nature. Counselling will help them to face and adapt to these problems and, eventually, their symptoms will be relieved—at least for the time being.

From these observations it should be clear that to practice obstetrics and gynaecology the student needs to be acquainted with the sensitivities, the hopes and aspirations, the embarrassments and setbacks that form the basis of women's emotional response. These reactions vary considerably from woman to woman, and this variation must be accepted and respected. At all times, a judgemental approach must be avoided. It also has to be realised that quite often it will not be easy to define the border between normal and abnormal.

Above all, good doctors in any specialty must be patient listeners and when, after the examination, conclusions have been reached, then their not inconsiderable authority must be used to sustain the women's hope, confidence and courage.

Young medical men and women, and many older ones as well, often fail to appreciate, that, in the end, the most effective therapeutic aid that we have at our command is the power of our mind. This power, in turn, is dependent upon the establishment of an effective rapport between the doctor and the patient, which inevitably takes time to establish, but once established, can sustain miracles—or at least what sometimes passes as miracles.

Norman Morris   *June, 1988*
Emeritus Professor of Obstetrics and Gynaecology
University of London

1

Approach to the Patient

Patients approach a doctor in the hope of a cure for their ills. Diagnosis is the first stage of the process, and is both a science and an art. The *science* is the reasoning which promotes the correct conclusions based on the facts assimilated from a good history and clinical examination, including the assessment of both positive and negative findings. The *art* is the skilful collection of these facts, and is learned and mastered only with much practice. All diagnoses are based on the three firm foundations of history, physical signs and the results of necessary investigations. The first two of these will be considered in more detail.

THE HISTORY

History taking is of paramount importance. The ability to obtain a good history is partly based on instruction, partly imitative and partly acquired by experience.

It is essential to hear the woman's story in her own words in order to learn the exact nature of her complaints. Each individual symptom should be dealt with in detail; the date and mode of onset, subsequent progression, exacerbating and relieving factors, previous treatment, etc. The symptom of pain must always be carefully considered and its site, nature, severity, duration, frequency, periodicity, radiation and relation to menses, micturition, defaecation and fetal movements, should all be recorded. She should not be allowed to leapfrog from one symptom to another before a complete account of each individual symptom has been rendered. Leading questions should be kept to a minimum, but may be necessary to elucidate the full story in a logical pattern. Direct questions may yield important information quickly, but should not suggest an answer. Once the voluntary history is complete, direct questioning is used for the assessment of the remaining systems and the student

should be familiar with the essential questions for each system.

Having dealt with the general aspects of history taking which are applicable to any specialty, the woman with gynaecological symptoms will now be specifically considered.

History of the Gynaecological Patient

Many women of differing age, social class and culture find it difficult to discuss gynaecological and sexual matters. The doctor must adopt a tactful, understanding and unhurried approach to gain the full confidence of the patient. It is often best to obtain general information first such as age, marital status, number of children, obstetric, family and social history, to allow the woman time to settle. She should then be encouraged to tell the story in her own words with gentle guidance to encourage the taciturn and direct the garrulous. As with all clinical documentation, the details should be recorded in a clear, precise manner.

Presenting complaint(s)

Often there are two or more symptoms and these should be enumerated to allow the doctor a clear picture in his/her mind of the facts which must subsequently be recorded in more detail. It is useful to note how long the symptoms have been present and record them in the woman's own words: (1) heavy periods for 6 months; (2) vaginal discharge for 3 years; (3) heavy feeling down below for 5 years. It is often of value to note which symptom is the most troublesome.

History of presenting complaints. Each symptom enumerated above should now be dealt with in detail and interrelated to each other and/or bodily functions where appropriate, e.g. pelvic pain and menstruation; uterovaginal prolapse and urinary symptoms. The features of any pain should be recorded as previously outlined.

Remaining gynaecological history

The following points should also be elicited as they will cast further light on the presenting symptoms or will bring out other possible problems:

1. Date of onset of last menstrual period, if not already noted.
2. Duration of menstruation.
3. Amount of blood loss — this may be recorded in terms of heavy, average or light, or by the amount of protection required.
4. The presence or absence of clots in the menstrual loss.
5. Length and regularity of menstrual cycle.
6. Age of menarche.
7. Age of menopause.
8. Dysmenorrhoea (pelvic pain associated with menstruation) — premenstrual, menstrual or both; site of the discomfort; severity; radiation; associated nausea; previous treatment.
9. Breast discomfort associated with menstruation.
10. Intermenstrual bleeding.
11. Postcoital bleeding.
12. Dyspareunia (pain on intercourse) — superficial (i.e. discomfort at the introitus or vaginal walls) or deep (i.e. pelvic pain experienced on full penetration of the penis).
13. Vaginal discharge — timing in relation to menstrual cycle; duration; character; amount; odour; irritation.
14. Pruritus — vulval irritation or itch.
15. Climacteric symptoms — hot flushes; dry vagina; irritability; insomnia; etc.
16. Contraception.
17. Urinary symptoms — frequency; dysuria; incontinence — stress or urge; nocturia; haematuria.
18. Bowel function — frequency; consistency and colour of stool; straining, pain on defaecation; blood or mucus per rectum.

PHYSICAL EXAMINATION

The thought of a physical examination is likely to cause anxiety due to embarassment and the fear of discomfort or pain. This is especially true for pelvic examination which is always performed last. The obstetrician/gynaecologist should approach the examination of the woman in a reassuring and gentle manner, remembering that she is not simply a carrier of pelvic organs but an entire human entity. An assessment of her general physical condition is required to provide valuable information as a background to her local pelvic condition. It is often of value to explain what is being done at each stage of the examination and to give a warning of anything which might be unexpected, such as pressure of the examining hand on the abdomen, the temperature of the bell of the stethoscope, vaginal speculum, etc.

An attendant nurse is essential during the examination. She can reassure the woman and, by allaying her fears, help her to relax. The nurse can also verify the correctness of the examination should the need ever arise in a medico-legal inquiry.

Ideally, the woman should be shown into an examination room. If this is not possible, she is left with the nurse to prepare for examination, which includes removal of all her clothes, although for antenatal appointments, this is unnecessary. A gown allowing easy access for examination should be available or she should be placed supine on a couch with two sheets covering her, one across the upper half of her body and the other across the lower half. This allows exposure of the part of the body to be examined, yet maintains a degree of modesty.

The order of examination will vary from one doctor to another, and the student should decide for him/herself which system to adopt and adhere to it thereafter. An orderly, logical approach will avoid missing important signs. On the other hand, the methods for elucidating clinical signs have stood the test of time and the student should be attentive in learning the correct methods from his/her peers. Inspection, touching, palpation and hearing are the cornerstones of physical examination. Leonardo's motto was *Sapere vedere* — learn to see things. As the woman walks into the examination room, an impression of height, weight, gait and body posture (kyphosis, lordosis) can be gained.

Examination of Head and Neck

The woman's facies, e.g. pallid, florid, cyanotic, is noted and the mucous membranes checked for the presence of anaemia. The eyes are observed for any suggestion of exophthalmos and any change in colour of the sclera. Any loss of normal texture, brittleness or excessive dryness of the hair should also be recorded. Lymphadenopathy is always important and the glands of the supraclavicular region, anterior and posterior triangles of the neck are examined. The thyroid gland is gently examined for asymmetry, enlargement or other irregularities, remembering that a slight, diffuse enlargement may occur in pregnancy. The tongue, tonsils and teeth require inspection, the latter being particularly important in pregnancy as any caries present will almost certainly worsen as pregnancy advances.

Examination of the Breasts

Breast examination is important in both obstetric and gynaecological examinations and should never be omitted. The breasts are first inspected with the patient sitting upright, her arms by her side. Their size, shape, and position of the nipples are compared. Prominent veins, retracted nipples, discharge from the nipples and prominent Montgomery's tubercles in the primary areola are noted. The woman is then asked to raise her arms above her head and the features outlined above are again checked. Any indentation or bulge in the contour of the breast or retraction of a nipple may indicate underlying pathology. The axillae are next examined, but this is only satisfactorily achieved if the pectoral muscles are relaxed. The woman should rest her forearm on the examiner's arm while the axilla is carefully palpated. She is then placed supine and the breast itself gently palpated with the flat portion of the fingers. This should be done systematically, starting with the upper inner quadrant and finishing with the upper outer quadrant. Finally, the nipple should be palpated and gently squeezed to release any secretion which might be present.

Examination of the Abdomen

In order to examine the abdomen properly, both the woman and the examiner must adopt the correct position. The former should be placed supine, as flat as is tolerable, with her arms at her sides. The examiner should be seated or on one knee, so that

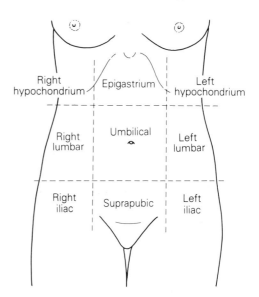

Fig. 1.1 *The regions of the abdomen.*

even pressure may be applied with the flat of the hand. The abdomen should be examined in sequence and is best divided into nine imaginary portions (Fig. 1.1). The sequence for the examination is inspection, palpation, percussion and auscultation.

Inspection allows assessment of the condition of the abdominal wall, and size and contour of the abdomen. Previous surgical wounds are noted as are any motile phenomena, such as movement with respiration, visible peristalsis or pulsation.

Palpation is performed gently, noting the presence of superficial or deep tenderness and any rigidity of the abdominal wall. If pain is a presenting symptom, palpation should commence in the diagonally opposite region, so that the area of pain is palpated last. The viscera should be checked for enlargement of liver, spleen and kidneys, and abnormal masses are noted, specifically those arising from the pelvic viscera — bladder, uterus, ovaries. Site, size, shape, contour, consistency and mobility are recorded. Hernial orifices should be checked routinely.

Percussion may add confirmatory information in the case of enlarged viscera and tumours and is the only technique in most patients for establishing the presence of ascites.

Auscultation is used to confirm the presence and nature of bowel sounds.

It should be emphasised that abdominal examination is an essential part of the gynaecological examination and should never be omitted. Occasionally, a tumour arising from a pelvic viscus is only palpable per abdomen and it is not unknown for uterovaginal prolapse to be caused by the raised intra-abdominal pressure of ascites or an ovarian cyst.

The foregoing is of necessity a superficial and incomplete account of the general medical examination of a patient. However, the obstetrician/gynaecologist must be capable of performing such an examination correctly. Coexisting conditions will affect his/her patient throughout pregnancy or influence the anaesthetic and postoperative risks of the woman requiring surgery for a gynaecological complaint. No one can be expert at everything, but a proper examination allows for appropriate referral for advice. Examination of the respiratory, cardiovascular and nervous systems have been omitted and reference should be made to a textbook of medicine. The importance of neurological examination must never be forgotten. The woman presenting to the gynaecological clinic with urinary incontinence and is found to have saddle anaesthesia is most unlikely to have a gynaecological cause for her complaint.

The Pelvic Examination

As previously mentioned, the pelvic examination must be approached by the examiner in a reassuring and gentle manner in order to allow the woman to relax as much as possible. Adequate palpation of the pelvic viscera is extremely difficult, if not impossible, when the abdominal and pelvic musculature is contracted.

There are several positions which can be employed for the pelvic examination and each has its adherents for many and differing reasons. Only the two most commonly used will be described here.

The full dorsal position. This is the most commonly used position. The woman is place supine with the hips flexed and abducted as fully as possible, the knees flexed and the ankles or soles of the feet in apposition. The woman will feel much less exposed if the lower abdomen and upper thighs are covered with a sheet. This is the best position for inspection of the vulva, visualisation of the cervix with a bivalve speculum and for bimanual palpation of the uterus, fallopian tubes and ovaries. It is

of less value than the lateral position for inspection of the vagina and assessing uterovaginal prolapse.

Modified Sim's or left lateral position. The woman is placed on her left side and near the edge of the examining couch. The left leg is kept straight, extended at the knee, while the right hip and knee are fully flexed so that the leg is over the abdomen. It is valuable if the nurse can help support the right leg at the knee and also gently retract the right buttock upwards. The anus, perineum and posterior vulva can be inspected and, using a Sim's speculum, the vagina is easily visualised. This is the best position for assessing uterovaginal prolapse. Bimanual examination is possible, but not as satisfactory as with the woman in the dorsal position.

Inspection of vulva and perineum

Adequate lighting must be available for this part of the examination. Points to note are local hair growth; the state of the skin — erythema, excoriation, rashes; ulceration; tumours; development of external genitalia — hypotrophic or hypertrophic labia, clitoral hypertrophy; presence of excessive vaginal discharge; presence of haemorrhoids; and general appearance of the perineum, especially with any previous vaginal delivery. The woman is asked to strain down to detect any evidence of uterovaginal prolapse.

Speculum examination

Speculum examination is required to allow inspection of the vaginal tissues and cervix, and to assess any degree of uterovaginal prolapse. The woman should be told what is happening at each stage of the examination. The index finger and thumb of the left hand are used to gently separate the labia minora to expose the vestibule. The speculum, which should be at body temperature and slightly lubricated, is gently inserted in an oblique position and in a cephalad and posterior direction with a gentle rotating action to bring it to lie in the transverse axis of the vagina. A speculum should not be inserted with its blade(s) in the axis of the vulval cleft as pressure on the urethra and clitoral region is painful. The blades of a bivalve speculum should only be opened when the instrument is fully inserted. The woman can be told as the examiner gently opens the blades of the speculum that she might experience a little pressure. The cervix is usually easily visualised. If a cervical smear is required, it should be taken at this stage. Opinions differ as to whether the speculum should be lubricated when a smear is required, but it is our opinion that a little lubrication never causes problems in obtaining an adequate cervical sample and enhances patient comfort and continuing cooperation.

The cervix is inspected for size, colour, contour, evidence of previous damage, eversion, infection, polyps and discharge from the canal. The finding of an irregular, injected, granular-looking cervix requires further diagnosis by cytology and possibly colposcopy.

The speculum is then withdrawn slowly and the vaginal walls inspected as they come into view. Colour, erythema, petechiae, ulcerations and adherent discharge are noted. If the woman has been examined in the dorsal position, an impression of the degree of any uterovaginal prolapse may be formed if she is asked to bear down as the speculum is removed. If prolapse is present, the woman may then be examined in the modified Sim's position using a Sim's speculum and the degree of prolapse assessed more accurately.

If vaginal infection is suspected, swabs for culture are obtained from the posterior vaginal fornix and the endocervical canal during the speculum examination. A urethral swab is also sometimes of value and should be taken once the speculum has been removed.

Bimanual vaginal examination

It should be stressed that this part of the examination requires two hands, each assuming equal importance. Most gynaecologists use their gloved right hand for the vaginal examination and the left as the abdominal counterpart. After the labia minora have been parted using the left hand, one finger of the lubricated gloved hand is introduced, passing upwards and backwards. As previously mentioned, pressure on the posterior vaginal wall and rectum is much less uncomfortable than pressure on the urethra and anterior vaginal wall. Once the woman has started to relax the muscles around the vagina, and it is clear that vaginal capacity is adequate, a second finger may be gently introduced. Slight pressure exerted by the abdominal hand brings the pelvic viscera into easier reach of the vaginal fingers.

The cervix is palpated for size, consistency,

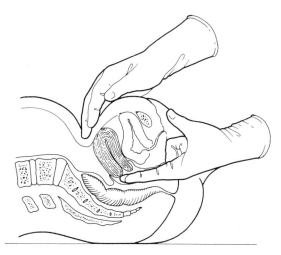

Fig. 1.2 *Bimanual examination, step 1. Two fingers are gently inserted into the vagina. The consistency and symmetry of the cervix are noted. The uterus is then elevated towards the abdominal wall to enable the size of the uterus to be ascertained. (Modified from A.S. Duncan, 1955. In British Gynaecological Practice, 1st edn., A. Bourne, ed. Philadelphia: Davis.)*

contour, lateral lacerations and mobility. It should be moved in both anteroposterior and lateral directions to ascertain that such movement causes no discomfort (Fig. 1.2) If there is sharp pelvic pain related to cervical movement, this is called excitation pain.

The uterus must then be palpated between the hand on the abdomen and the fingers in the vagina. The vaginal fingers should move the cervix backwards to rotate the fundus of the uterus downwards and forwards. The abdominal hand is placed just below the umbilicus and gradually moved lower until the fundus is caught against the fingers in the anterior fornix (Fig. 1.3) If the uterus remains impalpable, then it is in a retroverted position and may be felt by the vaginal fingers when placed in the posterior fornix (Fig. 1.4) The uterine size, shape, contour, regularity, consistency and mobility are noted, along with any tenderness.

The abdominal hand is now moved to the left iliac fossa and the vaginal fingers to the left lateral fornix (Fig. 1.5). This allows palpation of the left adnexa. Features such as thickening, tenderness, ovarian outline, mobility, and the presence of a mass should be noted. The procedure is then repeated on the right side. It should be noted that normal fallopian tubes are rarely, if ever, palpable and often normal ovaries are not felt.

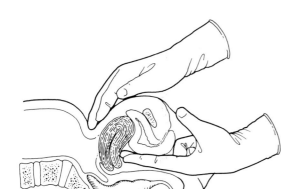

Fig. 1.3   *Bimanual examination, step 2. The vaginal fingers are moved into the anterior fornix and the body of the uterus is palpated. Size, contour, consistency and mobility are noted.*

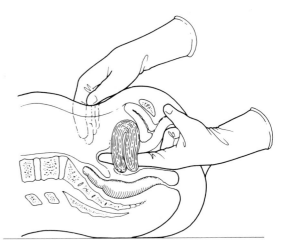

Fig. 1.5   *Bimanual examination, step 4. The vaginal fingers are moved to one of the lateral fornices and the abdominal fingers are moved towards the ipsilateral iliac fossa. The two are then approximated as closely as possible and the intervening tube and ovary palpated.*

Rectal examination

Rectal examination may replace vaginal examination in children or in adults who are *virgo intacta*. It can prove a useful adjunct to vaginal examination, especially in the assessment of the uterosacral ligaments, pouch of Douglas and outer portions of the broad ligaments. Occasionally, a combined rectovaginal examination, with the index finger in the vagina and the middle finger in the rectum, is of value for assessing lesions of the rectovaginal septum or bowel.

COMMUNICATION

When the examination is complete, the woman dresses and there should then follow an explanation, in terms that can be understood, of the findings, the diagnosis and its implications and any investigations or treatment that are required. It is well known that much of what a doctor tells a patient is immediately forgotten and some points may require reiteration. She should then be encouraged to ask questions and these should be answered patiently, honestly and clearly. There will be times when the news is not good and such situations will be briefly considered further with both patient and doctor in mind.

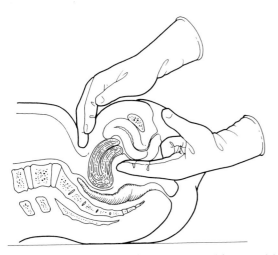

Fig. 1.4   *Bimanual examination, step 3. If the tips of the vaginal and abdominal fingers meet when performing step 2, it can be concluded that the uterus is retroverted or, less commonly, axial. The vaginal fingers are then moved to the posterior fornix. Contour, symmetry, consistency and mobility of the corpus uteri are assessed.*

Bimanual examination should impose no significant discomfort. If a painful lesion is encountered, extreme gentleness is required and the woman must never feel that she has been needlessly hurt by the examination.

The Approach to Difficult Situations

Situations arise in every practitioner's lifetime when events will be difficult for both doctor and patient to discuss. Obstetric and gynaecological practice is no exception. What should be done when an ultrasound examination reveals an abnormal fetus? How should we deal with the parents whose baby has died in the first few days of life or has survived with a congenital anomaly or has suffered cerebral damage? Should we tell the truth to the woman with gynaecological malignancy? Views on these subjects vary greatly among all those concerned with patient care and among patients themselves. Only a brief consideration is possible here, but may provide an introduction for further thought.

The ability of the doctor to provide comfort while imparting bad news will, to a large extent, depend on the doctor's own reactions and feelings. The art of communication with the dying patient remains a difficult and uncertain area, often inducing insecurity and anxiety, and may lead to doing nothing in such a situation. Such feelings may be enhanced by a fear of being blamed by the patient as the cause of her illness, rather than acceptance as the healer, soother or comforter. A patient's reaction to bad news is often difficult to predict, and the need for knowledge of how to deal with the consequences of the news we break to an individual enshrines a universal criterion of all medical practice. Fear of expressing emotion may also prove restricting, as all our clinical training is directed to encourage a calm approach, even in emergencies, and to stifle any emotional response invoked by the situation or the individual patient. It is necessary to learn to show sincere sympathy. Junior doctors commonly express the fear of incomplete knowledge, and not knowing all the answers is a real handicap when facing difficult situations. All confidence can be totally undermined. While ignorance should not be condoned, it is worth remembering that often the patient realises that the answers to his/her questions are unknown, or even does not want the answers, but simply needs someone to listen. The skill of talking to patients about difficult matters is an acquired talent. Those who do it often and do it well, should be encouraged to teach the rest of us. Guidance as to how to relate to parents suffering bereavement due to loss of pregnancy or a child is given in Chapter 15.

The aim in all these situations is broadly to provide the best possible degree of health for the woman in mind and body. This requires patience and commitment by all those involved and perhaps reflects the vocational element of 'medical' practice.

FURTHER READING

Jenkins D. (1986). *Listening to the Gynaecological Patient's Problems*. London: Springer Verlag.

2

The Reproductive Organs: Structure and Function

EMBRYOLOGY

Ovary

Primitive germ cells are first apparent in the endoderm of the yolk sac from which they migrate to the gut and through the mesentery to the genital ridge on the medial aspect of the mesonephros. The primitive gonad consists of the thickened coelomic epithelium of the genital ridge, the underlying mesoderm and the germ cells (oogonia). By 5–6 weeks, the epithelium has grown inwards as a series of gonadal cords. Further development of these cords obliterates the mesenchymal elements. The epithelial elements and oogonia proliferate vigorously up to 14 weeks; the predominance of cortical tissue distinguishes the early ovary from the testis. From this stage, stromal cells develop from the mesenchyme in the hilum and spread peripherally. When the process is complete, the primary oocytes are surrounded by a ring of epithelial granulosa cells embedded in the stroma. The identity of the gonad is apparent by 7 weeks in the testis and a little later in the ovary.

During the process of formation of the primary oocytes, the germ cells enter the diplotene stage of the prophase of the first meiotic division. They remain in this stage until ovulation occurs, which may be decades later. The number of germ cells reaches a maximum of 7 million in each ovary at 15–20 weeks, falling to 2 million at birth and 400 000 by puberty.

The early ovary is attached to the inguinal fold and uterus by a fibromuscular band, the gubernaculum, along which it is drawn to its definitive site. The cranial part of the gubernaculum becomes the ovarian ligament and the caudal part becomes the round ligament. The lower end of the gubernaculum is associated with a peritoneal projection, the processus vaginalis, which may persist in the labia majora as the canal of Nuck.

Uterus and Fallopian Tubes

The paramesonephric (müllerian) duct develops on the lateral aspect of the mesonephros at 5–6 weeks and extends caudally to reach the urogenital sinus at 9 weeks (müllerian tubercle). At 8 weeks both the müllerian and the wolffian ducts are present and sex differentiation begins. In the female, the wolffian ducts degenerate due to a lack of testosterone. The lower portion of the müllerian ducts fuse to form the uterus and cervix, while the upper portions remain separate as the fallopian tubes. In the male, the müllerian system degenerates under the influence of a glycoprotein inhibitory factor from the Sertoli cells of the testis; the 'müllerian inhibiting factor', which is locally active. Remnants of the wolffian duct system may be evident as cysts in the vagina (Gartner's duct) or the broad ligament (parovarian cysts).

Vagina

Paired sinovaginal bulbs on the posterior aspect of the urogenital sinus fuse with the lower end of the müllerian ducts to form the vaginal plate. This consists of solid epithelium which grows rapidly and then becomes canalised at 16–18 weeks.

External Genitalia

The primitive cloaca becomes divided by a transverse septum which fuses with the cloacal membrane at 7 weeks. The anterior part is the urogenital sinus, and on the external surface there is a conical projection, the genital tubercle. Proliferation of the mesoderm leads to formation of the genital folds medially and the genital swellings laterally. At this point, 10 weeks, male and female development is identical.

Normal female development does not depend on gonadal hormones: instead, it is a 'neuter' state, which occurs in the absence of the testis. The testis has three endocrine effects: (1) secretion of müllerian inhibiting factor; (2) secretion of testosterone which directly promotes wolffian development; and (3) secretion of testosterone which is converted to dihydrotestosterone by 5–α–reductase in the external genitalia and promotes male development at this site.

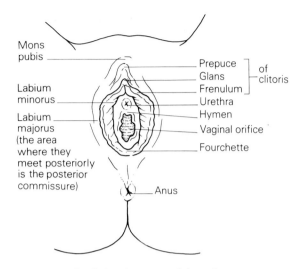

Fig. 2.2 *Anatomy of the vulva.*

ANATOMY

A simplified diagram of the female reproductive organs in shown in Fig. 2.1.

Vulva

The vulva comprises the mons pubis, the labia majora and minora and the clitoris and overlaps with the vaginal vestibule (Fig. 2.2).

Before puberty, the *mons pubis* is flat, the labia majora are small and the vaginal orifice is virtually occluded by the hymen.

At puberty, the fatty pad of the mons pubis develops, labia majora and minora enlarge considerably, the vaginal orifice becomes bigger and the hymen provides a partial barrier to the vagina.

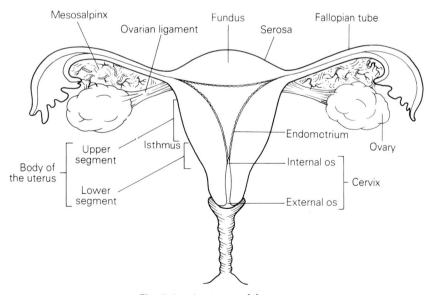

Fig. 2.1 *Anatomy of the uterus.*

Pubic hair grows with the upper margin being the upper edge of the mons pubis.

Labia majora

The labia majora form the lateral boundary of the vulva and extend from the mons pubis to the perineum. Their medial aspects consist of stratified squamous epithelium with hair follicles, a thin layer of smooth muscle (tunica dartos), a layer of fascia, adipose tissue and large numbers of sweat and sebaceous glands. They contain numerous nerve endings, some of which are free (pain sensitive), while others are in the form of corpuscles (e.g. Meissner). The nerve supply comes from the abdomen — the ilioinguinal and genitofemoral nerves; the buttocks — the posterior femoral cutaneous nerves; and the pelvis — the pudendal nerves. The arterial supply comes from the internal and external pudendal arteries which form a circular rete. The venous drainage forms a plexus with extensive anastomoses to surrounding areas. During pregnancy, these veins can become very distended, causing a vulval varicocele. If damaged at delivery, severe haemorrhage will occur. The lymphatic drainage is to the superficial subinguinal nodes, thence to the deep subinguinal nodes and the external iliac chain. The deeper tissues of the labia majora, together with the posterior third of the skin drain both anteriorly along the route described and posteriorly to the rectal lymphatic plexus and thence to the internal iliac chain.

The lymphatic drainage of squamous carcinoma of the vulva, and its spread to the inguinal glands should allow it to be readily detected. A radical vulvectomy for treatment of carcinoma of the vulva involves block dissection of the inguinal and occasionally the external iliac glands.

Labia minora

Labia minora are the folds of skin that overlap the vaginal vestibule. They split anteriorly to form two portions: one forming a hood or covering for the clitoris (prepuce) and the other passing ventrally to the clitoris as the frenulum. Posteriorly, the two labia minora meet at the fourchette. They consist of stratified squamous epithelium with hair follicles, sebaceous and sweat glands, and a thin layer of smooth muscle continuous with the tunica dartos. The epithelium is keratinised on the lateral surface, but changes to a mucous membrane on the medial side. The nerve endings are similar to, but less abundant than those of the labia majora and the nerve supply is similar to that described. The arterial supply again comes from the rete of the labia majora with an additional component from the dorsal artery of the clitoris. The venous drainage is again the same as that for the labia majora, with an additional superior connection to the vaginal plexus.

Clitoris

The clitoris consists of a small body of erectile tissue (the crura of the clitoris) covered by the prepuce. The nerve endings are similar to those of the labia and the nerve supply arises from the terminal branch of the pudendal nerve. The arterial supply is the dorsal artery of the clitoris, which is a terminal branch of the internal pudendal artery.

Both labia minora and clitoris are highly sensitive with a rich vascular and nerve supply. They are, therefore, important erogenous areas for sexual stimulation before and during intercourse. Ritual circumcision as practised still in some parts of Africa involves the removal of both labia minora and the clitoris during infancy.

Perineum

The perineum is bounded by the levatores ani muscles above, by the vulva and anus below, and by the pelvic outlet (subpubic angle, ischiopubic rami, ischial tuberosities, sacrotuberous ligaments and coccyx) laterally. It is divided into a urogenital triangle anteriorly and an anal triangle posteriorly. There is a superficial fascia of fat and a deeper membranous fascia (Colles), which extends over the pubis and into the anterior abdominal wall as the fascia of Scarpa.

Urogenital triangle

The urogenital triangle contains the termination of the vagina and urethra, the crura of the clitoris (erectile tissue) surrounded by the ischiocavernosus muscles, the bulb of the vestibule (erectile tissue) surrounded by the bulbocavernosus muscles, Bartholin's glands, the urogenital diaphragm and the superficial and deep perineal pouches.

Urogenital diaphragm (triangular ligament). The urogenital diaphragm is a sheath of muscle enclosed between two triangular fascial membranes. The muscle is formed by the deep transverse perineal muscle and fibres from the sphincter urethrae. The superior fascial layer is the thin fascia bridging the gap between the anterior portions of the levatores ani. The inferior fascial layer is tough and fibrous. The urogenital diaphragm is penetrated by the urethra and vagina and the glands and bulb of the vestibule lie inferior (superficial) to it (Fig. 2.3).

The ability to contract this muscle is important in preventing stress incontinence of urine. Young women who develop mild stress incontinence after childbirth are often helped by pelvic floor exercises which strengthen all the muscles, but particularly the perineal muscles.

Muscles of the perineum

The ischiocavernosus muscle arises from the medial aspect of the inferior ischial ramus and ensheaths the crus clitoridis. It compresses the crus and, by blocking the venous outflow, promotes erection of the clitoris.

The bulbocavernosus muscle originates in the perineal body, where it interdigitates with the external anal sphincter. It surrounds the bulb of the vestibule and is inserted into the body of the clitoris.

The superficial transverse perineal muscle radiates from the perineal body to the ischial ramus.

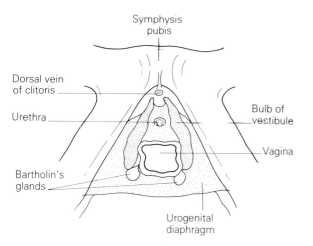

Fig. 2.3 *The urogenital diaphragm viewed from below. The urogenital diaphragm lies in the urogenital triangle which is the anterior portion of the perineum.*

The deep transverse perineal muscle has the same origin and insertion, but lies deep to the inferior fascia of the urogenital diaphragm.

Perineal body

This is a fibromuscular mass into which the bulbo-cavernosus, transverse perineal, external anal sphincter and levator ani muscles insert.

The integrity of the perineum is important in maintaining the distance between vagina and anus, and in preventing prolapse of the posterior vaginal wall (rectocele). It is damaged at childbirth by incision (episiotomy) or by tears. Failure to repair these adequately leads to an inadequate perineum, with consequent faecal soiling of the vagina and encouragement of rectocele.

Superficial perineal pouch

This is a potential space between the inferior fascia of the urogenital diaphragm and the fascia of Colles. It contains the Bartholin's glands and superficial transverse perineal muscles.

Deep perineal pouch

This is a potential space between the two fascial layers of the urogenital diaphragm and contains the membranous urethra surrounded by the external sphincter and deep transverse perineal muscles.

Damage to the urogenital diaphragm and deep perineal pouch can contribute to shortening of the urethra. Ascending urinary tract infection, particularly cystitis, can become common, especially after intercourse. A short urethra also contributes to stress incontinence of urine.

The blood supply of the perineum is largely from the internal pudendal artery, and vein. Motor and sensory nerve supply is by the pudendal nerve, and anteriorly the genitofemoral nerve.

Vestibule, Bartholin's Glands and Vagina

Vestibule

The vestibule lies between the labia minora and the hymen. The hymen is a perforated membrane which after rupture consists of skin tags (carunculae hymenales). Anteriorly the vestibule includes the urethral orifice around which the periurethral glands of Skene open. The duct openings of the larger vestibular or Bartholin's glands are at 5 and 7 o'clock. The latter are arranged as lobules consisting of alveoli lined by a columnar epithelium. They produce a mucoid secretion in response to sexual stimulation. Blockage of the ducts following infection leads to mucoid retention cysts (Bartholin's cysts) or, if infected, an abscess which is very painful.

Deep to the vestibule on either side of the commencement of the vagina lies the bulb of the vestibule; a flask-shaped mass of erectile tissue covered by the bulbocavernosus muscles.

The skin of the vestibule is stratified squamous epithelium without hair follicles. The nerve endings are mostly free and the blood supply is an anastomosis between branches of the pudendal artery, the inferior haemorrhoidal artery and the azygous artery of the vagina.

Vagina

The vagina is 7–10 cm long; the posterior wall being 2 cm longer than the anterior. The anterior vaginal wall is in direct relation to the bladder and urethra throughout its length. Surgery of the anterior vaginal wall, therefore, always carries a risk of urethral and vesical damage. At the level of the junction between urethra and bladder are the pubocervical ligaments (*see below*). The upper quarter of the posterior vaginal wall is related to the intraperitoneal cavity or pouch of Douglas. The middle half of the posterior vaginal wall is related to the rectum, while the lower quarter is separated from the anal canal by the anal sphincters and perineal body. The lateral relations of the vagina are shown in Fig. 2.4.

The vagina has an extensive blood supply with contributions from the uterine artery, the inferior vesical arteries, the terminal branch of the internal iliac artery, the haemorrhoidal arteries and the dorsal artery of the clitoris. All of the above anastomose to form the anterior and posterior azygous arteries which pass down the midline of the vagina. The good blood supply helps to provide vaginal lubrication by means of exudate. The vagina is also a distensible structure allowing the passage of the fetal head without excessive trauma.

Lymphatic drainage of the vagina is as follows:

1. *Upper:* via the cervical channels to the external iliac nodes;
2. *Middle:* to the hypogastric nodes;
3. *Lower:* to the hypogastric nodes and via the vulva to the inguinal nodes.

Those nodes are affected in the spread of carcinoma of the vagina or carcinoma of the cervix involving the vagina.

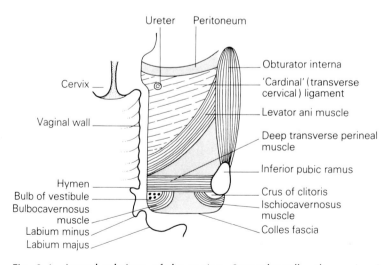

Fig. 2.4   *Lateral relations of the vagina. Superolaterally, the vagina is supported by transverse cervical ligaments. In its midposition it is surrounded by the medial fibres of the levator ani muscle. Inferiorly, it penetrates the urogenital diaphragm.*

Bony Pelvis

The pelvis consists of a saucer-shaped false pelvis which is situated above the pelvic cavity (true pelvis). The latter is of great significance and it is through here that the fetus passes during delivery. The true pelvis is a curved bony canal, the posterior wall (the sacrum) being considerably longer than the anterior (pubic symphysis) (Fig. 2.5).

The pelvic inlet is oval in shape with a shorter anteroposterior diameter between the sacral promontory and the back of the pubic symphysis (11 cm) and a longer transverse diameter (13.5 cm) (Fig. 2.6). The pelvic brim forms the inlet of the true pelvis and the fetal head passes through this when it engages in late pregnancy or early labour. Engagement of the fetal head is said to have occurred when the widest diameter of the fetal skull (biparietal) has passed through the pelvic brim. The transverse diameter (13.5 cm) is the maximum diameter of the pelvic brim and thus the largest diameter of the fetal head normally passes through this easily.

The curve of the sacrum allows the midcavity of the pelvis to be capacious and circular in outline with a diameter of 12 cm in all directions.

The pelvic outlet is diamond shaped and is bound by the ischopubic rami anteriorly and the sacrotuberous ligaments and sacral tuberosities poster-

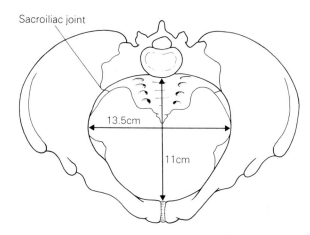

Fig. 2.6 *Mean diameters of the pelvic inlet.*

iorly. The anteroposterior diameter of the outlet is taken from the lower border of the symphysis pubis to the bottom of the sacrum and the transverse diameter is between the ischial tuberosities (Fig. 2.7). Thus the pelvis is wider from side to side of the brim than from front to back at the outlet. The relationship of pelvic shape and size to the passage

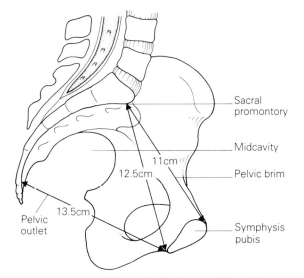

Fig. 2.5 *Saggital view of the bony pelvis. The true conjugate from the sacral promontory to the top of the symphysis pubis measures 11 cm. The diagonal conjugate (12.5 cm) is measured to the bottom of the symphysis. The anteroposterior diameter of the outlet is shown.*

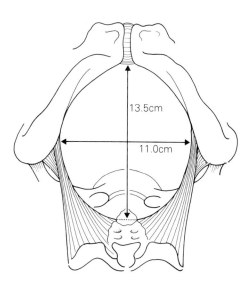

Fig. 2.7 *Dimensions of the diamond-shaped pelvic outlet. The anteroposterior diameter is measured from the bottom of the symphysis to the end of the sacrum and not to the end of the coccyx.*

of the fetus during labour is described in Chapter 10.

The bony pelvis is made up of the hip bone and the sacrum. The hip bone itself consists of three separate bones: the ilium, the ischium and the pubis. These are joined by bone in the adult, but they are separated by cartilage in children. These three bones converge on the acetabulum (Fig. 2.8). It can be seen that the ilium forms the false pelvis and iliac crest and this bone articulates with the sacrum, forming the major non-mobile sacroiliac joint. The pubic bone consists of a body and two rami as does the ischium. The rami of these two bones fuse to form the obturator foramen.

The sacrum consists of five vertebrae joined by bone in the adult and cartilage in children. There are four sacral foramina communicating with the sacral canal. The upper border of the pelvic surface is the sacral promontory.

During pregnancy, the angle of the pelvis increases and there is a lordosis to compensate for the anterior shift of the woman's centre of gravity. Ligaments become looser, and so sacroiliac discomfort, and less commonly discomfort at the pubic symphysis, particularly on movement, can be troublesome. The laxity is designed to facilitate childbirth and is brought about by oestrogen and relaxin-induced changes in collagen structure and density.

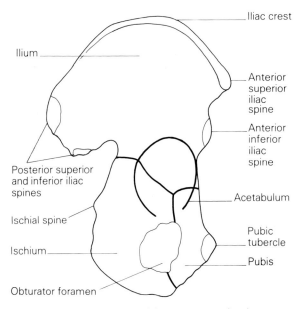

Fig. 2.8   *Lateral view of the innominte (hip bone).*

Uterus

The uterus is about 7.5 cm long and consists of a body, a constricted portion known as the isthmus (which includes the internal os) and a narrow terminal part called the cervix. The portion lying above the opening of the fallopian tubes is known as the fundus. The cervix penetrates the vaginal wall and is thereby divided into a supra- and infravaginal portion. The uterus lies between the bladder and the rectum in the peritoneal cavity. Removal of the uterus always involves dissection of the bladder from its lower part and cervix, so the operation carries risks of trauma to the bladder. It is separated from the rectum by the upper part of the pouch of Douglas.

The external cervical orifice (external os) is circular in nullipara but becomes transverse and fissured as a result of childbirth. The axis of the cervical canal is directed obliquely posteriorly and inferiorly, while the uterus is anteflexed and anteverted. Laterally the uterus is related to the broad ligaments and the uterine arteries.

The uterus has a remarkable capacity for enlargement during pregnancy. The isthmus elongates and its cavity becomes absorbed into the general uterine cavity to form the lower uterine segment. As further enlargement takes place, the upper part of the cervix is also incorporated into the thin lower segment. The uterus increases in weight only during the first half of pregnancy and its further enlargement in volume is achieved by thinning out of the uterine walls.

The main blood supply to the uterus is from the uterine artery which may arise directly from the internal iliac or in common with another of its branches, usually the superior vesical artery. The uterine artery crosses the tranverse cervical ligament (*see below*) and thereafter passes anterior to and above the ureter at about 1.5 cm from the lateral vaginal fornix. Care must be taken when clamping the uterine artery during hysterectomy not to clamp or cut the ureter. The uterine artery then ascends in a tortuous course between the two layers of the broad ligament on the lateral border of the uterus, giving out branches to the myometrium and anastomosing at the superior angle with the terminal portion of the ovarian artery. As mentioned above, the uterine artery also gives off a branch to the upper part of the vagina. The main lymphatic drainage of the uterus is to the external and internal iliac group of lymph nodes, although some lymphatics in the upper part of the uterus pass directly to the lateral aortic nodes following the ovarian blood supply. A few small branches run with the round ligament to the superficial inguinal nodes.

Fallopian Tubes

The fallopian tubes lie in the upper margin of the broad ligament and are 10 cm long. The abdominal opening is at the base of a trumpet-shaped expansion with a fimbriated edge, the infundibulum; one of the fimbriae of the infundibulum may form a small vesicle or hydatid. From the infundibulum, the succeeding parts of the tube are the relatively wide tortuous ampulla, cord-like isthmus and the uterine or intramural portion. The blood supply is from the uterine and ovarian arteries through the mesosalpinx. Sterilisation procedures and reversal of these are most effective if performed in the isthmic portions of the tubes. There is some form of physiological sphincter at the ampullary-isthmic junction which is thought to regulate the passage of the ovum through the tube. Tubal ectopic pregnancies frequently occur in the ampulla or ampullary-isthmic region of the tube. Rupture of the tube is less likely in the ampulla than if the pregnancy is in the narrow isthmus. Tubal occlusion for sterilisation purposes is best done at the isthmus.

Ovaries

The ovary is an almond-shaped organ attached to the posterior surface of the broad ligament, a fold of the ligament called the mesovarium and occupies the ovarian fossa on the wall of the pelvis. The fossa is bound anteriorly by the lateral umbilical ligament (obliterated umbilical artery) and posteriorly by the ureter and internal iliac vessels. In early fetal life the ovaries lie in the lumbar region near the kidney.

The surface of the ovaries is covered with a layer of cuboidal cells, which is the germinal epithelium, and beneath this there is a thin layer of condensed connective tissue, the tunica albuginea. The cortex contains the primordial follicles, corpora lutea and corpora albicans.

The primordial follicles consist of a central oocyte surrounded by a single layer of flattened follicular cells. After puberty some follicles develop each month to form primary, secondary and tertiary follicles.

The blood supply is from the ovarian artery, which is a branch of the descending aorta reaching the ovary in the infundibulo-pelvic ligament. There is a venous pampiniform plexus at the hilum of the ovary draining to the ovarian vein and then to the inferior vena cava with the renal vein on the left.

Female Urinary Tract

The female reproductive system cannot be fully understood without some mention of the urinary tract to which it is intimately connected.

Ureter

Each ureter is 30 cm in length and the abdominal part descends over the psoas muscle and is crossed by the ovarian vessels. It enters the pelvis in front of the external iliac vessels and the pelvic part follows the anterior border of the sacroiliac notch and runs above the levator ani muscle in the base of the broad ligament (parametrium) to the base of the bladder. In the parametrium the ureter lies below the uterine artery and above the lateral fornix of the vagina. It passes 2 cm lateral to the cervix (a point of importance in radiotherapy), and then turns medially in front of the vagina to follow an oblique course through the bladder wall.

The ureter is most liable to surgical trauma close to (1) the angle of the vagina, (2) the uterine artery in the base of the broad ligament, (3) the external iliac vessels at the posterolateral margin of the broad ligament.

Bladder

The bladder is a three-layered hollow, muscular organ with a peritoneal covering on the superior surface. The three layers consist of serous, muscular and mucous coats and the smooth muscle itself has internal and external longitudinal layers and a larger middle circular layer. The mucosa is a transitional epithelium which is loosely attached to the muscle, except over the trigone (the triangular area bounded by the orifices of the ureters and the urethra) where it is firmly attached. The trigone lies against the anterior vaginal wall and the cervix, and, consequently, at hysterectomy and anterior colporrhaphy, the bladder must be carefully resected from the underlying structures. Descent of the bladder through inadequate pubocervical fascia causes stretching of the anterior vaginal wall and the presence of a bulge or lump in the vagina (cystocele).

Urethra

The female urethra is 4 cm long and is embedded in the anterior wall of the vagina running below and behind the pubic symphysis. Its opening is between the labia minora and behind the clitoris. The muscle layer is continuous with that of the bladder and there is no anatomical internal sphincter at this junction. As it traverses the deep perineal pouch, it is surrounded by the voluntary external sphincter which is supplied by the perineal branch of the pudendal nerve. Between the muscle and the mucosa is a thin layer of connective tissue which may play a part in maintaining continence.

Peritoneum, Muscles and Ligaments of the Pelvis

The peritoneum covers the uterus with the exception of the anterior part of the supravaginal cervix and the intravaginal cervix. From the anterior surface of the uterus, the peritoneum is reflected onto the superior surface of the bladder, forming the uterovesical pouch. From the posterior surface of the uterus, the peritoneum continues onto the upper–third of the vagina before it is reflected onto the anterior rectal surface, forming the rectovaginal

pouch (or pouch of Douglas). The lower extremity of this pouch is attached to the perineal body by connective tissue of the rectovaginal septum (Fig. 2.9).

Broad ligament

From the lateral borders of the uterus, two layers of peritoneum on each side are reflected to the lateral pelvic walls forming the broad ligaments. These peritoneal folds include loose connective tissue referred to as parametrium which merge inferiorly with extraperitoneal connective tissue. The upper lateral border of the broad ligament forms the infundibulopelvic fold and contains the ovarian vessels in their course from the side wall of the pelvis. The ovary is attached to the posterior layer of the broad ligament by a short double fold of the peritoneum — the mesovarium — and the portion of the broad ligament above this is the mesosalpinx. The top of the broad ligament envelops the fallopian tubes. Below and in front of the fallopian tube is the round ligament, and below and behind it is the ovarian ligament connecting the ovary to the uterine cornu, which are all enclosed within the broad ligament.

Vestigial remnants of the mesonephric bodies and ducts (wolffian ducts, duct of Gartner) are contained within the broad ligament. Remnants of the mesonephric body lie above and lateral to the ovary (epoophoron and hydatid of Morgagni) and between the ovary and uterus (paroophoron).

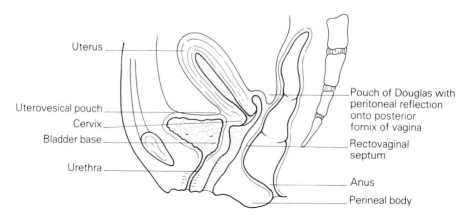

Fig. 2.9 *Saggital section of the pelvis to show the peritoneal reflections over the bladder, uterus, posterior vaginal fornix and rectum.*

Round ligament

The round ligament attaches to the uterine body below and in front of the fallopian tube. It is 12 cm long and passes through the broad ligament to the lateral wall of the pelvis, where it crosses the psoas muscle and external iliac vessels. It hooks round the inferior epigastric arteries to the deep inguinal ring, passes through the inguinal canal and fans out into the labium majus. It is composed mainly of fibrous tissue with some smooth muscle at the uterine end and some striated muscle at the labial end. It undergoes considerable hypertrophy during pregnancy, often causing mild pain on movement within the inguinal canal.

Ligaments formed from pelvic fascia

The connective tissue covering the levator ani is condensed into musculofibrous bands in three areas: (1) the transverse cervical ligament (cardinal ligament) arising from the arcuate line on the side wall of the pelvis; (2) the pubocervical ligaments arising from fascia over the pubic bone and passing around the bladder neck; and (3) the uterosacral ligaments (posterior part of the cardinal ligaments) arising from the sacral promontory. All three ligaments insert into the upper vagina and supravaginal cervix, and are important in supporting the pelvic viscera and the uterus, the cardinal ligaments being very important. Their apposition in front of the amputated cervix to support and antevert the uterus is the main part of the Manchester repair operation. Buttressing of the pubocervical fascia to raise and support the urethro-vesical angle, initially by sutures and subsequently by fibrous tissue, is the main purpose of the anterior vaginal surgical approach to stress incontinence.

Blood, Lymphatic and Nervous Supply

Blood supply

The blood supply of the pelvis is shown in Fig. 2.10. The aorta divides at the level of the fourth lumbar vertebra, and the common iliac artery at the level of the lumbosacral intervertebral disc. Continuing vessels leave the pelvis through the obturator foramen (obturator artery), behind the inguinal ligament (femoral artery), and through the greater sciatic foramen (superior and inferior gluteal arteries; internal pudendal artery). The internal puden-

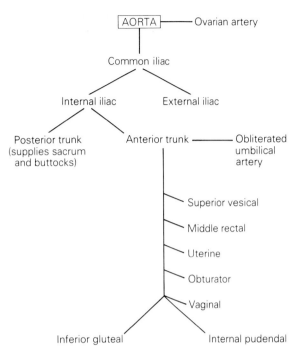

Fig. 2.10 *The arterial supply of the pelvis — diagrammatic.*

dal artery curves around the back of the ischial spine and enters the perineum through the lesser sciatic foramen and pudendal canal.

Lymphatic drainage

The lymphatic drainage of the pelvis begins as plexuses in the individual organs and generally follows the line of the blood vessels. Major and fairly constant groups of nodes include the common iliac, the external iliac, which drain the inguinal group, the internal iliac, the obturator, and the median and lateral sacral nodes.

Lymphatic drainage of the ovary is to the para-aortic nodes; of the body of the uterus to para-aortic iliac nodes and inguinal nodes; of the cervix to the iliac nodes and para-rectal nodes; and of the vagina to iliac and inguinal nodes.

Nerve supply

The parasympathetic nerve supply to the pelvis emerges as myelinated, preganglionic nerves with the ventral rami of S 2 and S 4 to constitute the pelvic splanchnic nerves. The ganglia are situated in the walls of the organs supplied. Motor or inhibitory fibres supply the rectum, bladder and erectile tissue of clitoris; vasodilator fibres supply the ovary and uterus.

The sympathetic nerve supply to the pelvis arises from the sympathetic nerve trunks, which have four ganglia in the lumbar region and a similar number anterior to the sacrum. The origin of the pelvic sympathetic fibres is from T 11 to L 2. From the ganglia, grey rami communicantes pass to the lumbar and sacral spinal nerves while other fibres form the hypogastric plexus from which further plexuses radiate to the various pelvic organs.

Stimulation of somatic afferent fibres from the external genitalia or adjacent skin causes vasodilation through the parasympathetic fibres of the pelvic splanchnic nerves.

Muscles of the Pelvis

We have already dealt with the muscles of the perineum (p. 11). The remaining muscle mass — the levator ani — is extremely important in obstetrics and gynaecology, as this forms the pelvic floor or diaphragm. The levator ani muscles arise on each side of the pelvis from the line which passes backwards from the posterior surface to the superior ramus of the pubis. This line then passes over the internal surface of the obturator foramen (arcus tendineus) to the ischial spine, forming the origin of the levator muscle and from here the fibres sweep inferiorly and posteriorly to interdigitate with each other in the midline. As they sweep downwards and backwards, they surround the vagina and then insert into (1) the preanal raphe where some fibres make a contribution to the perineal body; (2) the wall of the anal canal where fibres blend with the deep external sphincter muscle; (3) the postanal or anococcygeal raphe, where again the muscle meets its fellow from the opposite side and (4) the lower part of the coccyx (Fig. 2.11). The medial borders of each levator muscle have sphincteric action, and contraction partially occludes the vagina. The nerve supply to the levator ani muscles is from the third and fourth sacral nerves.

The most medial portion of the levator ani is referred to as pubococcygeus muscle and it is this portion that is inserted in front of the rectum. The next portion is the puborectalis and this is inserted into the rectum and into the first part of the raphe

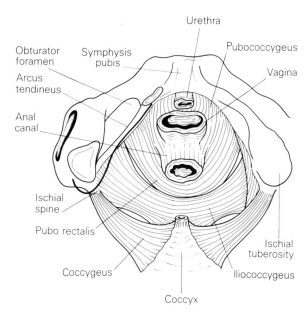

Fig. 2.11   *Inferior view of the levator ani muscles.*

behind the rectum. The most posterior portion is the iliococcygeus and this is inserted into the remainder of the posterior raphe and into the coccyx itself. Because the fibres of the levator ani run downwards as well as backwards, the pelvic diaphragm as a whole is funnel-shaped. Paradoxically, contraction of the abdominal wall with increased abdominal pressure, as in straining or coughing, relaxes the levator muscles. Thus during straining, the puborectalis muscle is relaxed and the angle between the rectum and anus is diminished.

MICROSTRUCTURE OF THE REPRODUCTIVE TRACT
(Excluding pregnancy)

Mucosa of the Fallopian Tube

The fallopian tubes are lined by a single layer of columnar epithelium with three types of cell: ciliated, secretory and resting ('peg'). The secretory cells are found throughout the tube, but are most numerous at the isthmic end; they develop microvilli and become secretory at midcycle. Pelvic inflammatory disease leads to deciliation of the tube, particularly the ampullary portion. This retards tubal transport of the fertilised oocyte and leads to an increased incidence of tubal ectopic pregnancy.

Fallopian tube secretions contain pyruvate, which is an important substrate for the embryo. They contain less glucose, protein and potassium than serum. Further understanding of the biochemistry of oviduct fluid is important in relationship to failure of implantation.

Endometrium

The endometrium is composed of a basal layer and a stroma covered by columnar epithelium. The latter forms uterine glands which extend through the stroma into the basal layer. The columnar epithelium includes ciliated cells, which are most numerous near the opening of the glands, and secretory cells with microvilli which are fully developed during the secretory phase. After menstruation, regeneration of the epithelium takes place from the epithelium at the base of the endometrial glands.

Following menstruation, the endometrium enters the proliferative phase. Under the influence of oestrogen, the epithelium proliferates and the endometrium reaches a thickness of 5 mm. Towards midcycle the arterioles take on a spiral form and subnuclear aggregates of glycogen appear in the epithelium. During the luteal phase, there is slight further thickening of the endometrium due to vascular proliferation, oedema of the stroma and accumulation of secretion in uterine glands. The glands become tortuous and vacuoles of glycogen push the nuclei to the luminal surface. After about Day 20, these vacuoles move to the surface and are discharged. Predecidual changes occur in the stroma: the stellate cells become rounder and accumulate lysosomes.

In the final stage of the cycle, the coiled arterioles constrict and the superficial zone becomes avascular. There is a loss of interstitial fluid, leucocytic infiltration of the stroma and extravasation of blood as the superficial layers become necrotic. The blood enters the lumen, but does not clot. The underlying basal layer remains intact, as do the bases of the glands. Levels of $PGF_{2\alpha}$ in the endometrium rise during the luteal phase and exceed PGE_2 by 25 : 1 at the time of menstruation. The former constricts spiral arterioles while the latter relaxes them. An altered ratio in favour of vasodilatory compounds such as PGE_2 may be a factor in the aetiology of menorrhagia.

Cervix

The cervix is lined by secretory columnar epithelium arranged as branched glands. This epithelium undergoes only minor changes during the menstrual cycle. The cervical mucus becomes profuse and clear under the action of oestrogen before ovulation. It produces a ferning pattern on drying, exhibits 'spinnbarkeit' (by Day 14 of the menstrual cycle a single thread may be drawn out to 8 cm) and has an alkaline pH. Towards midcycle the cervical fluid becomes more hydrated. The macromolecules of glycoprotein condense into 'micelles' which form a network of channels through which sperm swim. Once progesterone secretion begins, the cervical mucus becomes thick, opaque, highly cellular and less abundant, as a result of increased binding between the glycoprotein filaments.

Vagina

The wall of the vagina consists of three layers: a mucous membrane, a muscular coat (circular and longitudinal) and a thin connective tissue covering. Striated fibres of the bulbocavernosus and levator ani muscles form sphincters. The stratified squamous epithelium has three layers: a basal layer of cuboidal cells, an intermediate layer, which is rich in glycogen, and a superficial zone of flat cornified cells with small nuclei. The underlying lamina propria contains collagen and elastic fibres and a rich nerve and blood supply. The superficial zone is best developed at midcycle, as reflected by a high karyopyknotic index. This is much lower during the luteal phase when the vaginal smear contains many more leucocytes.

The pH is normally acid owing to conversion of glycogen to lactic acid by Doderlein's lactobacillus. Increase in vaginal pH to 5 or more is often associated with pathogenic infection, presumably due to reduction in numbers of lactobacillus. Vaginal fluid has a higher potassium and lower sodium concentration than plasma.

FUNCTION

Sexual Intercourse

The stages of physiological response to sexual stimulation are similar in both sexes, namely excitement, plateau, orgasm and resolution.

During the excitement stage in the woman, there is vasodilation and congestion of the clitoris, causing erection, and congestion of the labia minora and majora. Vaginal exudate increases. In the male, penile erection and contraction of the dartos muscle, tightening the scrotum and elevation of the testes, occurs.

During the plateau phase, these changes become more pronounced and, in addition, the length and diameter of the vagina increase, the introitus gapes and the uterus may rise out of the pelvis. Further lubrication occurs from the secretions of the Bartholin glands, and from the pre-ejaculatory emission of mucus.

Orgasmic phase is short and consists of strong pelvic movements in both sexes. In the woman, there are uterine and vaginal contractions, and in the male, expulsive penile contractions occur expelling the seminal fluid along the urethra.

The resolution phase varies in length depending on the intensity of orgasm and whether further stimulation is taking place. It is usually more rapid in the male than the female in whom repeated orgasms are more readily possible.

The physiological responses described are initiated and maintained by the autonomic nervous system, so some drugs or damage to the sacral parasympathetic nerve may affect the response.

Vaginismus

This is a psychologically induced spasm of perineal muscles and vagina making penetration difficult and painful or impossible. It may have had its origins in physical pain, such as an episiotomy scar, but often it is psychological, and sympathetic counselling may be of benefit.

Failure of orgasm

This has no effect on reproductive function. It is usually due to an unharmonious relationship, lack of adequate stimulation or general debility. If it becomes a real problem to the woman, she should seek counselling for herself and her partner.

Premature ejaculation

This is quite a commen male problem, usually due to sexual inexperience, anxiety or, occasionally, some more deep seated psychological problem.

Failure of ejaculation

This is usually psychological in origin. Both this and premature ejaculation are amenable to treatment using appropriate stimulating techniques.

Impotence

This can be primary due to a physical or congenital disorder, or secondary due to physical or psychological stress. Identification of these causes can lead to cure. Occasionally, temporary inflatable splints can be used to allow intercourse to take place. Intermittent drug therapy to increase arterial flow into the penis and reduce venous outflow is under investigation.

Sexual assault

Occasionally, doctors other than police surgeons are asked to see a woman who claims to have been sexually assaulted. Such women are usually deeply emotionally shocked, and should be treated with great sympathy and gentleness, but also with frankness.

After a history has been taken, a thorough examination of all clothing and all parts of the body in a good light is essential. All parts of the body should be examined for signs of violence, with particular attention to the thighs, buttocks, introitus and vagina. Swabs or aspirates should be taken for the presence of seminal fluid and for infection. Finally, prescription of a postcoital contraceptive in the form of a double dose of combined oral contraceptive on two consecutive days should be considered. Detailed notes must be taken of the entire examination, in case these are later legally required.

Micturition

This involves a complex coordinated interaction of bladder and pelvic muscles. As the bladder fills, it maintains a relatively constant tone in the muscle wall. Ultimately the increased intravesical pressure stimulates the sensory fibres in the pelvic splanchnic nerves. Through the efferent fibres of the same nerves, the bladder contracts while the urethra relaxes. Relaxation of the perineal muscles is caused by the pudendal nerve arising from the same segment of the spinal cord. Urine in the urethra stimulates sensory fibres in the pudendal nerve, which maintain the reflex until the bladder is empty. In addition to this basic spinal process, sensory impulses via the pelvic and hypogastric plexuses reach the thalamus and cerebral cortex. The higher centres exert inhibitory control on micturition.

Defecation

Defecation is similar in its control to micturition. Sensory fibres accompanying the pelvic splanchnic nerves carry afferent impulses from a distended rectum. This stimulates the parasympathetic fibres of the same nerves arising from S 2, 3 and 4, which causes a peristaltic wave to pass through the descending colon. Simultaneously the anal sphincters relax unless there is cortical inhibition.

FURTHER READING

Philipp E., Barnes J., Newton M. eds. (1980). *Scientific Foundations of Obstetrics and Gynaecology*, 3rd edn. pp. 86–176. London: Heinemann Medical.

Smout C.F.V., Jacob E., Lillie E.W. (1969). *Gynaecological and Obstetrical Anatomy*, 4th edn. London: H.K. Lewis.

3

The Menstrual Cycle

The menstrual cycle is the term used to describe the monthly cycle of physiological events which prepare the female for pregnancy and culminate in menstruation should pregnancy not occur. On average it takes 28 days from the onset of one menses to the next, with a range of 21–35 days for normal cycles.

Menstruation follows abrupt changes in oestrogen and progesterone which, in turn, are influenced by the hypothalamic pituitary output.

The endocrinology of the menstrual cycle is complex as there are three levels (hypothalamus, pituitary and ovary) of endocrine function. Trophic hormones are produced at each level and there are control feedback mechanisms (positive and negative) exerted by the pituitary and ovarian hormones. Negative feedback occurs when a rising level of the induced hormone progressivly inhibits the production of its stimulatory trophic hormone. Positive feedback occurs when a rising level of hormone stimulates the further production of the trophic hormone, i.e. oestradiol rise in midcycle stimulating the LH surge. Finally, the ovarian steroids act on the target organ, the uterus, through the classical steroid receptor proteins exerting their effect on the nature and function of the uterine cells.

This chapter will consider the hormonal factors responsible for ovulation, the events in the uterus throughout the cycle and mechanisms of menstruation. It will then consider bleeding abnormalities due to dysfunction of endocrine control, causes of absence of bleeding and finally menstrually related symptoms such as dysmenorrhoea and premenstrual syndrome.

HYPOTHALAMIC–PITUITARY–OVARIAN AXIS (Figs. 3.1–3.3)

The hypothalamus secretes a decapeptide, Gonadotrophin Releasing Hormone (GnRH). It has a half-life of only a few minutes and is secreted in rapid pulses, the amplitude and frequency of which can be varied. During the menstrual cycle, GnRH secretion varies, as measured by the resultant luteinising hormone (LH) pulses. These occur at roughly 90 min intervals during the follicular phase, increasing in frequency to 60 min intervals at midcycle, subsequently slowing down to 120 min intervals in the luteal phase. GnRH secretion is under the influence of the catecholaminergic neurones. Those with noradrenaline as the neurotransmitter are facilitatory, while those with dopamine are inhibitory. GnRH exerts its effect on the anterior pituitary, arriving by means of the hypophyseal-pituitary portal vasculature. It acts to increase synthesis, storage, activation and secretion of the gonadotrophins — luteinising hormone (LH), and follicle stimulating hormone (FSH). GnRH activity is modulated partly by itself, by stimulating the formation of its own receptors, and partly by short feedback loops from the pituitary, but mainly by the ovarian steroids — oestrogen and progesterone (*see below*).

The anterior pituitary secretes LH and FSH from the gonadotrophic cells in a pulsatile fashion in response to GnRH. They act to stimulate ovarian activity directly. LH and FSH secretion is modulated by the pattern of GnRH secretion, and by oestrogen and progesterone. Oestrogen and progesterone are secreted by the ovary. Oestrogen acts on the hypothalamic-pituitary unit by inhibiting FSH secretion (negative feedback), while having little effect on LH secretion, except at midcycle (Fig. 3.2), when high levels of oestrogen (probably in a specific pattern only) induce the LH surge. Progesterone feedback at midcycle enhances the LH surge, and is mainly responsible for the FSH surge (positive feedback). In the luteal phase, high levels of progesterone act with oestrogen to inhibit gonadotrophin secretion (Fig. 3.3).

Other hormones that affect this axis are prolactin and androgens mainly in pathological states. Prolactin has not been found to have any function in the

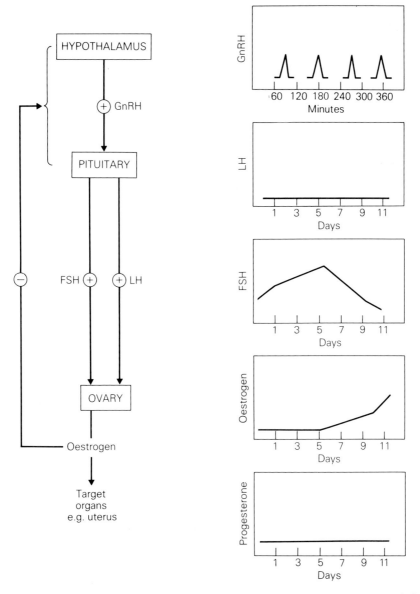

Fig. 3.1 *Hypothalamic–pituitary–ovarian axis. Follicular phase. The oestradiol rise inhibits FSH secretion in the midfollicular phase.*

normal menstrual cycle. It is under hypothalamic inhibitory control via dopamine (Prolactin Inhibitory Factor). Prolactin is responsible for its own regulation via positive feedback on the hypothalamus causing further dopamine release. It is subject to marked diurnal variation; highest concentrations are found during sleep and lowest levels during the late morning. Its secretion is also enhanced by stress. Thyrotrophin releasing factor also stimulates

prolactin secretion, although the physiological significance of this is unclear.

MECHANISM OF ACTION OF THE STEROID AND TROPHIC HORMONES

The mechanism of action of the steroid hormones is similar irrespective of the target organ. The steroid

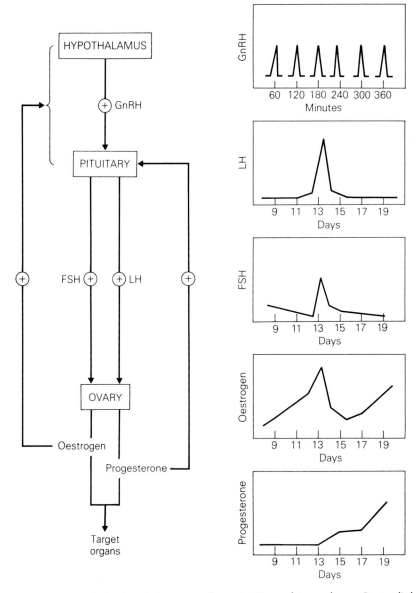

Fig. 3.2   *Hypothalamic–pituitary–ovarian axis. Preovulatory phase. Oestradiol positively feeds back on the hypothalamic-pituitary unit to initiate the LH/FSH surge. Oestradiol secretion subsequently drops, while progesterone secretion gradually commences.*

crosses the cell membrane, binds to a cytoplasmic receptor protein and this complex is then transferred across the nuclear membrane to the nucleus. The complex with an additional activating factor then binds to nuclear DNA, resulting in synthesis of specific messenger RNAs. These are then transported to the ribosomes where protein synthesis

takes place. The major regulator of the process is the activity of intracellular receptors. The target cells of the ovarian steroids contain oestrogen receptors. Oestrogen stimulation causes the proliferation of further oestrogen receptors (*upregulation*) as well as the synthesis of progesterone and androgen receptors (*priming*). Progesterone and androgens

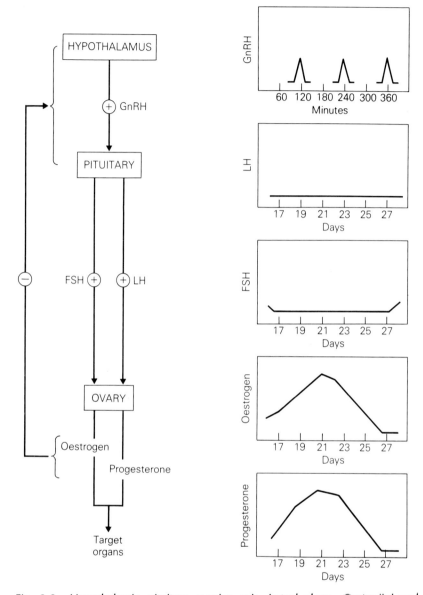

Fig. 3.3 *Hypothalamic–pituitary ovarian axis. Luteal phase. Oestradiol and progesterone inhibit FSH and LH secretion by the pituitary. At the end of this phase the levels of oestradiol and progesterone have declined, allowing a rise in FSH.*

cause a decrease in intracellular oestrogen receptors (*downregulation*).

The trophic hormones, such as the gonadotrophins may act via the cyclic-AMP pathway. The hormone binds with its specific receptor on the cell surface, thereby activating adenyl cyclase, and hence increased conversion of ATP to cyclic-AMP. The cyclic-AMP is then bound, and the whole complex activates a protein kinase which, in turn, catalyses the phosphorylation of a number of cellular enzymes which changes their catalytic activity. For example, phosphorylation of cholesterol esterase results in increased rates of release of cholesterol (the precursor of the steroid hormones) from cholesterol esters which act as an intracellular storage form.

Prostaglandins which are present in all cells may also stimulate adenyl cyclase activity and thus alter rates of steroid hormone synthesis and other intracellular events.

OVARIAN CYCLE

The ovarian cycle usually culminates in the development to maturity of one egg, nurtured prior to ovulation within a follicle. Following ovulation, this same follicle becomes a different functional unit, the corpus luteum, serving to maintain the environment necessary to allow implantation and very early development of the embryo.

The ovarian cycle can be divided into:

1.   Follicular development;
2.   The ovulatory process;
3.   The luteal phase.

Follicular Development

Follicular development, though a continuous process, can for the purposes of description be considered in three phases.

Very early follicular development

It takes about 10 weeks for a primordial follicle, which is an oocyte arrested in the diplotene stage of meiotic prophase and surrounded by a single layer of granulosa cells, to develop into a potential preovulatory follicle. This is a follicle capable of undergoing complete maturation, provided it receives appropriate gonadotrophic stimulation (Fig. 3.4). The stimulus for the continuing development of a pool of primordial follicles is unknown, although it seems to be independent of pituitary control.

Each month a few hundred primordial follicles will start to grow. Most will undergo atresia, while only a few will be at the peak of development at the appropriate time to be able to respond to gonadotrophins and thereby progress to the next phase.

Early follicular development

Continued follicular development is dependent upon FSH and LH secretion. The relationship between the ovarian cycle and the pituitary-ovarian axis can be summarised as follows:

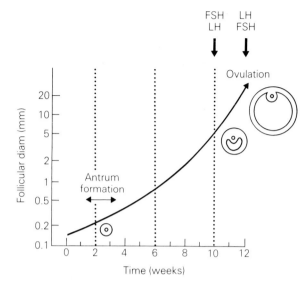

Fig. 3.4   *Development of a follicle destined to ovulate.*

1.   Perimenstrual FSH rise stimulates follicular development.
2.   The developing follicles secrete oestrogen.
3.   Oestrogen exerts a negative feedback on FSH secretion, causing it to decline.
4.   High midcycle oestrogen levels exert a positive feedback on LH and FSH secretion, causing the midcycle gonadotrophin surge.
5.   The gonadotrophin surge initiates the final stages of follicular maturation, culminating in ovulation.
6.   The follicle now becomes the corpus luteum.
7.   The corpus luteum secretes both oestrogen and progesterone, which inhibit gonadotrophin secretion by negative feedback.
8.   Oestrogen and progesterone levels decline at the end of the life of the corpus luteum, allowing the perimenstrual rise of FSH.

The follicle destined to ovulate in any given cycle, along with a cohort of similarly mature follicles, reaches the developmental threshold of its ability to respond to gonadotrophins about 1–2 days prior to the onset of menses in that cycle.

The regression of the corpus luteum, along with a concomitant decrease in its steroid output, removing its negative feedback, allows the rise in pituitary FSH secretion. It is this FSH rise which enables the developing follicles to take the quantum leap to continue the final phases of development.

By this stage the follicles have undergone the following morphological changes:

1. Fluid has appeared between the granulosa cells and coalesced to form a fluid-filled antrum.
2. The oocyte has enlarged and become surrounded by the zona pellucida, a mucopolysaccharide layer. It, in turn, is surrounded by a dense layer of granulosa cells, the cumulus oophorus.
3. The granulosa cells have proliferated.
4. The differentiation of the theca from the surrounding stroma (i.e. external to the basement membrane). The theca interna is well vascularised, while the theca externa forms a fibrous layer.

The avascular granulosa cells are the only unit to contain FSH receptors, and hence the only layer able to respond to this hormone. The theca interna contains LH receptors, and since it is well vascularised, responds to the relatively low, but ever present, circulating LH.

Under LH stimulation, the theca is able to synthesise androgens, mainly androstenedione and testosterone from cholesterol. FSH causes induction of granulosa cell aromatase — the key enzyme system involved in the synthesis of oestrogens (oestrone and oestradiol) from thecal androgen. Oestrogen production is reflected in the serum and follicular fluid levels of this hormone. Under FSH stimulation, the granulosa cells also acquire LH receptors (Fig. 3.5).

Oestrogen further sensitises the granulosa cells to FSH, as well as acting with FSH to increase granulosa cell proliferation, thereby increasing the total number of FSH receptors.

Late follicular development

It has already been stated that there are a cohort of follicles developing, of which only one is destined to be selected as the ovulatory follicle for the following reasons:

1. Because of negative feedback by oestradiol on the hypothalamic-pituitary axis, FSH secretion rapidly diminishes.
2. Only one follicle is able to continue to respond to the decreasing FSH stimulation, because the dominant follicle has the largest number of granulosa cells, and hence the largest number of FSH receptors.

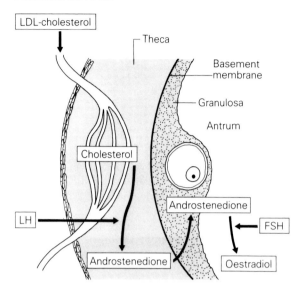

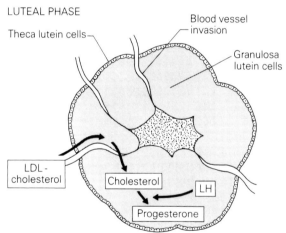

Fig. 3.5 *Ovarian steroidogenesis in the follicular and luteal phases. (Adapted from S.G. Hillier and E.J. Wickings, 1985. In* The Luteal Phase. *S.L. Jeffcoate, ed. Chichester, New York: Wiley.)*

3. The lead follicle contains the largest number of the recently acquired LH receptors and so is able to respond to LH stimulation.
4. Thecal vascularity is markedly increased, thereby allowing more gonadotrophin to permeate through and reach the receptors.

The dominant follicle is recognised as the largest follicle present in either ovary, measuring about 2 cm in diameter and containing about 6 ml follicular fluid, just prior to ovulation.

While the main function of the follicular phase is to allow these intraovarian events to take place, the secretion of oestrogen is the primary stimulus for a number of target organs, particularly the uterus.

Ovulation

Preovulatory phase

LH is the chief hormone responsible for initiating the ovulatory process. The lead follicle has had prior priming with LH receptors in response to FSH stimulation.

The onset of the LH surge is the trigger which programmes the preovulatory follicle into a timed and orderly sequence of events culminating in ovulation. Concomitant with the LH surge is a smaller FSH surge. After the gonadotrophin surge has been initiated, there is a dramatic and precipitate drop in serum oestradiol levels. This is probably due to downregulation by LH of its own receptors in the theca cells, thus depriving the granulosa cells of the necessary androgen substrate.

Progesterone also inhibits further granulosa cell proliferation. The signal for the initiation of the midcycle gonadotrophin surge is unclear. It is thought to be related to the pattern of oestradiol secretion which, under these circumstances, assumes a form of positive feedback on LH secretion. Serum oestradiol rises steadily and reaches a peak. The LH surge is triggered as the oestradiol level approaches or attains its maximum (Fig. 3.2). It appears that LH production in order to reach a surge requires 2–3 days of sustained and incremental oestradiol priming at a critical level. Progesterone at low, but increasing, levels may act synergistically with oestrogen to enhance the surge. It seems likely that other factors are also involved.

As a result of the LH surge, specific cytoplasmic and nuclear events take place. Cytoplasmic changes include a marked increase in protein synthesis, particularly the proteolytic enzymes involved in lysis of the follicular wall. $PGF_{2\alpha}$ levels in follicular fluid also increase. Oestrogen levels decline and progesterone increases as the granulosa cells, under the influence of LH, switch to progesterone production. Nuclear maturation involves the progression of the chromosomes through the remainder of the first meiotic division, culminating in equal chromo-somal, but unequal cytoplasmic division, with one cell (the secondary oocyte) taking nearly all the cytoplasm. The remaining chromosomes are discarded as the first polar body. The chromosomes are then arrested for a second time, this time in metaphase of the second meiotic division. Ovulation will occur with the oocyte in this state. Premature oocyte maturation is thought to be prevented by a local inhibitory factor in the follicular fluid, known as inhibin. However, it has not been isolated as yet. The LH surge overcomes this local inhibitory factor.

The mechanism for shutting off the LH surge is unknown. There is a depletion of pituitary LH due to downregulation of GnRH receptors in the pituitary, and exhaustion of the stored LH. There may also be a negative feedback loop between the pituitary and the hypothalamus. In addition, there is a loss of the positive feedback of oestradiol following its precipitate fall, combined with the increasing negative feedback of progesterone.

Ovulation

Follicular rupture with escape of the oocyte depends upon degenerative changes in the expanding and thin follicular wall. There is enhancement of the activity of the proteolytic enzymes, such as collagenase. Prostaglandins, particularly $PGF_{2\alpha}$, play a significant role by activating these enzymes and by increasing ovarian contractions which could increase the intrafollicular pressure. The site of follicular rupture is called the stigma. Tubal and ovarian motility ensure that the tubal fimbriae sweep over the ovarian surface to take in the freshly ovulated egg.

It is imperative that follicular maturation and the gonadotrophin surge coincide appropriately. The trigger for ovulation occurs as a result of hormonal feedback from the developing follicle. Only after the follicle has reached the appropriate stage of maturity will the positive oestrogenic feedback trigger the LH surge, thereby ensuring precise synchrony.

Luteal Phase

Progesterone is the main hormone of the luteal phase. Normal luteal function is dependent upon optimal follicular development. The formation of sufficient numbers of LH receptors predetermines the degree of luteinisation and hence its subsequent functional capacity. It is also dependent upon adequate vascularisation so that cholesterol substrate can be transported in order to synthesise progesterone.

Luteinisation of the developing follicle occurs before ovulation in response to the LH surge. This is reflected in a significant rise in serum progesterone prior to ovulation. Luteinisation may even occur in the absence of follicular rupture, with entrapment of the egg — the so-called luteinised unruptured follicle syndrome.

After ovulation, the follicle gives rise to a new anatomical structure, the corpus luteum. The granulosa cells become larger and stained with a yellow pigment (lutein) and are now known as the granulosa-lutein cells. The theca also differentiates to contribute to the corpus luteum, the theca-lutein cells. Capillaries, probably in response to a trophic stimulus secreted by the granulosa-lutein cells, penetrate through the basement membrane. They invade the granulosa layer, ultimately reaching the central cavity, now vacated by the follicular fluid after ovulation, often filling it with blood. Cholesterol, carried mainly within low density lipoproteins (LDL), combines with specific receptors to be taken up by the granulosa-lutein cells. It is now available as substrate for progesterone synthesis (Fig. 3.5). This process along with the synthesis of both oestrogen and progesterone is dependent on continued gonadotrophic stimulation.

Oestrogen is synthesised in the same way as in the follicle, as FSH is able to reach the granulosa-lutein cells in significant quantities due to the increased vascularity.

Corpus luteum function is twofold: it provides the hormonal stimulus for the target organs, specifically the uterus; it also regulates the ovarian cycle. Progesterone depletes local oestrogen receptors. It also acts synergistically with oestradiol to inhibit, by negative feedback, gonadotrophin secretion. As a result, FSH and oestradiol-dependent follicular growth is inhibited.

The corpus luteum reaches peak activity about 7 days postovulation. This is coincident with peak vascularisation, and is therefore reflected in peak serum progesterone and oestradiol levels in the luteal phase. The corpus luteum declines rapidly 9–11 days postovulation. The next menses occurs 14 days postovulation. Variability in cycle length is due mainly to differences in the length of the follicular phase.

Luteal regression or luteolysis involves ischaemia and cell death, resulting in a fall in progesterone secretion. The whitish scar tissue thus formed is called the corpus albicans. The main hormone responsible for luteolysis is oestrogen, though the mechanism is uncertain. Oxytocin can be detected in the late corpus luteum. This has the effect of inhibiting conversion of cholesterol to pregnenolone, thus switching off progesterone production. It also reduces luteal blood flow, leading to ischaemia. However, the mechanism for initiation of luteolysis in the human has still to be defined.

Regression of the corpus luteum is inevitable unless pregnancy supervenes. Should pregnancy occur, rising beta hCG levels are detectable around 12 days postovulation. HCG maintains the corpus luteum steroid output until about the 10th week of pregnancy.

OVARIAN FUNCTION

Menarche

Follicles are first seen in the fetal ovary during the 25th week of gestation. From its inception, the follicles in the ovary are continuously undergoing development and atresia, though the steroid output of the ovary is minimal. Prior to puberty the ovary grows slowly in size. The menarche is defined as the age at which the first menstrual bleed takes place. It indicates that there is sufficient overian activity to have secreted some oestrogen to induce uterine development and to have caused bleeding. It does not signify fertility as, during the first two years, the cycles are mainly anovulatory.

The menarche occurs fairly late in the pubertal process. Puberty starts initially with a growth spurt, followed by the development of the secondary sex characteristics, such as breast development, pubic hair and the development of the external genitalia. The onset of menarche requires the prior maturation of the hypothalamic–pituitary–ovarian axis. At birth, there are low plasma levels of gonadotrophins as a result of the high levels of circulating maternal steroids. This is followed by a rebound rise in the gonadotrophin levels, until about 2 years of age. FSH then becomes very sensitive to the negative feedback effect of oestrogen. This is coupled with an inherent repression of GnRH secretion. After the age of 8, the central inhibition of GnRH assumes greater importance. This results in very low gonadotrophin levels until puberty when LH and FSH levels gradually rise. The first indication is a marked increase in magnitude and frequency of GnRH pulses at night, leading to similar pulses of the gonadotrophins. In late puberty, daytime pulses also become apparent, until gradually the adult pattern of GnRH pulsatility is reached. A maturation of the feedback mechanisms is also involved, as the negative feedback effect of oestrogen diminishes during puberty, allowing increased FSH and LH secretion for the same amount of oestrogen. The pituitary's sensitivity to GnRH also increases during puberty. This may be due in part to a self-priming effect, and in part to the rising oestrogen levels. The positive feedback effects of oestrogen and the ability to have a gonadotrophin surge is a relatively late process.

Over the past 150 years, the average age of the menarche has declined from 17 years to 13 years, the normal range now being 10–16 years. This decline can be attributed to improved health care and a rise in socio-economic standards, as the body weight at menarche has remained remarkably constant, 45–47 kg. It seems that a critical weight needs to be attained to allow activation of the hypothalamic-pituitary axis.

UTERINE CYCLE

The ovarian cycle determines the pattern of ovarian hormones measurable in the blood. The most important, but by no means the only target organ of these hormones, is the uterus.

Changes in the Uterine Body

Myometrium

Myometrial activity is inversely related to progesterone secretion. During menstruation, the uterus actively contracts with a greater frequency and strength than found in labour as a result of stimulation by locally released prostaglandins. After menstruation, there is a slow decline in activity during the follicular phase until there is almost no spontaneous activity at midcycle. This quiescence is maintained until the late luteal phase. If pregnancy supervenes, the myometrium remains inactive.

Uterine blood flow

Uterine blood flow correlates positively with the pattern of oestrogen secretion. Blood flow through the uterus is least during menstruation and the early follicular phase. There is then a marked increase with a peak just before ovulation, followed by a slight decrease and a secondary peak in the luteal phase. The flow then decreases prior to menstruation.

Endometrial changes (Figs. 3.6–3.10)

The proliferative phase. This is under oestrogenic control. Oestrogen stimulates the production of its own receptors, thus enhancing its own effect (upregulation). It also causes production of progesterone receptors, priming the endometrium, to enable it to respond to progesterone in the luteal phase. Without oestrogen priming, progesterone has no influence on the endometrium.

Within 48 hours of menstruation ceasing, the surface of the endometrium is covered by epithelial outgrowths from the remnants of glands in the basal part of the tissue. The rapid growth of the endometrium is seen mostly in the glands, which start as straight tubular structures (Fig. 3.6), but become increasingly long and convoluted. The gland cells are low columnar cells with centrally placed nuclei showing considerable mitotic activity (Fig. 3.7). The stromal cells similarly increase in number. These are small, spindle-shaped cells with very little cytoplasm. Except for a brief period of transient stromal oedema in the midfollicular phase, the stroma becomes compact and syncytial-like. The glandular epithelium thus extends onto the surface to link one segment with another, showing pseudostratification.

The blood supply to the endometrium is twofold: the basal layer is supplied by straight arteries; the glands are supplied by coiled spiral arteries, forming three capillary plexuses — one just below the surface epithelium, a second surrounding the glands, and a third within the stroma. A network of veins drain into the venous sinuses.

During proliferation, the endometrium grows from approximately 0.5 mm to 5 mm in height — a tenfold increase. This is in part due to new tissue growth and in part to stromal expansion.

The secretory phase. Following ovulation, progesterone becomes the dominant hormone,

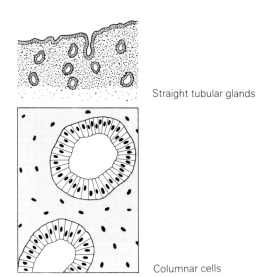

Straight tubular glands

Columnar cells

Fig. 3.6 *The endometrium in the early proliferative phase.*

although oestrogen is secreted in levels comparable to the follicular phase. Under the influence of progesterone, endometrial growth ceases, and the tissue now enters its functional stage as it prepares to accept the embryo.

The glands are convoluted and dilated with secretions. They commence secretory activity with subnuclear vacuoles appearing (Fig. 3.8). These gradually come to lie in the apical part of the gland before discharging their contents into the lumen of the gland. The secretions consist mainly of glycogen, sugars, amino acids, mucus and enzymes, such as alkaline phosphatase. By the end of the week following ovulation, the secretory process is finished and the glands appear exhausted (Fig. 3.9). Meanwhile, nuclear mitotic activity has declined considerably.

The spiral arteries are more prominent, becoming increasingly coiled. This is mainly due to their continuing growth, while the endometrial height has remained relatively static.

The changes in the late secretory phase will depend on whether implantation has taken place.

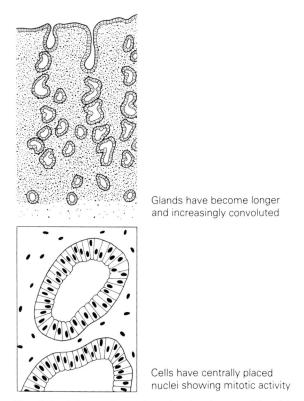

Glands have become longer and increasingly convoluted

Cells have centrally placed nuclei showing mitotic activity

Fig. 3.7 *The endometrium in the late proliferative phase.*

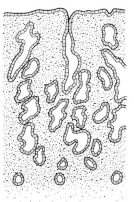

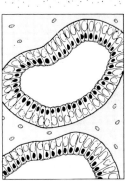

Glands are convoluted and dilated with secretions

Cells have apical nuclei and basal vacuoles

Fig. 3.8 *The endometrium in the early secretory phase.*

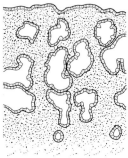

Marked decrease in tissue
height. Glands exhausted
of secretions

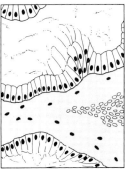

Cells show basal nuclei.
Vacuoles have discharged
their contents into the lumen.
Breakdown of spiral arteries
in the stroma

Fig. 3.9   *The endometrium in the late secretory phase.*

Implantation. Glandular secretory activity is reawakened, while the superficial stromal cells become large and polyhedral with cytoplasmic extensions, forming a strong compact layer, the stratum compactum. This overlies loose oedematous stroma, surrounding the tightly coiled spiral arteries, the stratum spongiosum. The basal layer remains unchanged with the spindle-shaped stromal cells surrounding the straight arteries, stratum basalis. This histological appearance describes the uterine decidual reaction to pregnancy and is known as the Arias-Stella reaction (*see* p. 54).

Non-implantation. A similar pattern is seen initially (pseudodecidualisation). However, in the absence of implantation and continued gonadotrophic support to maintain the steroid output of the corpus luteum, there is first a modest, then a marked reduction in tissue height. This causes a tighter coiling of the spiral arteries, similar to a spring being compressed. This buckling causes stasis and ischaemia. The spiral arteries undergo rhythmic constriction and relaxation, each wave longer and more profound than the previous one, eventually leading to blanching of the endometrium. This activity is probably under local prostaglandin control. PGE_2 causes relaxation of vascular smooth muscle, and $PGF_{2\alpha}$ causes vasoconstriction. Even more powerful are prostacyclin (PGI_2) as a vasodilator and inhibitor of platelet aggregation, and thromboxane A_2 as a vasoconstrictor. These substances are all synthesised in the endometrium and in the spiral arteries themselves. Their balance may be important in causing vasospasm.

In the 24 hours prior to menstruation, there is marked ischaemia and stasis. These stimuli further increase the local release of prostaglandins. White cells migrate into the stroma, red cells leak into the interstitial spaces, and thrombin-platelet plugs appear. Further thromboxane release occurs from the platelet plugs.

Menstruation. Interstitial haemorrhage occurs as a result of the breakdown of the superficial arterioles and capillaries. The generalised ischaemia weakens the structure of the superficial layers of the endometrium. The non-viable tissue formed as a result of cell and vascular necrosis is extruded into the endometrial cavity and contributes to the menstrual flow. This process continues until the basal layer is reached, where a natural cleavage plane is formed. Here the straight arteries maintain the blood supply and hence integrity of the basal layer, and in this way the layers superficial to the basal layer are shed (Fig. 3.10).

Menstrual flow is limited and eventually stops due to the vasoconstriction of the spiral arteries and the formation of thrombin-platelet plugs. Resumption of oestrogen secretion by the developing follicle induces healing and new tissue growth. Menstrual blood does not normally coagulate, and does not contain fibrin, probably as a result of proteolytic and fibrinolytic enzymes secreted by the damaged endometrial cells. Within 12 hours the endometrial height has shrunk from 4 mm to about 1 mm.

Changes in the Uterine Cervix

Oestrogen causes relaxation of the muscles of the cervix and increased stromal vascularity and oedema. Collagenase is activated and the tightly bound collagen bundles are largely dispersed into a loose matrix of collagen and stroma. It is softer to the touch, and eversion of the external os can be seen prior to ovulation. Under progesterone influence, the muscles retract and the stroma becomes more compact and the collagen matrix

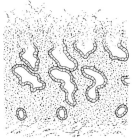

Loss of integrity of the endometrial surface. Glandular collapse

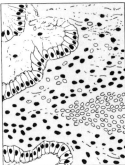

Cellular infiltration particularly red and white blood cells

Fig. 3.10 *The endometrium during menstruation.*

reforms. The cervix is therefore firmer and the external os becomes tighter.

Cervical epithelium

The endocervical canal is about 3 cm long and is lined with columnar epithelium. The epithelium is thrown into complex folds, with extensive gland formation, known as crypts. Groups of cells in each crypt secrete different types of mucus, namely E and G mucus. The former is produced in response to oestrogenic stimulation. E mucus has a very high water content (98%), and a network of long polypeptide macromolecules, lying parallel to each other and linked by carbohydrate sidechains. The channels thus formed are up to 5 microns in width and allow easy sperm migration. G mucus is produced under progesterone influence. It consists of a meshwork of polypeptide strands with increased carbohydrate linkages, with much smaller spaces between the macromolecules, and with reduced water content.

Clinically, E mucus is seen as a copious, clear watery secretion, which stretches easily for up to 8 cm between two glass surfaces (spinnbarkeit test). Under the microscope, the mucus is acellular, and on drying, the dehydration reveals strands of mucus forming a ferning pattern. G mucus is scanty,

cloudy and tacky. Microscopy reveals the presence of cells and the absence of ferning. The function of the cervical mucus is to assist the passage of sperm deposited in the vagina at the appropriate time. It, along with the uterine isthmus, acts as a major reservoir for sperm. The mucus plug would also seem to serve to protect against the passage of infection.

Other Physiological Changes during the Menstrual Cycle

Fallopian tube

Oestrogen increases epithelial activity with increased ciliation and secretory activity. Progestogenic effects are the reverse of this. Progesterone also decreases muscle activity.

Vagina

Oestrogens increase mitotic activity in the surface columnar epithelium and cause keratinisation. These cells have a small pyknotic nucleus and abundant cytoplasm. Under progesterone influence, the nucleus becomes larger and vesicular. A vaginal smear shows cells clumped together and folded in on themselves, as opposed to the single flat cells seen during oestrogen stimulation.

Breast

Although oestrogenic and progestogenic changes have been shown, these are not marked until the premenstrual period. At this time there is connective tissue oedema and hyperaemia. This is responsible for the increase in breast size and breast tenderness experienced during this period.

Skin

Changes are sometimes seen during the premenstruum. There is an increase in skin pigmentation, especially around the mouth, forehead, the nipple areolae and the linea nigra. Progesterone also causes constriction of the sebaceous gland ducts, thus exacerbating acne in sufferers.

Body temperature

Small rises in progesterone will cause a rise in basal body temperature. Progesterone or its metabolites act directly on the thermoregulatory centre in the hypothalamus to raise the temperature between 0.2°C and 0.6°C.

Thyroid function

The only change is the expected slight rise in the basal metabolic rate secondary to the rise in temperature in the luteal phase.

Adrenal function

Aldosterone is secreted in larger amounts during the luteal phase, probably in direct response to progesterone.

Symptomatic changes

During the premenstrual phase, from ovulation to the onset of menstruation, many women experience a feeling of bloatedness, breast tenderness, and a change of affect, particularly depression and irritability. It seems that at least 50% of women experience these symptoms to some degree and hence they may be considered 'physiological'.

DISORDERS OF THE MENSTRUAL CYCLE

Menstruation depends upon an intact hypothalamic-pituitary axis, normal ovarian function, a functionally responsive uterus and an intact outflow tract, i.e. cervix and vagina. A disturbance of any one of these components may result in disordered menstrual function.

The main symptom groups are:

1. Absent or scanty bleeding
2. Heavy and/or frequent bleeding
3. Painful periods
4. Premenstrual syndrome.

Symptoms related to the menstrual cycle often have considerable emotional and psychological overlay, which may be due to a central effect on the hypothalamus, altering its function, or to a colouring of the perception of the symptoms.

Amenorrhoea and Oligomenorrhoea

Primary amenorrhoea means that a woman has never had a period, while secondary amenorrhoea is the absence of uterine bleeding for 6 or more months. Oligomenorrhoea is scanty, infrequent uterine bleeding occurring every 6 weeks or more. If menstruation has not occurred by the age of 17, this is abnormal and the patient should be investigated.

The most common cause of amenorrhoea is pregnancy, and this diagnosis should always be considered.

Amenorrhoea implies either a problem with the uterus and outflow tract, or profound depression of the ovarian steroids.

Oligomenorrhoea implies an ovulatory disorder, but with a small amount of ovarian steroidogenesis to cause some endometrial proliferation and either breakthrough bleeding, as occurs with low levels of oestrogen, or a withdrawal bleed, with removal of oestrogenic or progestogenic influence on the endometrium, with its subsequent shedding.

Primary Amenorrhoea

The aetiology and diagnosis of primary amenorrhoea can seem complicated. The process of making a diagnosis can be simplified if, by a physical examination, patients can be divided into three categories. These are:

1. those with normal female genitalia, but no breast development;
2. normal breast development, but absent uterus;
3. normal breast development, and an apparently normal genital tract.

The causes of the first two categories, together with the diagnostic steps needed to arrive at a conclusion are shown in Fig. 3.11. Hypogonadotrophic hypogonadism may respond to chronic GnRH administration, resulting in a normal pituitary response. There is no specific treatment for women with an abnormal karyotype or absence of the uterus. Removal of intra-abdominal testes in testicular feminisation, and occasionally removal of striate ovaries in gonadal dysgenesis, may be advisable because of the risk of malignancy.

If the initial physical examination is unremarkable, then the cause of primary amenorrhoea can arise from the hypothalmus or pituitary.

Hypothalamic causes

Primary hypothalamic dysfunction prevents a normal interaction between GnRH and gonadotrophins, and there is usually evidence of other hormonal abnormalities.

Hypothalamic dysfunction can occasionally follow trauma or infection such as encephalitis in childhood. In all these cases, oestradiol levels will have been always low, uterine development will not have taken place and there will be no withdrawal uterine bleeding following 5 days of oral progestogen therapy. There may be bleeding following oestrogen priming.

Isolated GnRH deficiency is caused by an unknown malfunction of the rhinencephalon causing anosmia as well as amenorrhoea. It is known as Kallmann's syndrome. It responds to GnRH treatment. Colour blindness and mental retardation are sometimes associated.

Marked weight loss and severe stress as in anorexia nervosa can also cause hypothalamic dysfunc-tion. These cases will usually respond by having a withdrawal bleed following progestogen therapy. Cases of stress and severe weight loss occurring just prior to puberty may respond to alterations in the way of life and diet as well as to GnRH stimulation.

Cases of primary amenorrhoea due to hypothalamic causes will usually require prolonged GnRH administration in order to first prime the pituitary.

Pituitary causes

These include congenital hypopituitarism or pituitary tumours, although the latter are more likely to cause secondary amenhorrhoea. Patients with congenital hypopituitarism will present with other signs of pituitary dysfunction, such as failure to grow. Pituitary tumours are diagnosed radiologically by alterations to the pituitary fossa, and sometimes by altered visual fields due to pressure on the optic chiasma. The treatment of hypopituitarism is substitution of the deficient pituitary hormones where possible. Treatment of pituitary tumours, which are usually adenomas, is by surgical removal or ablation by radioactive implants. Small prolactinomas will usually respond to suppression by bromocriptine.

Cryptomenorrhoea

Failure to expel menstrual blood occurs when there

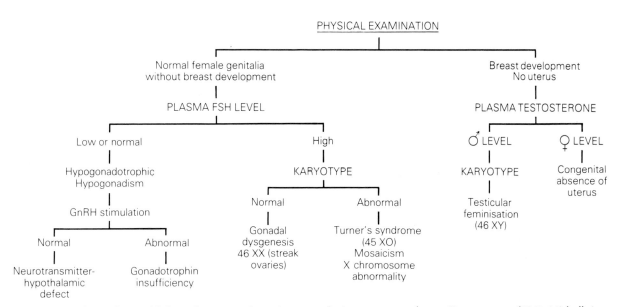

Fig. 3.11 *Scheme for establishing the cause of certain types of primary amenorrhoea. (By courtesy of D.R. Mishell, Jr. and V. Davajan, eds., 1979.* Reproductive Endocrinology in Fertility and Contraception. *Philadelphia: Davis.)*

is an intact hymen or septum just above the hymen closing off the vagina completely. This is easily detected on physical examination. The patient will be endocrinologically normal and anatomically otherwise normal.

Treatment is by surgical incision and drainage of the retained menstrual blood. Care must be taken to avoid introducing infection.

Congenital absence of the uterus

This may or may not be accompanied by other abnormalities of the genital tract, such as an absent vagina.

Secondary Amenorrhoea

It is helpful to consider the possible causes in two groups:

1. Disorders of the uterus and lower genital tract.
2. Anovulation.

Disorders of the uterus and lower genital tract

If the patient has menstruated or has oligomenorrhoea, then it can be assumed that the anatomy of the uterus and lower genital tract has been, or is, normal. Asherman's syndrome is amenorrhoea caused by uterine synechiae following curettage of the uterus in the pregnant state, e.g. following a miscarriage. Treatment by hysteroscopic division of adhesions is usually only attempted if the patient wishes to conceive. The responsivity of the uterus can be tested by giving a progestogen and waiting for a withdrawal bleed within the following 2–4 days. If this does not occur, then prior oestrogen priming may be necessary.

Anovulation

It follows that if the uterus is functionally intact, then the problem lies with the lack of appropriate sex steroid stimulation, as a result of anovulation. Failure to ovulate may be due to hypothalamic-pituitary-ovarian hypofunction or dysfunction.

Hypothalamic hypofunction. Hypothalamic failure is diagnosed by finding low circulating gonadotrophin levels. Treatment is either to give pulsatile GnRH or exogenous gonadotrophins.

Causes of secondary hypothalamic failure include:

1. *Stress, severe weight loss*, and *anorexia nervosa*. This group has disordered GnRH pulsatile secretion. Normal function is usually restored when the underlying cause is treated.
2. *Drugs*, such as the phenothiazines, methyldopa and cimetidine. They act by disturbing neurotransmission, in this case dopamine transmission.
3. *Tumours*, either within the hypothalamus such as a hamartoma, or outside, such as a craniopharyngioma.
4. *Miscellaneous causes* including tuberculosis and sarcoidosis. Irradiation may also cause hypothalamic failure.

Pituitary hypofunction. Pituitary failure is characterised by low levels of pituitary hormones and lack of response to hypothalamic releasing factors. Low gonadotrophin levels will result in atrophy of the ovaries and uterus — hence the term 'hypogonadotrophic hypogonadism'. Hypopituitarism may involve only the gonadotrophin secreting cells, which are usually the first cells to be affected by the presence of a space-occupying lesion, except in children, when growth hormone is the first to suffer. When other aspects of pituitary function are involved, the condition is called 'panhypopituitarism'.

A skull x-ray with coned views of the pituitary fossa is essential to identify and define any space-occupying lesion. Computerised tomography (CT scan) is currently the most accurate radiological investigation. Visual field testing is also essential due to the close approximation of the optic chiasma to the pituitary fossa. Classically, a pituitary tumour is said to cause bitemporal hemianopia.

Causes of pituitary failure include:

1. *Pituitary tumour.* This is the commonest cause of secondary hypopituitarism. The commonest tumour is a chromophobe adenoma. However, it may also be due to a functional tumour.
2. *Empty sella syndrome.* This is a radiological finding. It is due to leakage of cerebrospinal fluid into the sella tursica, exerting pressure on the pituitary gland, thus flattening it against other structures, and also onto the sella itself, causing bony erosion. Endocrine problems are usually very mild, despite the fact that gonadotrophin secretion is usually very sensitive to outside influences.

3. *Sheehan's syndrome*. Pituitary failure developing, following obstetric shock. The pituitary is particularly vulnerable to circulatory collapse in pregnancy. This condition is rare as almost total destruction of the gland is needed before pituitary failure ensues.
4. *Miscellaneous causes*, including internal carotoid artery aneurysm; tumours of the 3rd ventricle; radical ablative therapy following surgery or radiotherapy of a pituitary tumour and infections such as meningitis or tuberculosis.

Ovarian hypofunction. Ovarian failure occurs at the menopause. If it occurs before the age of 40, it is known as 'premature ovarian failure'. The diagnosis is made on finding elevated gonadotrophin levels in the postmenopausal range, due to the lack of negative feedback by oestrogen. The cause is unknown, but there is a genetic predisposition. It may occur as an autoimmune phenomenon. Histological examination of ovarian tissue may reveal the presence or absence of primordial follicles. In the former case, the condition is known as the 'resistant ovary syndrome', presumably resistant to FSH. The rare occurrence of spontaneous resumption of ovulation has been recorded in this group. There is no cure for this distressing condition and treatment is aimed at relieving the 'menopausal symptoms', with cyclical hormone replacement therapy.

Endocrine causes of hypothalamic-pituitary-ovarian hypofunction

Hyperprolactinaemia inhibits both LH and FSH release, although LH to a much greater extent. It acts at the hypothalamic level, probably by disrupting the hypothalamic dopamine system. A raised prolactin will feedback to stimulate dopamine release (Prolactin Inhibitory Factor). The dopaminergic neurones inhibit GnRH release. As a result, GnRH and gonadotrophin pulsatility is lost. Clinically, there is probably a spectrum of effect, ranging from an inadequate LH and progesterone production to complete suppression of the gonadotrophin levels and resultant amenorrhoea. However, raised oestrogens and androgens will stimulate prolactin release and this may confuse the picture.

Causes of raised prolactin levels include:

1. **Physiological:**
   Pregnancy
   Lactation
   Stress
   Marked diurnal variation; highest levels are seen during sleep
   Idiopathic.
2. **Pathological:**
   Prolactinomas. These are prolactin secreting pituitary tumours. They may be either macro- or microadenomas depending on their size (<1 mm in diameter is defined as a microadenoma). Like all pituitary tumours, they should be investigated as previously described. Treatment is either by ablative surgery, radiotherapy or with bromocriptine. Bromocriptine is a lysergic acid derivative. It is a dopamine agonist, binding specifically to dopamine receptors, thereby mimicking the inhibitory dopamine effects. Bromocriptine has established itself as the treatment of choice, perhaps combined with surgery for the larger tumours.
   Drugs. The commonest group of drugs that may cause hyperprolactinaemia are the phenothiazines. Others are methyldopa, reserpine, opiates, and benzodiazepams. They act either to deplete dopamine levels or to block dopamine receptors. Treatment is either to stop the drug or to add bromocriptine.
   Hypothyroidism causes raised prolactin levels indirectly. The subsequent raised hypothalamic thyroid releasing hormone (TRH) acts as a prolactin releasing factor. Correcting the hypothyroid state promptly returns the prolactin to normal.
   Other causes include tumours compressing the pituitary stalk, which may interfere with delivery of dopamine. There is also an association between 'post pill' amenorrhoea and a raised prolactin level.

Hyperadrenalism may result in sufficiently high circulating androgen levels to inhibit menstruation, as a result of feedback at the hypothalamic-pituitary level, though the precise mechanism is unclear. There are two usual clinical presentations.

1. *Cushing's syndrome*. The patient is obese and hirsute, with a plethoric complexion, in addition to the menstrual disturbance. She may complain of bruising and muscle weakness.
2. *Adrenogenital syndrome*. This describes an androgenised phenotype and female genotype — 46,XX. This is due to markedly elevated androgen levels in early life.

Biochemical confirmation of hyperandrenalism is by finding a raised dehydroepiandrosterone sulphate (DHEA-S) level, as the ovary (the only other site of androgen secretion) does not have the necessary sulphatase enzyme to convert DHEA to DHEA-S.

Causes include:
  Pituitary tumour (Cushing's disease);
  Congenital adrenal hyperplasia;
  21-hydroxylase enzyme deficiency, thereby preventing the conversion of 19-hydroxyprogesterone to cortisol, causing it to be converted to androgens instead.

Hyperthyroidism may also cause amenorrhoea, although the mechanism is unclear. Treatment will cause resumption of normal menstruation.

Hypothalamic–pituitary–ovarian dysfunction. Functional abnormalities of the hypothalamic-pituitary-ovarian axis will present as either amenorrhoea or oligomenorrhoea, depending on the severity of dysfunction.

Folliculogenesis is a complex phenomenon, depending upon appropriate endocrine signals and feedback mechanisms. Any disturbance of this system usually corrects itself. Occasionally a vicious cycle of events develop, culminating in Polycystic Ovary Disease (PCOD), also known as the Stein-Leventhal syndrome. This consists of obesity, hirsutism and infertility due to anovulation. These symptoms can be understood by considering the pathophysiology of the disease (Fig. 3.12).

Poor follicular development leads to decreased conversion of androgen substrate to oestradiol. The intraovarian effect of excess androgen is to directly inhibit further oestrogen production. The extraovarian effect is for the increased circulating androgen to depress levels of its own binding globulin — sex hormone binding globulin (SHBG). Androgen is also peripherally converted to oestrogen (oestrone) in fat. The increased levels of free testosterone and the oestrogen feedback on the hypothalamic-pituitary axis inhibit FSH secretion. Paradoxically this sensitises the pituitary to GnRH, selectively raising LH levels while depressing FSH levels. The increased pulsatile LH stimulates further ovarian androgen production, while aromatisation is depressed.

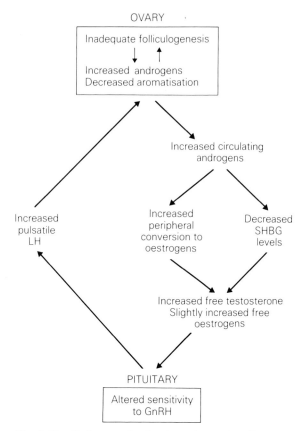

Fig. 3.12   *Pathogenesis of polycystic ovarian disease.*

The clinical picture will depend upon the severity and the duration of the dysfunction. The patient is hirsute because of the raised androgen levels. Anovulation results in the menstrual disturbance. The obesity may be an aetiological factor (*see below*), or be due to the anabolic effects of the raised androgens. Endocrine investigations reveal raised LH, depressed FSH and raised free testosterone levels. Ultrasound and laparoscopy will confirm large ovaries with multiple small cysts and a thick capsule, which can be confirmed on ovarian biopsy.

Causes of polycystic ovary disease include:

1. *Abnormal hypothalamic function.* PCOD can be seen around puberty. It is associated with daytime LH surges, as opposed to the usual night-time surges.
2. *Obesity.* Increased peripheral fat conversion of androgen to oestrogen results in constant ele-

vated oestrogen levels, thereby preventing an adequate perimenstrual FSH rise, and subsequent normal folliculogenesis.

3. *Congenital adrenal hyperplasia.* A very mild form may present in adult life. The diagnosis is made on finding raised 17α-hydroxyprogesterone levels. The dysfunction results from raised androgen levels. Treatment by dexamethasone will depress adrenal function, thus removing the underlying cause.
4. *A raised prolactin*, by the mechanism already described.

Treatment of PCOD depends on whether the patient wishes to conceive. If so, the principle is to raise FSH levels to stimulate follicular development. This is usually achieved with clomiphene, an antioestrogen which prevents oestrogenic feedback on the hypothalamic-pituitary axis, or by giving exogenous FSH, either in the pure form or with LH. Ovarian wedge resection is an old and effective treatment which has fallen out of favour, mainly because of the risk of adhesion formation. However, as microsurgical techniques are being used, wedge resection still has a place. If pregnancy is not desired, then cyclic progesterone therapy should be given to counteract the unopposed oestrogenic stimulation of the endometrium, with the theoretical risk of malignant change. Hirsutism and obesity may be specifically treated.

Abnormal Uterine Bleeding

Normal menstruation occurs every 28 days $\pm$ 7 days. The number of days of bleeding can vary from 2 to 8 days. The total average blood loss is about 60 ml, but ranges from 30 to 80 ml. Menstrual blood rarely clots.

Terminology for characterising the periods is best confined to describing the symptoms. Frequent periods are known as polymenorrhoea. Heavy periods are known as menorrhagia. Heavy and frequent periods are known as polymenorrhagia.

The presence of vaginal blood does not always signify uterine bleeding. It may be due to local causes in the vagina and cervix, e.g. cervical polyp. Haematuria or a urethral caruncle may present as 'vaginal' bleeding. Intermenstrual bleeding may be from the uterus or from non-uterine sources.

Abnormal uterine bleeding may be due to the following conditions (Fig. 3.13):

Local

1. Endometrial polyps.
2. Submucous fibromyomata. These are benign tumours of smooth muscle and fibrous tissue underlying the endometrium.
3. Foreign body, e.g. intrauterine contraceptive device.
4. Endometriosis. These are ectopic foci of endometrium usually within the pelvis.

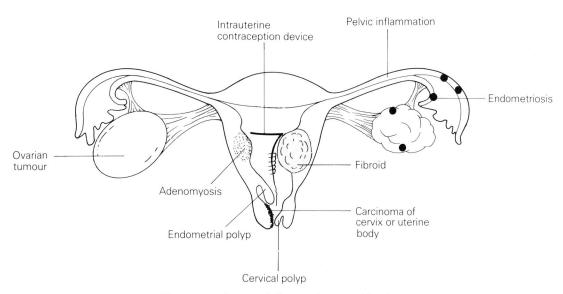

Fig. 3.13 *Causes of abnormal uterine bleeding.*

5. Adenomyosis. These are ectopic foci of endometrium within the uterine muscle.
6. Congenital abnormalities, e.g. bicornuate uterus.
7. Chronic or acute endometritis.
8. Carcinoma of the body of the uterus or cervix.

The last two causes may present with any pattern of abnormal bleeding. Carcinoma of the uterus or cervix should always be considered with any abnormal bleeding pattern. As a result, a cervical smear and uterine curettage are mandatory procedures to exclude malignancy. The other causes usually present with menorrhagia with or without prolonged bleeding.

Systemic disorders

1. Blood dyscrasias/clotting disorders
2. Liver disease
3. Renal disease
4. Severe anaemia.

Dysfunctional uterine bleeding

This may be defined as abnormal uterine bleeding not due to organic disease of the genital tract. It is a diagnosis of exclusion and encompasses a range of ovulatory disorders resulting in disordered menstruation. At the extremes of the reproductive age, disordered ovulation and abnormal menstruation are frequent. In these cases, patience and reassurance are all that is required. However, about 50% of all referrals for dysfunctional uterine bleeding are in the 20–40 age group.

Anovulation is the most common defect. Progesterone is not secreted in significant quantities and therefore the predominant hormonal environment is oestrogenic. The endometrium shows proliferative changes and excess vascularity. There is overgrowth of both the glands and the stroma. In this state, the endometrium is not stable and irregular shedding occurs, giving rise to episodes of prolonged, frequent and occasionally torrential bleeding (polymenorrhoea or polymenorrhagia). Endometrial hyperplasia should be monitored closely as it may represent a premalignant state, particularly if there is a glandular component. Oestrogen secreting ovarian cysts may also present with this picture.

Disordered ovulation may present with any pattern of abnormal bleeding, from premenstrual spotting to polymenorrhagia. Endometrial histology shows either a proliferative or a mixed proliferative and secretory picture, resulting in irregular shedding.

Management of dysfunctional uterine bleeding involves: (1) excluding other causes of vaginal bleeding; (2) trying to correct the underlying cause; (3) limiting the blood loss and establishing normal cycles. Uterine curettage and cervical cytology are mandatory. Endometrial histology will help to define the type of ovulatory disorder.

If the patient wishes to conceive, then the best approach is to stimulate follicular development by giving clomiphene citrate. If the patient does not wish to conceive, then prescribing the contraceptive pill, or a progestogen, will induce regular withdrawal bleeds. Menstruation may also be suppressed by giving continuous progestogen therapy. Danazol, an ethinyltestosterone derivative may also be used for this purpose. Other non-hormonal agents can be used either in addition to the above or as a first choice.

1. Prostaglandin synthetase inhibitors, such as mefenamic acid. Cyclo-oxygenase metabolites of arachidonic acid, namely prostaglandins E_2 and $F_{2\alpha}$ from the endometrium are increased towards the end of the luteal phase. In women with menorrhagia, the proportion of vasodilatory PGs such as PGE_2 compared with vasoconstrictor PGs ($PGF_{2\alpha}$) have increased compared with normal. The synthesis of prostacyclin by the endometrium has not been fully investigated.
2. Antifibrinolytic agents, such as aminocaproic acid or tranexamic acid.
3. Maintaining capillary integrity. Ethamsylate acts principally on the capillaries to maintain structural integrity of the walls, thereby reducing excessive capillary blood loss.

If medical treatment is unsuccessful, hysterectomy will be considered. The patient's attitudes and wishes are of paramount importance if this operation is not to lead to psychological sequelae (*see* p. 267).

Dysmenorrhoea

Dysmenorrhoea means painful periods of which there are two main forms.

Primary or spasmodic

This is a reflection of the extreme of the physiological spectrum. Cramping lower abdominal pains starting just before or with the menstrual flow and continuing during menstruation are characteristic. There are often associated gastrointestinal symptoms, such as nausea, vomiting or an increased number of bowel motions. The patient may also complain of headaches, feeling faint and symptoms of peripheral vasodilatation. The examination is essentially normal except during menstruation when the uterus is tender. The aetiology is thought to be related to excessive prostaglandin production, as the levels particularly of $PGF_{2\alpha}$ and its metabolites in endometrium, menstrual loss and peripheral blood have shown significant elevation in women with dysmenorrhoea.

Treatment is aimed (1) at either abolishing ovulation so that the endometrium becomes atrophic, usually by prescribing the pill, or (2) by giving drugs that inhibit prostaglandin synthesis, such as indomethacin, mefenamic acid or ibuprofen. Treatment is nearly always partially successful, but sometimes a combination of the above treatments may be required. If, however, the symptoms persist, then the patient should be investigated for a pathological cause (*see below*).

Secondary or congestive dysmenorrhoea

This usually presents in the older patient. She complains of a congested ache, with lower abdominal cramps, which usually start a few days, but can start up to 2 weeks prior to the menses, and are relieved at onset of flow. There may also be spasmodic dysmenorrhoea.

The most common causes are pelvic inflammatory disease, endometriosis, fibroids and the presence of an intrauterine contraceptive device. The most helpful investigation is a diagnostic laparoscopy. Treatment is aimed at the underlying cause. Suppressing menstruation in the case of endometriosis helps to cure the condition, but otherwise inhibiting ovulation does not help as the pain is associated with any type of menstrual loss. Antiprostaglandin agents may be of some help. In cases of severe endometriosis or uterine pathology, only surgery will be of significant benefit.

Premenstrual Syndrome

The premenstrual syndrome is a collection of differing signs and symptoms which occur only in the premenstruum, i.e. after ovulation and is relieved by menstruation. It is often misdiagnosed, is of unknown aetiology, and can be extremely debilitating and distressing. Most women at some time or other will experience some premenstrual symptoms. It is usually first reported by women in their mid-thirties. The main symptom groups are:

1. Feeling bloated and an increase in abdominal girth, occasionally with some weight gain. This is due to gaseous intestinal distension and generalised fluid retention.
2. Breast tenderness due to stromal oedema and hyperaemia.
3. Mood changes, particularly irritability, depression or aggression.

The aetiology of this multisymptomatic condition is unknown, though various theories have been put forward:

1. Oestrogen/progesterone imbalance, or a relative progesterone deficiency, which may lead to:
2. fluid retention due to raised aldosterone levels in the luteal phase. The renin-angiotensin system has also been incriminated;
3. raised prolactin levels, particularly regarding breast symptoms.
4. Prostaglandins, due to their ubiquitous nature, have also been implicated.
5. Central opiod levels decline in the premenstruum. One theory puts forward a withdrawal-like effect.
6. A neurotic personality.

None of these theories has been substantiated.

Treatment is largely empirical and is frequently no better than the average placebo response rate of 40%. It cannot be emphasised too strongly that there is a major need for psychological support, reassurance and explanation of the condition. Treatment can be symptomatic or general.

General treatments

1. The contraceptive pill has been prescribed to inhibit ovulation. It is not as effective as was previously hoped and the symptoms may return during the pill-free week, although it can be given continuously. The pill may also be contraindicated in the older patient.
2. Vaginal or rectal progesterone or oral synthetic

progestogens such as dydrogesterone are frequently used. Treatment is usually started on Day 12 of the cycle and continues for 2 weeks. In appropriate cases therapy can be very effective.
3. Alteration of prostaglandin levels, either decreasing them by giving antiprostaglandin agents, or altering their balance by giving evening primrose oil which is plentiful in linolenic acid, a precursor of prostaglandins.
4. Dietary changes such as a greater intake of vegetable fats, vitamins and various trace elements.

Symptomatic treatments

1. Feeling of bloatedness: a diuretic may be appropriate, particularly if weight gain has been recorded. Spironolactone is a specific aldosterone antagonist and is probably the most appropriate diuretic.
2. Breast tenderness: bromocriptine (a specific inhibitor of prolactin release) and Danazol are both effective.
3. Mood changes: Pyridoxine (vitamin B6) is involved in serotonin (5HT) metabolism. De-

creased levels of 5HT have been shown in the affective disorders. Pyridoxine from Day 14 of the cycle may be of some use. Anxiolytics such as the benzodiazepines may also be of benefit. However, it should be stressed again that reassurance and sympathetic support are the most important elements of therapy.

FURTHER READING

Baird D.T., Michie E.A., eds. (1985). *Mechanisms of Menstrual Bleeding*. New York: Raven Press. Serona Symposia Publications.
Johnson M., Everitt B. (1984). *Essential Reproduction*. Oxford: Blackwell Scientific Publications.
Speroff L., Glass R.H., Kase N.G. (1984). *Clinical Gynaecologic Endocrinology and Infertility*. Baltimore, London: Williams and Wilkins.
Tyson J.E., ed. (1978). Neuroendocrinology of reproduction. In *Clinics in Obstetrics and Gynaecology*, Vol. 5, No. 2. London: W.B. Saunders.
Wilson E.W., Rennie P.I.C. (1976). *The Menstrual Cycle*. London: Lloyd Luke.

4

Early Development

The development of the fetus begins with the process of fertilisation, a complex process involving the penetration of the oocyte by the spermatozoon.

FERTILISATION

Spermatozoa undergo a number of physiological changes during their course through the female genital tract before they are able to penetrate oocytes. The initial change is known as capacitation which involves changes in the plasma membrane induced by enzymes located in the acrosome region (Fig. 4.1).

This leads to the acrosome reaction, a process essential for fertilisation. The acrosome reaction involves structural changes, which start with swelling of the sperm head, followed by the fusion of the two outer membranes, releasing enzymes, which results in vesicle formation and loss of integrity of the acrosomal cap. As this degenerates, the acrosomal cap is lost, leaving the inner acrosomal membrane and nucleus exposed. The acrosome reaction usually occurs in the ampulla of the fallopian tube, where the oocyte is found soon after ovulation. There is an increase in motility of the sperm after the acrosome reaction has occurred.

The sperm (Fig. 4.2) now has to penetrate through several layers of the oocyte (Figs. 4.3 and 4.4). The outer layer of cumulus (corona radiata) is enzymatically penetrated (hyaluronidase) and this exposes the zona pellucida to which the sperm loosely binds. The zona is also penetrated with the

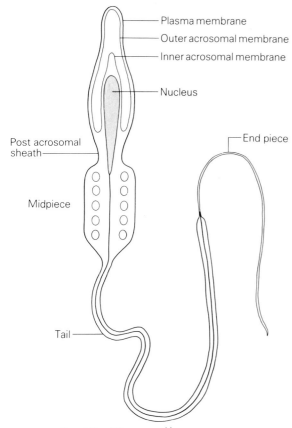

Fig. 4.1 *Diagram of human sperm.*

Plasma membrane
Outer acrosomal membrane
Inner acrosomal membrane
Nucleus
End piece
Post acrosomal sheath
Midpiece
Tail

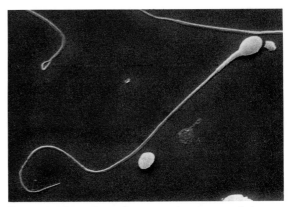

Fig. 4.2 *Scanning electron microscope of human sperm.*

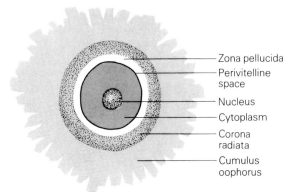

Fig. 4.3   *Oocyte and its surrounding layers.*

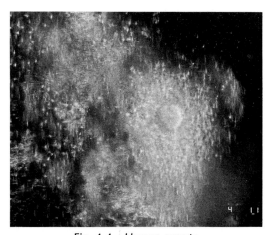

Fig. 4.4   *Human oocyte.*

aid of an enzyme, a protease known as acrosin, and the sperm enters the perivitelline space between the zona pellucida and the oocyte. More than one sperm may reach this space, but only one sperm fuses with the nucleus, activating the oocyte, and thereafter the development of the block to polyspermia (Fig. 4.5). The activated oocyte undergoes a meiotic division and discards 23 chromosomes as the 2nd polar body (having lost nuclear material as 1st polar in early ovum formation) and these chromosomes form the pronucleus, which fuses with the pronucleus from the sperm and the cell is ready to divide, with 46 chromosomes.

CLEAVAGE

This first mitotic division of the embryo occurs about 36 h after fertilisation resulting in a 2-cell embryo. By 48 h, it has cleaved again to reach the 4-cell stage (Fig. 4.6) and by 72 h it is at the 16–32 cell stage.

During this time, the embryo is moving down the fallopian tube by a combination of tubal ciliary and muscle action. The embryo is carried in tubal fluid which has a complex formulation of ions, proteins and steroid molecules, all of which are necessary to promote the ideal environment for embryo growth. Any damage to the fallopian tube, e.g. salpingitis, will interfere with tubal transport, as cilia will be destroyed, and the tubal environment may no longer be ideal. So, infertility can result from altered tubal physiology without tubal blockage.

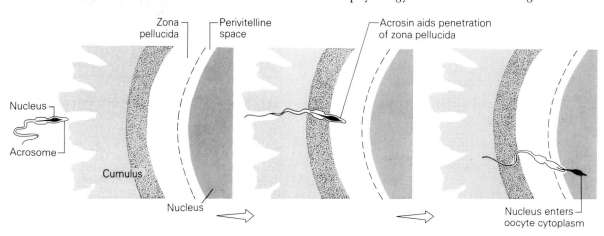

Fig. 4.5   *Fertilisation.*

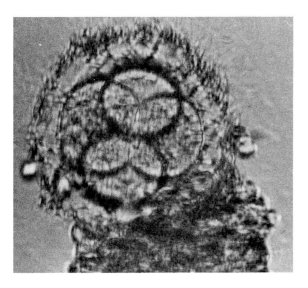

Fig. 4.6   *Four-cell human embryo.*

The human embryo enters the uterus about 3–4 days after ovulation, at about the 16–32 cell stage.

The Morula and Blastocyst

Cell division continues in the uterus until the 32-cell (morula) to 64-cell (blastocyst) stage. Cleavage is synchronous in the early stages, but by the morula stage, the division is much more haphazard. Eventually, individual blastomeres become indistinct, a process called compaction. This results in the formation of an outer layer of cells (the future trophectoderm) and the inner cells which are destined to become the inner cell mass. This then leads to blastocyst formation with secretion of fluid into the morula and the inner cell mass becomes eccentrically placed (Fig. 4.7).

The zona pellucida persists until this stage and now the zona opens (hatching) and the blastocyst is expelled.

IMPLANTATION

The uterus is primed by steroid hormone changes during the follicular and early luteal phase of the cycle and the blastocyst is now lying free in the

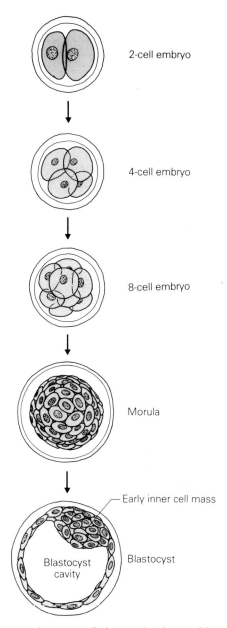

Fig. 4.7   *Embryonic cell division leading to blastocyst formation.*

uterine cavity in close approximation to the endometrium.

The endometrium has undergone several biochemical and physiological changes, resulting in changes in the secretions of the uterine glands. There is an increase in the cellular content of the stroma, an increased uterine blood flow and endometrial oedema. The role of the various uterine secretions and their influence on the blastocyst is still uncertain, but a role in implantation is probable.

The embryo also plays an active role in implantation (Fig. 4.8) and there are changes in the membranes which result in receptor formation, enabling the blastocyst to respond to external stimuli. The time when an embryo can implant is probably restricted to 1 or 2 days, and the rise in oestrogen and progesterone in the luteal phase is critical. The endometrial receptor for these steroids must be primed in order to facilitate implantation, and the proteins produced in response to this probably stimulate the embryo directly.

The human embryo implants by a process called interstitial implantation, becoming apposed to and then invading the endometrium. At the site of implantation, there is a change in capillary permeability which occurs about 24 h before attachment occurs. These changes may be due to histamine, released from uterine mast cells, or cyclic AMP.

There are three steps in implantation:

Apposition
Adhesion
Penetration

During apposition, the blastocyst becomes closely orientated to the endometrium, facilitated by microvilli on both the trophoblast and the endometrium. The process of adhesion involves interdigitation of the endometrial and trophoblastic microvilli and adhesion is further enhanced by the secretion of glycoproteins which have a 'sticky' nature. The final process of penetration involves the trophoblast, now firmly attached, growing between the endometrial cells and invading the endometrium. The erosion of the surface of the endometrium means that 2 days after apposition, the blastocyst is completely implanted. From the time of entering the uterus, the embryo has been secreting proteins, especially human chorionic gonadotrophin (HCG) which is released into the maternal circulation to maintain the corpus luteum.

As invasion proceeds, the trophoblast cells enter the local capillaries and spaces (lacunae) appear,

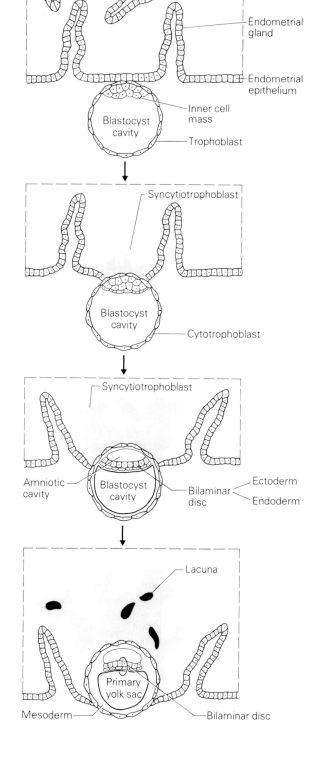

Fig. 4.8   *Implantation.*

filled with blood, which are the primitive intervillous spaces. The development of the trophoblast is not uniform, being most marked towards the decidual base of the blastocyst, which will become the placenta.

DEVELOPMENT OF THE EMBRYO

There are changes within the blastocyst during implantation. By Day 7 after ovulation, the cells of the outer layer of the inner cell mass become ectodermal cells and the inner layer, endodermal cells. One day later, the ectodermal layer becomes split and the space becomes enlarged to form an amniotic cavity. So by Day 10 postovulation, there is a two-layered inner cell mass, and two cavities, the amniotic cavity and the primary yolk sac.

By Day 11, there is active proliferation of cells from the inner surface of the trophoblast, which leads to separation of the ectoderm and the endoderm and the formation of an intermediate, mesodermal, layer.

The surrounding tissue is called the mesoblast; vacuolation occurs and two layers form, one lining the trophoblast and the other lining the embryo and yolk sac. The cavity is called the extra embryonic coelome and it separates the embryonic disc from the trophoblast except for the body stalk. The embryonic disc, by Day 16, is trilaminar (Fig. 4.9). The amniotic cavity continues to expand and by Day 50 completely surrounds the embryo and fuses with the chorion.

From this point, there are two separate entities to consider, the placenta and the fetus. The former will be described in Chapter 6.

Later Development of the Embryo

By Day 21, the embryo is ready to enter the somite stage of development which lasts 10 days. At this point it is a trilaminar disc consisting of layers of ectoderm, mesoderm and endoderm. The endoderm and mesoderm only remain in contact at two areas, the oral and cloacal membranes. During the invasion by mesoderm, an area of intense mitotic activity, called Henson's node, arises in the ectoderm and grows between the endoderm and ectoderm to form the notochord. The ectoderm spreads laterally on both sides and moves anteriorly to fuse

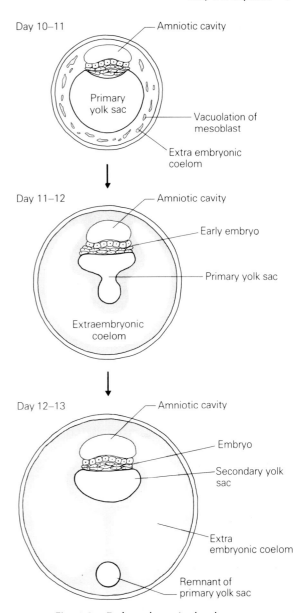

Fig. 4.9 *Early embryonic development.*

in the midline, taking mesoderm with it. The ectodermal tube forms the basis of the nervous system and the endoderm forms somites which become the vertebral column. There are usually a total of 25.

By the 7 somite stage, closure of the neural plate and cephalic enlargement have begun and by the 10 somite stage, three ventricles can be discerned. From this point onwards, differentiation and growth are rapid and embryogenesis occurs in a very fixed time scale.

The somite stage closes with the fusion of the distal ends of the neuropores and the formation of a well-defined umbilical cord and tail. The embryo is comma shaped at this stage.

The external changes from now on are much less rapid. During weeks 6–8, there is the development of forelimb buds and the arms, hindlimb buds and the legs, expansion of the brain, modifications to the tail, development of the face and eyes, so that by 8 weeks, the embryo has a human form and is now called a fetus.

CONGENITAL MALFORMATIONS

The fetus may be born with an anatomical abnormality, which may be microscopic or macroscopic, as a result of either primary maldevelopment or disordered normal development due to interference from an outside influence. It is estimated that 10% of human developmental abnormalities result from drugs, viruses and other environmental factors, and 20% of deaths in the perinatal period are attributed to congenital malformations.

Causes of congenital abnormalities are divided into genetic and environmental factors, although some abnormalities may occur as a result of genetic and environmental factors occurring together and this is called multifactorial inheritance.

Genetic Disorders

These are the largest group of anomalies and they are present in 1 : 200 newborn infants in some form or other. The chromosomes can be subjected to two kinds of change, numerical and structural. Either of these two types of alteration in chromosomes will initiate developmental changes which result in a characteristic phenotype, such as Down's syndrome.

Numerical disorders usually arise as a result of non-disjunction. Chromosomes normally exist in pairs and, if at the time of cell division the paired chromosomes fail to separate (or disjoin), then there is depletion of the total number of chromosomes. Normally, females have 22 autosomes (non-sex chromosomes) plus two X chromosomes, and males have 22 autosomes plus one X and one Y chromo-

some. Any deviation from the normal 46 chromosomes is called aneuploidy and the commonest problem is non-disjunction, such as Turner's Syndrome where the chromosome complement is 45 with one X chromosome missing. If a chromosome is missing, then the condition is called monosomy; for instance Turner's syndrome is called Monosomy X. If an autosome is missing the embryo almost always dies.

If three chromosomes are present instead of two, the condition is called trisomy and again the cause is usually non-disjunction, resulting in a germ cell with 24 instead of 23 chromosomes. The most common condition is trisomy 21 or Down's syndrome, in which three chromosome 21s are present. Other chromosomes are susceptible to trisomy; for instance, 18, 13, and 22, but they are less common. Trisomy may occur in the sex chromosomes and this is much more common. The incidence of these disorders, e.g. 47,XXX, 47,XXY (Klinefelter's syndrome) or 47,XYY is about 1:1000. Usually the greater the number of X chromosomes present, the greater the mental retardation; there is no effect of extra sex chromosomes on male or female characteristics.

It is possible for an individual to have a combination of cell lines and this is known as mosaicism. The malformations are usually less severe than the monosomy or trisomy forms, for example Turner Mosaic 45,X0/46,XX.

If a complete extra set of chromosomes is incorporated into the embryo, then it is known as triploidy and these embryos all spontaneously abort.

Structural abnormalities, on the other hand, are the result of chromosome breaks which may be induced by environmental factors, such as drugs, viruses, radiation, etc. The type of abnormality depends on what happens to the broken pieces.

Translocation is the transfer of a piece of one chromosome to a different chromosome. It does not necessarily result in abnormal development; for example translocation between chromosome 21 and 14 (robertsonian translocation) is phenotypically normal. Persons who have a normal phenotype, but have a translocation anomaly are called translocation carriers.

If a chromosome breaks and the piece is lost, this is known as deletion, e.g. deletion of the short arm of chromosome 5 results in cri-du-chat syndrome.

Malformations can be caused by mutant genes, such as achondroplasia, polydactyly, or they may occur *only* if these abnormal genes are present on both of the paired chromosomes, known as an autosomal recessive disorder, for example congenital adrenal hyperplasia. As these disorders are only manifest when two sets of chromosomes with a mutant gene unite, many carriers remain undetected.

Environmental Causes

Certain agents, called teratogens, may be responsible for inducing congenital malformations when the tissues and organs are growing, and they are most sensitive during the time of rapid differentiation. The critical period of human development depends on the tissue or organ concerned, e.g. the brain grows rapidly from the start of its development and for the first two years of life, but other organs are only rapidly developing from Days 15 to 60, and during this time teratogens may be lethal. Each organ has a critical time during which its development may be altered, and a teratogen may affect different developing systems at the same time (Fig. 4.10).

Drugs and chemicals as teratogens

Drugs vary greatly in their teratogenicity from severe, for example thalidomide, to mild, smoking.

While few drugs have been positively implicated in congenital abnormalities, the use of all drugs in pregnancy should be avoided if possible. Some examples of teratogens are shown in Table 4.1.

Table 4.1

Teratogen	Congenital malformation
Alcohol	Growth retardation Mental retardation Microcephaly
Androgens	Masculinisation of female fetus
Busulfan	Stunted growth, cleft palate, skeletal abnormalities
Lithium carbonate	Cardiovascular abnormalities
Methotrexate and other cytotoxic drugs	Multiple congenital abnormalities
Phenytoin Tetracyclines Warfarin	Mental retardation, growth retardation, bone and teeth abnormalities, cartilagenous abnormalities

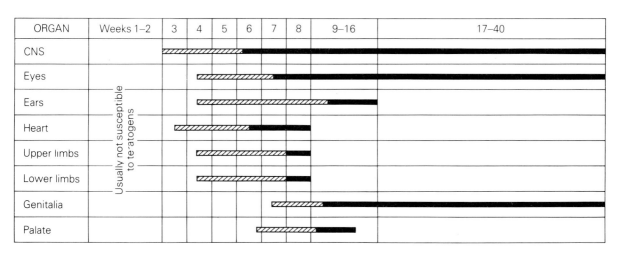

Fig. 4.10 *Critical periods of teratogenicity.*

Infectious agents

Three viruses are known to be teratogenic in man
(Table 4.2.)

Two other micro-organisms are known to be
teratogens (Table 4.3).

Table 4.2

Virus	Onset	Condition
Rubella virus		Cataract
	Early	Cardiac anomalies
		Deafness
Cytomegalovirus	Early	Most pregnancies abort
		Growth retardation
	Late	Mental retardation
		Deafness
		Cerebral calcification
Herpes simplex virus	Late	Microcephaly
		Mental retardation

Table 4.3

Micro-organism	Condition
Toxoplasma gondii	Microcephaly
	Microphthalmia
	Hydrocephaly
Treponema pallidum (syphilis)	Deafness
	Hydrocephalus
	Mental retardation

Radiation

Large amounts of ionising radiation can produce
congenital malformations and if the exposure
during early pregnancy is over 25 Rads, over a short
space of time, it is recommended that the pregnancy
be terminated. There is no evidence that human
congenital malformations have resulted from exposure to diagnostic levels of radiation. However, it is
prudent to minimise x-ray examination of the pelvic
region in pregnant women.

Multifactorial Inheritance

Most common congenital malformations are the
result of a subject who is susceptible to a disorder
being exposed to the appropriate dose of teratogen.
These traits tend to run in families, such as cleft lip,
neural tube defects, congenital dislocation of the
hip. What the teratogen is in these cases is under
investigation, but one theory is exemplified by the
use of multivitamins to prevent neural tube defects
recurring, the teratogen thought being to be the *lack*
of vitamins during development in susceptible subjects.

FURTHER READING

Edwards R.G., Fishel S. (1986). Ovulation, fertilisation, embryo damage and early development.
In *Scientific Foundations of Obstetrics and Gynaecology*,
3rd edn. Philipp E., Barnes J., Newton M. (eds).
pp. 212–23. London: Heinemann Medical.
Jones O.W. (1984). Reproductive genetics. In
Maternal Fetal Medicine. Creasy R.K., Resnik R.
(eds). pp. 3–92. Philadelphia: W.B. Saunders.

5

Abortion

The *Concise Oxford Dictionary* defines abortion as the 'act of giving untimely birth to offspring, premature delivery, miscarriage; the procuring of premature delivery so as to destroy offspring' (L. *abortus* — an untimely birth). To the physician, the terms 'abortion' and 'miscarriage' are synonymous, but to the patient the terms have different implications: abortion is an operation deliberately to end a pregnancy; miscarriage is an accidental, unwanted event in a woman's reproductive life. As either event can have long-term psychological sequelae, it is important for the physician to adopt an understanding attitude when interviewing gynaecological patients and preferably he should use the term 'miscarriage'.

In the UK, an abortion is a pregnancy which miscarries before 28 weeks' gestation, as dated from the first day of the last menstrual period. Beyond 28 weeks, termination of pregnancy is not legal, and events such as bleeding, loss of liquor or the onset of contractions, all of which before 28 weeks will be evidence of a threatened or inevitable abortion, after 28 weeks are called antepartum haemorrhage, rupture of the membranes and preterm labour respectively. Consideration is being given to reduce the gestation at which termination of pregnancy is legal.

SPONTANEOUS ABORTION

Spontaneous abortion is the miscarriage of a pregnancy without prior intervention before 28 weeks' gestation. A spontaneous abortion can occur in the first trimester (conception to 12 weeks), or in the second trimester (12–28 weeks). The incidence of fetal wastage is variously assessed at 15–24%, with 12% of spontaneous abortions occurring after 12 weeks. If late periods are taken into account, the rate of pregnancy loss may be much higher (Table 5.1).

Table 5.1
Predicted Future of an Individual Ovum

Sixteen per cent of ova do not divide.

Fifteen per cent of ova are lost during various preimplantation stages in the first postovulatory week.

Twenty-seven per cent of ova abort during implantation in the second postovulatory week.

Ten-and-a-half per cent of ova surviving the first missed menstrual period, subsequently abort spontanteously.

(After Opitz *et al.*, 1979. *Postgraduate Medicine*; **65**, 247.)

Now that intensive care units within Special Care Baby Units (SCBU) are able to save babies of 26 weeks' gestation or less, a modification in the law governing abortion is required. This would have relevance to the requirements for the notification of still-births, and therefore late abortions would gain statistical significance. Under Section 11 (1) of the Births and Deaths Registration Act 1953, a Stillbirth Certificate must be delivered to the Registrar of Births and Deaths within 42 days of the stillbirth occurring. Section 41 of the same Act defines stillbirth as follows: 'Stillborn means a child which has issued forth from its mother after the twenty-eighth week of pregnancy and which did not at any time after being completely expelled from its mother breathe or show any other signs of life, and the expression "stillbirth" shall be construed accordingly.' A child which has breathed or shown any other sign of life, such as beating of the heart, pulsation of the umbilical cord or definite movements of voluntary muscles, is considered as liveborn for registration purposes.

A spontaneous abortion may progress through different stages:

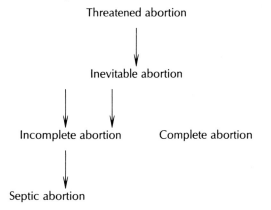

In addition, a pregnancy may end in a 'missed abortion', or a blighted ovum.

Threatened Abortion

Threatened abortion is a very common gynaecological emergency, which usually presents as vaginal bleeding during a pregnancy of less than 28 weeks' gestation. The bleeding is usually light and, if pain is present, it is usually likened to period pain, and localised to the suprapubic region and/or the low back and sacral area.

The haemorrhage is due to the separation of the syncytiotrophoblast, and later the placenta, from the uterine wall. The blastocyst with syncytiotrophoblast at the embryonic pole erodes the secretory endometrium to form an implantation cavity in the decidua. Cytotrophoblast and mesoderm containing fetal blood vessels grow into the syncytiotrophoblast in which lacunae containing maternal blood have formed. The lacunae become the inter-

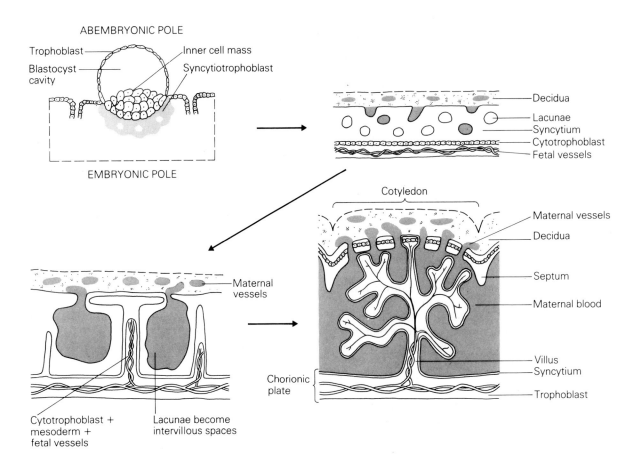

Fig. 5.1   *The development of the placenta.*

villous spaces, and the in-growths containing the fetal blood vessels become the villi (Fig. 5.1).

After 28 weeks' gestation, haemorrhage may be due to placenta praevia or placental abruption. The former is painless and the latter is painful. These causes of haemorrhage may, of course, occur before 28 weeks, but at this earlier stage of pregnancy no distinction is made between them.

Aetiology

When discussing almost any subject in obstetrics, aetiological factors may be divided into maternal and fetal. Maternal factors are local or systemic. Local factors are mainly concerned with uterine abnormalities — congenital or acquired, including cervical incompetence — which will be discussed later (*see* p. 57). Systemic factors come under three headings:

Infection
Drug ingestion
Progesterone deficiency.

Infections, especially those causing a high temperature, such as malaria, can cause spontaneous abortion, but common virus infections can cause abortions by killing or severely damaging the developing embryo/fetus. Syphilis, cytomegalovirus (CMV), toxoplasmosis, listeriosis, and brucellosis are all possible causes of recurrent/habitual abortions.

Any drug given to the mother is able to cross the placenta to some extent, unless it is broken down or changed during its passage. Placental exchange of substrates between mother and fetus is established by the fifth week of pregnancy: substances of low molecular weight diffuse freely across the placenta, driven mainly by a concentration gradient. There is no placental barrier, but what is important is whether the rate of transfer and quantity transferred is sufficient to produce significant concentrations within the fetus. Teratogenic effects of drugs usually appear as anatomical malformations and these are dose and time related, the fetus being most at risk during the first trimester. The mechanisms of teratogenesis are poorly understood: they may affect maternal tissues with indirect effects upon the fetus, or they may exert a direct effect on embryonic/fetal cells causing specific abnormalities. Drugs may affect the placenta, thereby interfering with fetal nutrition. Currently, there is concern about the delayed effects of drugs given during pregnancy: daughters of women given diethylstilboestrol in pregnancy are at increased risk for developing vaginal adenosis and adenocarcinoma of the vagina.

Management

There is little that doctors can do for the patient threatening to abort, except to try to relieve anxiety by counselling that usually the outcome is favourable and that the threatened abortion is unlikely to harm the fetus. Bed rest, with or without sedation, is the traditional method of management. One attitude is that it doesn't matter what the woman does, if she is going to abort, she will — if not, then the threat will settle. Hospital admission is usual, though a good explanation to the patient and her partner may well reassure them enough to allow management at home, especially if domestic commitments make hospital admission difficult. Progestogens have been used in the management of threatened and recurrent abortion, but there is no definite proof that they are effective. If used, only those drugs which do not masculinise the fetus should be given, e.g. dydrogesterone.

A positive pregnancy test is encouraging. If urinary HCG titres can be obtained, the pregnancy test can provide an early indication of pregnancy failure, and help to distinguish between a threatened abortion and a missed abortion. Ultrasound scan of the uterus can confirm fetal viability, in which case the prognosis is good. It may show a cause for the bleeding, such as the failure of one pregnancy in a twin gestation. It may also distinguish between a blighted ovum/missed abortion. However, fetal echoes may not be seen on an early scan, and then a repeat scan should be performed about 2 weeks later.

If the woman has not booked for antenatal care, her blood group and rhesus factor should be determined while estimating the haemoglobin. Transplacental haemorrhage can occur and the risks of rhesus immunisation should be reduced by giving anti-D immunoglobulin, 50 µg i.m.

Inevitable Abortion

Inevitable abortion means that the pregnancy cannot be saved, no matter what treatment is undertaken. The woman has regular painful contractions, which she may liken to period or labour pains, and often complains of severe back pain localised to the sacrum. This is very suggestive of cervical dilatation. Uterine pain is always referred to areas of skin supplied by branches of the first lumbar nerve. Corpuscular nerve endings in the region of the endocervix may act as stretch receptors.

There is usually vaginal bleeding and there may be a history of loss of amniotic fluid. Vaginal examination reveals an open cervix.

Management

The management of a suspected inevitable abortion is summarised below:

1. Vaginal examination to confirm cervical dilatation.
2. Haemoglobin estimation and blood group determination. Serum should be saved in case of need of crossmatching.
3. Surgical evacuation of uterus under general anaesthesia using vacuum aspiration or sponge forceps and blunt curette. Excessive curettage, particularly with a sharp curette, must be avoided as it will damage the basal layers of endometrium and cause fibrous adhesions leading to oligomenorrhoea or amenorrhoea (Ashermann's syndrome).

Following evacuation of retained products of conception (ERPC), the patient's anti-D and contraceptive requirements are determined. The products should be sent for histopathological examination to confirm a pregnancy by demonstrating the presence of chorionic villi and sometimes fetal parts. Occasionally, fetal parts are not seen, only atypical endometrial changes called the Arias-Stella reaction in which there is considerable variation in nuclear size, numerous mitoses, nuclear hypertrophy, local enlargement of glandular cells with loss of cell boundaries, increased quantities of cytoplasm with vacuolisation, loss of cellular polarity and nuclear lobulation (Fig. 5.2).

The reaction is probably due to hormonal over-stimulation and is suggestive of ectopic pregnancy, which must be a differential diagnosis in any woman presenting with lower abdominal/pelvic pain, a period of amenorrhoea and vaginal bleeding.

● *An important practical point:*
   If an ectopic pregnancy is suspected, establish an i.v.

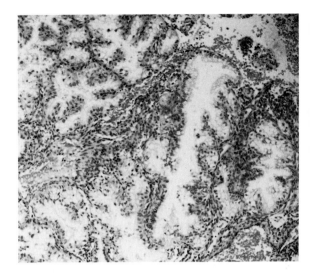

Fig. 5.2   *Photomicrograph of the Arias-Stella reaction.* (H & E x 100)

infusion with a large cannula prior to performing vaginal or rectal examination, as such an examination may rupture a tubal pregnancy, producing bleeding and consequent profound shock in the patient. Resuscitation in such cases should be with whole blood rather than crystalloid.

Spontaneous first trimester abortion is common, and medically is a straightforward condition to treat. However, it must never be forgotten that, for the woman, the process is a tragic loss even in early pregnancy, and there is always some degree of grief through which she must pass. Realisation of this, sympathetic treatment, and encouraging advice for the future are essential ingredients of the management of these patients.

Incomplete Abortion

By definition, in an incomplete abortion, some of the products of gestation have been passed and others are retained within the uterus. This situation can lead to very severe vaginal bleeding requiring rapid rescuscitation and management.

Management

It may be necessary to delay a full clinical history. The salient points are that there has been unprotected intercourse (not always admitted), plus a period of amenorrhoea, ending in the onset of vaginal bleeding and cramping lower abdominal pains likened to contractions or severe dysmenorrhoea. The woman may be shocked. After establishing an intravenous infusion, which may initially be a crystalloid with Syntocinin added (20 i.u/500 ml), and obtaining blood for haemoglobin estimation and crossmatching, inspect the vagina with a Cuscoe speculum. An i.m. injection of Ergometrine 500 μg may be given, but it should be remembered that this contracts the cervix as well as the uterus. Products are often seen in the external os. These should be quickly removed with sponge-holding forceps, whereupon the bleeding usually subsides and the situation comes under control. The patient can now be fully clerked and admitted, and properly prepared for general anaesthesia and the evacuation of the products of conception from the uterine cavity as described on p. 59. The products of conception are sent for histopathology not only to document the patient's ability to conceive, but also to exclude trophoblastic disease.

Again, the importance of sympathetic handling of these women who are undergoing an emotionally disturbing experience must be emphasised. Counselling as to the possible cause (although this is rarely known) and advice about future pregnancies both before discharge and subsequently, if necessary, is also essential.

Postoperatively, anti-D and contraceptive requirements are checked as above. It may be felt necessary to prescribe prophylactic antibiotics, such as tetracycline or penicillin and metronidazole. An haemoglobin estimation will determine the need for further transfusion. The patient should be discharged on oral iron if the haemoglobin is less than 11 g/dl, and the level checked 6 weeks later.

Complete Abortion

Complete abortion implies that the whole of the conceptus has been passed. Clinically, this is indicated by the cessation of pain and bleeding, and may be confirmed by ultrasound scan of the uterus.

Management

By using ultrasound to confirm the diagnosis of complete abortion, an unnecessary curettage may be avoided. Some clinicians believe that all spontaneous abortions are incomplete, and on this basis

arrange for all patients to undergo evacuation. However, it would seem preferable, if ultrasound facilities are available, to try to avoid a general anaesthetic and curettage with their attendant risks. As before, anti-D γ globulin should be given and contraception requirements are determined before the patient is discharged.

Septic Abortion

Septic abortion is a serious complication of spontaneous or induced abortion, not necessarily criminally induced. It may complicate procedures such as amniocentesis, cervical cerclage and evacuation of retained products of conception. Necrotic products of conception provide good culture medium for organisms, the most commonly found being *Escherichia coli*, aerobic haemolytic and non-haemolytic plus anaerobic streptococci, *Staphylococcus aureus*, and the anaerobes *Clostridium welchii*, *Clostridium tetanii* and the bacteroides. The infection is usually confined to the products and the uterine cavity, and is manifested by an offensive purulent or pinkish discharge from the cervix and vagina, pelvic and abdominal pain, pelvic and suprapubic tenderness, cervical excitation, signs of peritonitis and pyrexia which, if severe, is accompanied by rigors. Severe infections with *E. coli* and *Proteus mirabilis* may be complicated by Gram-negative endotoxic shock due to inadequate return of blood to the heart, because of peripheral pooling secondary to the vasodilation produced by the endotoxin. The patient's extremities are warm and flushed, the blood pressure low, and the pulse rapid. Rigors should alert the attendants to the possibility of imminent endotoxic shock. Anaerobic gas-forming organisms may cause gas gangrene of the uterus. The infection can spread via the portal system to the liver.

Management

The priorities in the management of septic abortion are:

1. Treat the infection
2. Empty the uterus

The choice of antibiotics for treating the infection is discussed below. How the uterus is emptied depends on the period of gestation. In some circumstances, such as gas gangrene of the uterus, hysterectomy may be required.

Antibiotics are best given i.v. initially; blood is obtained when the i.v. infusion is established, and is sent for full blood count, blood biochemistry, to provide a base-line for renal function, blood culture and clotting studies, the latter because severe endotoxic shock may be complicated by disseminated intravascular coagulation (DIC) (*see* Chapter 8). Swabs are taken from the discharge for aerobic and anaerobic culture.

A chest x-ray may be useful if septic emboli are suspected, and a plain abdominal film may show gas in the uterus or subphrenic gas if the uterus has been perforated.

When septicaemia is present, cefuroxime, gentamicin and metronidazole are given i.v. A central venous pressure line should be inserted as part of the management of shock. Hydrocortisone should be given, 1 g i.v. and repeated 1 h later if necessary. A urinary catheter will allow an hourly assessment of urine output. In the absence of septicaemia, intravenous cefuroxime and rectal metronidazole will provide adequate therapy until bacterial sensitivities are available. When the patient has improved, i.e. the temperature and pulse have returned to normal, the antibiotic course can be completed with oral medication. Treatment in an Intensive Care Unit may be required initially.

The uterus should be evacuated within 8 h of starting treatment. When the uterus is not much larger than the non-pregnant state, this is easily performed by curettage, although the risks of perforation are greater as the uterus may be softer. Suction curettage may be required, and some authorities will evacuate a uterus of 16-week size by this method. Thereafter, to 28 weeks, an abortion will be induced chemically with a syntocinon or prostaglandin i.v. infusion. Uterine evacuation is performed following the abortion.

Blood loss should be rapidly replaced, using the central venous pressure as a guide. If DIC is present, platelets, fibrinogen and plasma may be required, in addition to replacing the blood loss.

Subsequent secondary infertility due to tubal infection and damage may follow a septic abortion.

Missed Abortion

A missed abortion occurs if a fetus dies or fails to develop (blighted ovum) before 28 weeks' gestation

and the pregnancy fails to abort. The diagnosis can be made on clinical grounds: the patient may no longer feel pregnant; the breasts are less tender; and, if she has reached the stage where fetal movements have been felt, these have stopped. On examination, the uterine size/fundal height is much smaller than the dates suggest. The diagnosis can be confirmed by ultrasound scan. The clinician may want to confirm the diagnosis by a pregnancy test, but continuing physiological activity by the trophoblast may give a positive result. Estimating titres of urinary HCG and watching them fall will aid confirmation of the diagnosis.

Management

Current practice is to evacuate the uterus as soon as possible under as aseptic conditions as possible because, theoretically, there is a great risk of sepsis by virtue of the fact that a lot of necrotic tissue is being incubated at body temperature. A further reason is the avoidance of DIC, which may occur if the uterus is left unevacuated for more than 1 month. These considerations were important in the past when inactivity was a method of management. Infection is still a problem, and vaginal examination should be avoided once the diagnosis has been made. Prostaglandins have simplified the management of this condition in those women in whom the uterus is above 14-week size and thus unsuitable for vaginal suction ERPC. Prostaglandins can be used to induce abortion by the intravenous or extra-amniotic route. These methods are described below in the section on therapeutic abortion (*see* p. 60). Prostaglandin vaginal pessaries are also effective. Prophylactic antibiotics may be given as part of the procedure. Extra-amniotic and vaginal prostaglandins may be used in conjunction with i.v. syntocinon. It is a wise precaution to check the clotting screen if the fetus has been dead for more than a month.

● *One further note of caution:*
   In the first trimester, ultrasonography may mistakenly diagnose an anembryonic pregnancy. There is nothing to be lost by repeating the examination 2 weeks later and confirming the findings.

Recurrent (Habitual) Abortion

If a woman has three or more consecutive spontaneous abortions, she is said to have recurrent abortion. The cause may be maternal (congenital or acquired), or fetal. It has been shown statistically that when a patient has had three or more consecutive abortions, the prognosis for a subsequent pregnancy is poor and that a recurring aetiological factor must be suspected. If a couple have one normal living child, the prognosis for carrying to term is markedly improved.

These women have experienced great emotional trauma of grief and disappointment. They are therefore especially anxious, stressed and vulnerable with strong feelings of reproductive inadequacy. They thus need particularly sympathetic care and counselling.

A specific cause for habitual abortion is found in approximately 63% of cases. The causes may include genetic, hormonal, anatomical or immunological abnormalities, infections or chronic systemic diseases.

Genetic

There is evidence of genetic defects in 50–60% of spontaneous first trimester abortions. Approximately 1–5% of couples with habitual abortion have an abnormal karyotype. Therefore as part of the management of first trimester recurrent abortion, both partners should have chromosome studies. One survey showed that in 10% of couples with habitual abortion, one or other partner had an abnormal chromosome.

Hormonal

It is now no longer considered that thyroid disorders are associated with recurrent abortion, but the rare patient will respond to appropriate thyroid therapy. Similarly, there is no definite evidence to suggest that low serum progesterone is responsible for first trimester abortion.

Anatomical

A uterine abnormality has been shown in 10–15% of patients with recurrent abortion, which may be congenital, such as a unicornuate or septate uterus, or acquired such as fibroids. Congenital anomalies may be minor, such as a septate uterus, or major with two uterine horns, each with a cervix — bicornuate, bicollis. Such anomalies arise because

of varying degrees of failure of fusion of the müllerian ducts. In such patients an i.v. urogram should be performed to exclude abnormality of the urinary system, which occurs in 5% of such patients.

Submucous fibroids and fibroid polyps may exert an effect by acting as foreign bodies in the uterine cavity or they may interfere with the uterine blood flow. The endometrium covering a fibroid may be deficient. Excessive curettage can cause Ashermann's syndrome, in which the cavity of the uterus is denuded of endometrium and heals by the formation of fibrous synechiae between the walls.

Cervical incompetence. The stroma of the cervix consists mainly of connective tissue. As one gets nearer to the internal os, there is an increasing proportion of smooth muscle cells. At the internal os, the muscle layers of the myometrium — the outer longitudinal layer and the inner layer with fibres running in all directions — hypertrophy, forming a sphincter. This sphincter may be rendered incompetent by cervical lacerations occurring during normal and abnormal childbirth. Nonobstetric damage may occur as a result of forced instrumentation at vaginal termination of pregnancy or simple dilatation and curettage.

Recurrent abortion in the second trimester may be due to cervical incompetence. The standard methods for demonstrating this are by hysterocervicogram, or by passing cervical dilators under general anaesthesia.

An hysterocervicogram should be performed premenstrually. The reason for this is that, under the influence of progesterone in the second half of the menstrual cycle, the internal os becomes tight and, therefore, radiographic evidence of widening of the canal is of significance. The x-ray is performed by inserting a cannula into the cervix and injecting a radio-opaque dye, usually 'Urographin'. A steel screw-in cannula has been used for this in the past, but more modern vacuum cannulae are less traumatic and more comfortable for the patient.

This same technique is used to demonstrate uterine and tubal abnormalities. If cervical incompetence is present, a funnel shape with a wide canal is seen. If a Hegar dilator of 6 mm diameter or more can be passed through the cervix without resistance, then incompetence is present. During pregnancy the diagnosis is based on shortening and dilatation of the cervix detected by vaginal examination, and can be made by ultrasound examination of the internal os. In pregnancy, a non-absorbable suture encircling the cervix is inserted, the two eponyms commonly associated with this being Shirodkar and McDonald. In the Shirodkar operation, a thick tape suture (Mersilene) is inserted under the cervical skin at the level of the junction of the cervix and the anterior fornix usually at about 12 weeks from the last menstrual period. The knot may be tied anteriorly or posteriorly and is removed either at the onset of labour or at 38 weeks, or at the time of caesarean section. In McDonald's operation, which is easier to perform, a non-absorbable nylon suture is inserted, like a purse-string, around the cervix at the same level and tied tightly (Fig. 5.3). Recently, the value of the procedure of cervical cerclage has been called into doubt. These studies show evidence of an association with serious adverse effects such as preterm rupture of the membranes, more hospitalisation and more frequent puerperal pyrexia due to infection probably caused by the suture.

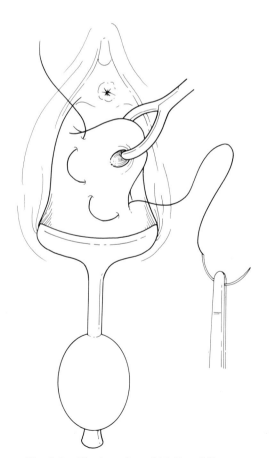

Fig. 5.3   *The insertion of McDonald's suture.*

Immunological

It may be that the mother exerts an immune response to the cell membranes of the trophoblast, which have discreet antigens, and thereby exerts an immune response on the fetus/embryo which, because it may not stimulate maternal protecting factors, is rejected. Despite the fact that recurrent abortion is not uncommon, an immunological cause has not been proven. A recent review of the causes of recurrent pregnancy loss only failed to identify the cause in a few couples. Some authors have found evidence for protective antibodies to HLA-linked paternal antigens in that they were present in 22 of 27 first trimester pregnancies compared with 1 out of 10 women having a spontaneous abortion. Another paper, which looked specifically for an abnormal immune response to paternal lymphocytes in women who had suffered recurrent abortion, found no evidence for such an abnormal response. lending less credence to the theory that a defective immunological response is involved in problem pregnancies. Despite this, it has been known for a long time that, using immunological mechanisms, abortion can be produced in laboratory animals. Couples with recurrent abortion have been treated in a paired sequential double blind trial of immunological treatment with purified lymphocytes prepared from their husband's blood. In those women so treated, 17 out of 22 had successful subsequent pregnancies, compared with 10 out of 27 women who were given their own lymphocytes.

Infection

Definite evidence that infection causes recurrent abortion is lacking. Toxoplasmosis is thought to cause abortion by invading the placenta and transplacentally infecting the fetus, but a positive dye test for the organism is positive in the same percentage of control cases as in habitual aborters. More significantly, *Mycoplasma* has been cultured from 31% of spontaneous abortions, but from only 5% of therapeutic abortions. Other agents implicated in recurrent abortions are *Chlamydia*, *Listeria monocytogenes*, syphilis and herpes simplex.

Systemic diseases

Diabetes mellitus is not thought to be a cause of recurrent abortion, although it is associated with a higher rate of congenital abnormality. Any systemic disease which affects uteroplacental blood flow may

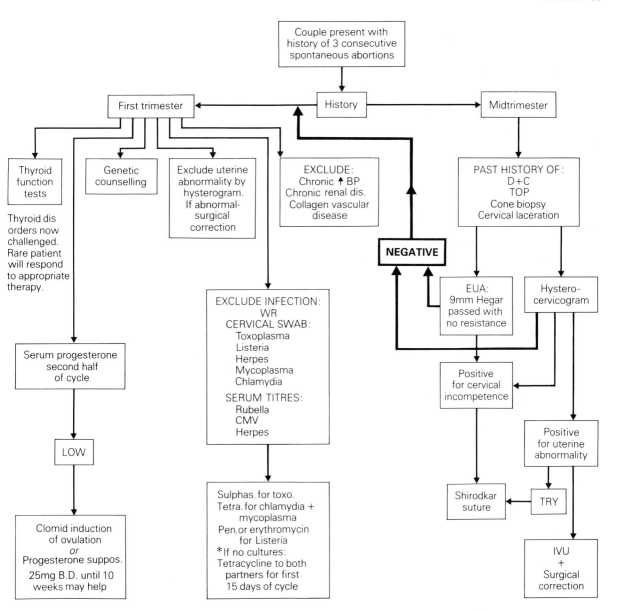

Fig. 5.4 *Evolution and management of habitual abortion. (Modified from A. de Cherney and M.L. Polan, 1984. Brit. J. Hosp. Med; **31.4**: 261–8.)*

be associated with recurrent abortion, e.g. lupus erythematosus, associated with a 40% abortion rate, and collagen vascular diseases. Chronic hypertensive disorders and renal disease are also implicated.

Management

The aim of management of recurrent abortion is to identify the aetiological factor and then to rectify it if possible. A logical approach to the problem is mandatory (Fig. 5.4).

Evacuation of Retained Products of Conception (ERPC). Mention of the operation of ERPC has already been made, p. 55. This is usually performed under general anaesthesia, but can be performed under local anaesthesia, such as paracervical block. Strict sterile precautions must be observed. The instruments used are shown in Fig. 5.5.

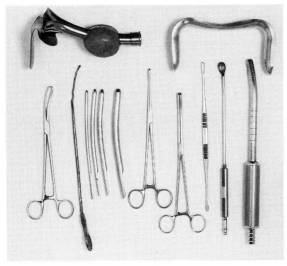

Fig. 5.5   *The instruments for ERPC on a trolley ready for use.*

Cervical dilatation is not required in the case of an incomplete abortion but, for missed abortion and some cases of septic abortion, the cervix must be dilated enough to accept sponge holding forceps. Ideally, dilatation should not be forced beyond Hegar 9 mm.

During the evacuation, ergometrine 150–250 µg may be given i.v. to reduce bleeding. By producing sustained uterine contraction, the uterus becomes firmer and less liable to perforation. However, ergometrine can cause postoperative vomiting, especially if given in doses of 500 µg. The most likely cause of persistent bleeding is the fact that the uterus still contains products of conception.

Postoperatively, it may be wise to give prophylactic antibiotics to prevent sepsis leading to salpingitis and tubal damage with subsequent adverse effects on fertility. Blood loss should be replaced, and oral iron used to replenish depleted stores. As mentioned previously, no woman should be discharged from hospital until it is known whether or not she requires anti-D immunoglobulin.

Contraceptive requirements should be ascertained and supportive counselling provided. Patients need to talk with their doctors who should

be prepared to answer a multitude of questions including: why did it happen? why me? and will it happen again?

To reduce the risk of postabortion infection, the patient should be advised to avoid intercourse until a normal period has been seen. Evidence that folic acid and vitamin C in therapeutic amounts can reduce the incidence of recurrent neural tube defects may form the basis of advising patients to boost levels of these agents prior to conception.

THERAPEUTIC ABORTION

This is one of the most commonly performed operations in the world. The ratio of therapeutic abortions to live births in some developed countries can be as high as 1 : 1.

Indications for therapeutic abortion are almost always social, namely the inability of the mother or couple to cope with a further pregnancy in their particular situation. Therapeutic abortions for medical reasons alone are virtually unknown.

Preoperative Work-up

In addition to history taking and confirmation of the pregnancy, the work-up should include a haemoglobin estimation (with Sickle-test if necessary), blood grouping and a cervical smear. If the preoperative period is viewed as a counselling and screening session, then the rubella titre, syphilis serology and endocervical bacteriology should be assessed. Contraceptive advice should be given before as well as after the operation and if the termination of pregnancy (TOP) has been performed for reasons of fetal abnormality, the couple should be offered genetic counselling.

Methods

Suction termination of pregnancy

Suction termination of pregnancy is a simple method of abortion which is currently the most common method of termination of pregnancy in developed countries.

It is the cervical dilatation which causes the pain during abortion. Pain from the cervix is carried by the nervi erigentes (S 2,3), which pass along the base of the broad ligament from the pelvic side wall. They enter the cervix just above the vault of the vagina, so that local anaesthetic injected at two or three sites around the cervix can block pain impulses. Local anaesthesia is suitable for suction termination up to 8–10 weeks' gestation, and is safer than general anaesthesia. If a small 4–6 mm Karman curette is used, cervical dilatation is not usually required, and the procedure may be performed without anaesthesia.

Cervical dilatation is a prerequisite to the standard procedure. Dilatation should be slow and gentle and, although the amount of dilatation required may be determined by the size of the uterus, in general the cervix should not be dilated beyond 10 mm. The risk at this stage of the procedure is of tearing the cervix with subsequent cervical incompetence. The need to dilate the cervix mechanically can be reduced by using laminaria tents inserted into the cervix the night before the operation, or by using intravaginal prostaglandin analogue pessaries. The latter have been shown to be effective when inserted 3–4 h before the operation. The laminaria tents and their modern equivalents work by absorbing water from their surroundings and expanding. As they expand they stretch the cervix, prostaglandins are produced and the cervix dilates. Prostaglandins work by softening the cervix, so that no force is required when dilating the cervix. After cervical dilatation, a suction curette, of which there are several types, is used to remove the products of conception.

Prostaglandin termination of pregnancy

Midtrimester abortions can be dangerous, and are unpleasant for the medical attendants and patient. The surgical risks rise steeply after 13 weeks, and the main indication for such terminations should be fetal abnormality, which is usually diagnosed in the second trimester, abortion being delayed by the need to confirm the diagnosis. Routine amniocentesis is offered to women who will be around 37 years of age at delivery. This is performed at about 16 weeks' gestation, and the chromosome analysis may take 3–4 weeks. A neural tube defect may be detected earlier on ultrasound scan permitting a first trimester termination of pregnancy, but in those centres where women are screened with maternal serum α-fetoprotein estimations at 16

weeks, confirmation of the diagnosis may require a further 2 weeks.

Prostaglandins may be given by the intra-amniotic or extra-amniotic route and, in Europe, have replaced chemicals such as saline, glucose and urea which were given intra-amniotically. Prostaglandins (PGs) are long chain fatty acids derived from the essential unsaturated fatty acids, linolenic, arachidonic and eicosapentanoic acids. PGEs and PGFs act on the female reproductive system to stimulate contraction of the gravid uterus. PGE_2 also softens the cervix and so is a marginally better compound to use. Both PGE_2 and $PGF_{2\alpha}$ are involved in the mechanism of labour, and they are found in the menses being partly responsible for dysmenorrhoea. The use of PGs for procuring midtrimester abortions is safer than the surgical techniques.

Technique. PGE_2 in tylose gel can be injected into the extra-amniotic space under aseptic conditions. Occasionally, a second injection, 8–10 h after the first is required. Solutions containing PGE_2 are infused down an indwelling Foley catheter either manually every hour, or by automatic syringe pump until the abortion has occurred. Often the first sign of this is the passage of the catheter with the balloon inflated. Although syntocinon is not essential to make the method more efficient, some practitioners do use simultaneous infusions of the agent, 20 iu added to one litre of infusion solution. It is important to avoid water intoxication with syntocinon, which has antidiuretic hormone-like properties.

Following injection of the solution or gel, painful contractions may start within 15–30 min. Adequate analgesia should be given. Pethidine with an anti-emetic is appropriate; promethazine, an antihistamine with sedative properties, is commonly used.

Ergometrine 500 µg is given to avoid haemorrhage, which can be severe when products are retained, i.e. an incomplete abortion.

As an alternative, prostaglandin E_2 or $F_{2\alpha}$ can be administered intra-amniotically. After an injection of local anaesthetic into the anterior abdominal wall overlying the gravid uterus, a needle is passed into the amniotic cavity and about 100–200 ml of liquor is removed. The volume removed is replaced with a prostaglandin solution containing 10 mg of PGE_2. This may need repeating in 12–24 h. In the past, other solutions have been used: hypertonic saline, which has been associated with maternal death from changes in salt concentration in the blood and cerebral haemorrhage in the base of the brain; glucose, which has been associated with intrauterine infections and with the consumption coagulopathy/DIC; urea, which has been associated with DIC but is considered to be safer than hypertonic saline, and which may be used with intra-amniotic PGE_2. The urea solution contains 80 g urea in 200 ml 5% Dextrose.

An infusion of oxytocin can be used to supplement the action of intra-amniotic prostaglandin solutions, the amount infused being titrated against the uterine effect.

Haemorrhage as a result of incomplete abortion, and postoperative considerations, are as previously described.

Hysterotomy

Hysterotomy is the surgical opening and emptying of the uterus via an abdominal incision. It is associated with a higher incidence of morbidity and mortality than other methods of midtrimester abortion, and has, therefore, been largely replaced. A supposed advantage is that it can be combined with sterilisation, but current opinion holds that sterilisation is better performed, psychologically and technically, at least 6 weeks after a termination, spontaneous abortion or delivery. Also, sterilisation adds to the complications of the procedure, and has a higher failure rate.

A lower segment hysterotomy, technically very similar to a lower segment caesarean section, is to be preferred to the classical midline uterine incision (Fig. 5.6). Great care must be taken to avoid contaminating the abdominal wound with decidua, as endometriosis of the scar can result. This seems to be peculiar to hysterotomy.

The complications of hysterotomy are anaesthetic and surgical, the latter being haemorrhage, infection and pelvic vein thrombosis. The scars may weaken the uterus with subsequent rupture in labour. It is an obsolete procedure.

Menstrual regulation

This term is a euphemism for very early termination of pregnancy, whereby a woman ensures that her period occurs on time when she has reason to suspect that she may have conceived in the preceding 2 weeks. Essentially, the endometrium is aspirated at the time at which menstruation would have occurred, so that if conception has occurred, the conceptus is aspirated, or finds that there is no endometrium in which to embed.

Insertion of copper-bearing intrauterine contraceptive devices after intercourse or shortly after a missed period has also been used to procure an abortion, as have progestogens and combined oral contraceptives. In the latter case, two tablets of a preparation containing levonorgestrel 250 µg and ethinyloestradiol 50 µg are taken within 72 h of intercourse, and a further two tablets 12 h later. If menstruation has not occurred within 3 weeks of the course of tablets, the patient should see her GP.

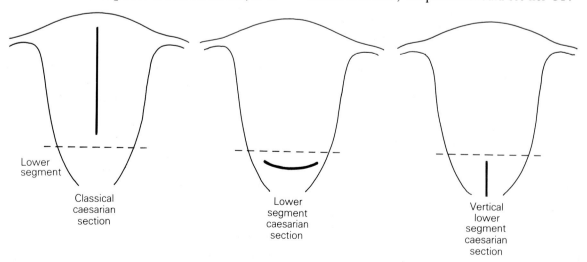

Lower segment

Classical caesarian section

Lower segment caesarian section

Vertical lower segment caesarian section

Fig. 5.6   *Uterine incisions.*

Complications

Whether performed in the first or second trimester, the complications of therapeutic abortion are similar. The earlier an abortion is performed, the safer.

Summarised, the complications of a surgical termination of pregnancy are:

Uterine perforation
Haemorrhage
Infection
Embolism
Anaesthetic risks
Damage to cervix
Rhesus isoimmunisation
Infertility
Psychological

Future obstetric performance as determined by the length of labour, blood loss in labour, and the incidence of instrumental delivery is unaffected by previous terminations.

Uterine perforation

This can occur with the uterine sound, cervical dilator, or the curette. Sounding the uterus is unnecessary and, by avoiding this procedure, the incidence of perforations will be reduced. Laparotomy is required if one is aware of perforation. The overall incidence is approximately 1 : 1100.

Haemorrhage

This is a rare complication, and very few hospitals crossmatch blood for a first trimester abortion. It is more of a risk with midtrimester abortions and, after expulsion of the fetus, bleeding may be very rapid, due to incomplete separation or expulsion of the placenta. These cases should have two units of whole blood crossmatched and instantly available on the ward, and they should always have an i.v. infusion established with a wide bore cannula (16 or 14 FG) in a large vein. The veins on the back of the hand are not ideal.

Infection

Infection and pyrexia are said to have occurred if the patient has a temperature of 37.8°C on two occasions. An MSU and high vaginal swabs should be taken and antibiotics commenced, usually a penicillin or cephalosporin and metronidazole, the latter orally or rectally. In one series of 1000 cases, pyrexia occurred in 30 cases. No organisms were isolated in 17 of these. The early resumption of intercourse may increase the chance of developing postoperative pelvic sepsis. Antibiotics do have a role in prophylaxis. An American study using 4 day courses of tetracycline started before the termination showed that the treated group had two-thirds of the complications and a quarter of the hospital admissions of the untreated group.

Pulmonary embolism

Pulmonary embolism from deep vein thrombosis can follow any surgical procedure, particularly if complicated by infection, and in the past it was mainly embolism which was responsible for mortality after hysterotomy and hysterectomy for a termination of pregnancy. Thrombosis and embolism are relatively less common in the young.

Anaesthetic

The anaesthetic complications are the same as those for any other elective operation.

Damage to the cervix

Previous termination of pregnancy may feature in the history of a woman with proven cervical incompetence, but most women are equally likely to cite a straightforward D & C as the only past history. If proven, a Shirodkar suture may be of benefit in subsequent pregnancies.

Rhesus immunisation

This should not occur as the anti-D requirement should be determined preoperatively, and if required should be given postoperatively. The risk of maternal immunisation in a full term rhesus positive pregnancy is about 1 : 8; the risk after a spontaneous abortion about 2–4%. The incidence related to termination is uncertain. In one series of 25 rhesus negative women followed up for 4 months after the operation, and not given anti-D, only one had become immunised.

Infertility

This is unlikely to occur after a termination unless infection occurs. In one series, only 5 out of 1132 women followed up for up to 5 years after the operation complained of secondary infertility.

Psychological effects

Postabortion psychosis is virtually unknown. Feelings of guilt or shame are reported, but these may reflect the attitudes of the doctors doing the survey. One survey of 73 000 terminations of pregnancies in the USA revealed only 16 major psychiatric disorders, including two suicides and five depressions. In Hungary, where legal terminations are more common than births, it is almost impossible to find a psychiatric admission precipitated by a termination. However, some patients may have mixed feelings in a subsequent pregnancy, with some degree of guilt.

Postoperative Management

Anti-D immunoglobulin should be given if the patient is rhesus negative. The standard dose is 250–500 units by i.m. injection.

Rubella immunisation should be offered if the patient is not rubella immune. The woman's contraceptive requirements should be determined and a clear record kept of her wishes and the actual arrangements made.

FURTHER READING

Decherney A., Polan M.L. (1984). Evaluation and management of habitual abortion. *Brit. J. Hosp. Med* **31; 4:** 261–8.

Hern W.M. (1984). *Abortion Practice*. Philadelphia: Lippincott.

Mowbray J.F., Lidell H., Underwood J.L., Gibbings C. *et al.* (1985). Controlled trial of treatment of recurrent spontaneous abortion by immunisation with paternal cells. *Lancet*; **i:** 941–4.

Potts M., Diggory P., Peel J. (1977). *Abortion*. London: Cambridge University Press.

Power D.A., Mason R.J., Stewart G.M., Catto G.R.D. *et al.* (1983). The fetus as an allograft: evidence for protective antibody to HLA-linked paternal antigens. *Lancet*: **ii:** 701–4.

6

Anatomy and Physiology of Normal Pregnancy

From the beginning of the menstrual cycle, changes occur in a woman's body which prepare her for the demands of pregnancy. After fertilisation, the physiological systems of the mother continue to adjust so that the metabolic demands that the fetus imposes on the mother are anticipated. This allows for a large margin of safety, thus ensuring the safety of the fetus in terms of growth and development and of the mother in terms of metabolic adaptation.

CARDIOVASCULAR SYSTEM

Blood Volume

Blood volume increases almost linearly during pregnancy to plateau about the 32nd week of gestation at levels 50% above those found in non-pregnant women. The early increases are caused by an expansion of plasma volume of about 40% (1250 ml), brought about by the retention of sodium due to the activation of the renin-angiotensin aldosterone system. An alternative explanation is that the osmoregulatory and thirst centres are influenced, so that there is an increased intake of water which brings about the expansion of the plasma volume. Red cell mass increases by 240–400 ml during the second half of pregnancy, which is an average of approximately 20% above the non-pregnant mean. Due to the fact that the increase in plasma volume occurs earlier than that of the red cell mass, there is haemodilution. This is minimal in women with adequate iron stores, who can synthesise the additional amounts of haemoglobin required, but in those with inadequate reserves, there will be a considerable drop in haemoglobin concentration (2–3 g/l).

Cardiac Output

One of the first changes in the cardiovascular system to occur in pregnancy is an increase in cardiac output to 4–5 l/min which is in response to an increase in blood volume. This begins early in the first trimester and by midpregnancy increases by approximately 40% above non-pregnant levels. The early increases in cardiac output are mainly brought about by an increase in stroke volume, but this falls in the latter half of pregnancy, and so cardiac output is maintained by an increase in the heart rate. The belief that cardiac output fell in the later stages of pregnancy was probably due to the fact that measurements of cardiac output were performed on women lying in the supine position. It is now known that this will lead to a fall in cardiac output, because the uterus compresses the vena cava and, as the collateral circulation through the vertebral veins is inadequate, the venous return is reduced. Cardiac output is increased during the first trimester, continues to increase during the second and is relatively static thereafter. The change in cardiac output occurs before there is an increase in oxygen consumption (Fig. 6.1) and this is borne out by the fact that the arteriovenous oxygen difference decreases early in pregnancy and only returns to non-pregnant levels by the beginning of the third trimester.

Blood Pressure

Paradoxically, despite the increases in both plasma volume and cardiac output, blood pressure does not rise during pregnancy but, in fact, shows a slight fall due mainly to a fall in diastolic blood pressure. The

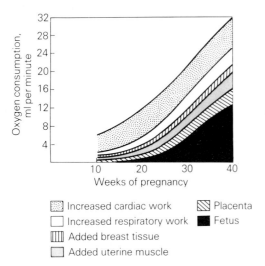

Fig. 6.1   *Components of increased maternal oxygen consumption during pregnancy. Cardiac output and respiration have increased prior to the added oxygen consumption of the placenta and fetus. (Adapted from F.E. Hytten and I. Leitch, 1971.* The Physiology of Human Pregnancy. *London: Blackwell Scientific Publications.)*

fall in diastolic blood pressure is greatest during the second trimester, after which it rises progressively to reach non-pregnant values slightly before term. The fall is due to a decrease in peripheral vascular resistance, which may be a consequence of the local production of vasodilatory prostaglandins. Evidence for this comes from the fact that, as early as the 10th week of pregnancy, the maternal vasculature becomes refractory to the pressor effects of infused angiotensin II, an event which can be reversed by the administration of prostaglandin synthetase inhibitors. Diastolic blood pressure has been found to correlate with maternal plasma angiotensin II levels during pregnancy, indicating that the renin-angiotensin system, modulated by vasodilator prostaglandins, may be important in the regulation of blood pressure during pregnancy.

Blood Flow

The increase in cardiac output is distributed between the kidneys, skin, breasts, uterus and other, as yet undetermined, sites. The increase in uterine blood flow occurs later than the increases in

blood flow to the kidneys and skin, and is probably due to the changes in the spiral arteries and through the release of vasodilators. Consequently, low doses of angiotensin II infused i.v. lead to an increase in uterine blood flow and not a fall as in other tissues.

It is interesting to speculate that the increases in skin and renal blood flow are brought about in readiness for the increased need to remove heat and metabolic waste that occur during pregnancy.

Femoral venous pressures increase during pregnancy. This may be due to compression of the

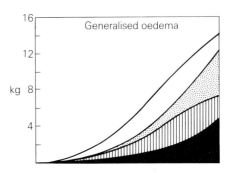

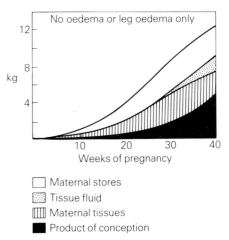

Fig. 6.2   *Components of maternal weight gain during pregnancy. Oedema in the absence of hypertension is not pathological and reflects increased permeability of connective tissues due to oestrogenic stimulation and decreased colloid osmotic pressure. Increased intravascular pressure may also play a role in lower limb oedema due to increased venous pressure resulting from increased intrapelvic pressure. (Adapted from F.E. Hytten and I. Leitch, 1971.* The Physiology of Human Pregnancy. *London: Blackwell Scientific Publications.)*

inferior vena cava and iliac veins by the increasing weight of the uterus or by hydrodynamic obstruction due to the outflow of blood from the uterus at relatively high pressures. Evidence for the former hypothesis has been obtained by cineangiographic photography in which constrictions of the inferior vena cava were observed with the pregnant women lying supine. Normally, compression of the vena cava does not represent a problem during pregnancy, due to the development of a collateral circulation through the azygous and vertebral venous systems which circumvent the constriction. However, in some women this system fails to develop properly and, as a result, they suffer from the supine hypotensive syndrome. The increased venous pressure as well as increased peripheral flow and vasodilatation in the legs may contribute to the increased incidence of lower limb oedema, varicose veins of the legs and vulva and haemorrhoids (Fig. 6.2).

Haemostasis

Bleeding time and prothrombin time are shortened during pregnancy and this is accompanied by a big increase in fibrinogen as well as increases in factors VII, VIII and X with smaller increases of factors IX and XII and prothrombin. At the same time, there are decreases in fibrinolytic substances. Platelet number and function are thought to be unchanged by pregnancy. The quantitative increases in factors involved in coagulation do not necessarily imply a hypercoagulable state, but there is evidence from animal work that activation of the coagulation system is quicker during pregnancy, and this probably contributes to the shorter bleeding time.

Anatomical Changes

There is an increase in the size of the heart, which may be due to a combination of hypertrophy and increased diastolic filling. The heart also changes position during pregnancy, being pushed upwards by the elevation of the diaphragm and rotated forwards. The changes in position of the heart lead to changes in the electrocardiograph, with a shift of the electrical axis of the heart of approximately 15°

to the left, although this may change towards the end of pregnancy.

RESPIRATORY SYSTEM

There is an increase in ventilation in pregnancy, which is principally due to an increase in tidal volume with little change in respiratory frequency. The increase in tidal volume may be caused by the central action of progesterone on central and/or peripheral chemoreceptors, although the exact nature of this action is not clear. In the latter half of pregnancy, there is a decrease in the expiratory reserve volume, residual volume and thus functional residual capacity of approximately 20%. As a consequence of this, mixing and distribution of gas in the lungs is more efficient during pregnancy, leading to increased efficiency in gas exchange. Various other tests of pulmonary function, such as maximum breathing capacity, timed vital capacity and pulmonary diffusing capacity have been found to be unchanged by pregnancy.

If the changes in respiration are indeed attributable to the actions of progesterone, then they would be expected to start from the point of the first missed period. Women in early pregnancy often comment upon changes in respiratory pattern. The growth of the fetus and placenta accounts for almost half of the increased demand for oxygen in the latter stages of pregnancy. The rest of the increased oxygen consumption is due to an increase in cardiac and respiratory work and an increase in uterine muscle and breast tissue.

Because of hyperventilation, arterial and alveolar P_{CO_2} falls to a value of 30.5–31 mmHg compared to a non-pregnant mean of 37–39 mmHg. Plasma pH is maintained by a fall in the levels of plasma bicarbonate.

Anatomical Changes

There is an increase in chest size during pregnancy which most pregnant women notice as a flaring of their lower ribs. The subcostal angle increases during pregnancy from a value of approximately 68° in early pregnancy to 103° in late pregnancy. The diaphragm is elevated by about 4 cm and this is accompanied by breathing becoming more diaphragmatic than costal during pregnancy.

Exercise during Pregnancy

That the physiological systems of the mother are not compromised by the added demands of the fetus is illustrated most clearly in the physiological responses of pregnant women to exercise. Experiments have shown that in exercises which rule out the effect of weight, oxygen consumption is increased to the same extent in pregnant women who exercised regularly when compared pre- and postpartum. Pregnant women who do not exercise regularly accrue greater oxygen debts while using the bicycle ergometer, but this may be simply due to inefficiency which results from mechanical hindrance of the increased size of the woman, a feature which disappears with training. The onset of respiratory responses to exercise is accelerated during pregnancy and the cardiac output increases to a greater extent. Because of the reduced peripheral resistance, blood pressure stays at non-pregnant levels despite the greater increase in cardiac output.

The fetal response to light exercise before the 35th week is a transient mild bradycardia, but after this point a transient and more pronounced tachycardia is seen. The degree of fetal tachycardia is reduced in pregnant women who exercise regularly.

There is, therefore, little evidence to suggest that being pregnant inhibits the ability of women to perform exercises. The cardiovascular and respiratory systems respond in such a way as to more than provide for the needs of both the mother and the fetus.

RENAL FUNCTION

Effective renal plasma flow, blood flow and glomerular filtration rate are all increased from early in pregnancy to a value approximately 50% greater than non-pregnant values. Earlier studies on these parameters showed a fall towards term, but this is because there is a reduction in renal arterial blood flow due to mechanical compression of the renal arteries by the pregnant uterus in the supine position.

In response to water loading or deprivation, pregnant women are able to produce dilute and concentrated urine to the same extent as non-pregnant women, but plasma osmolality is maintained at approximately 9 mosmol/kg lower than in non-pregnant women.

Pregnant women excrete greater quantities of amino acids and certain sugars (glucose, lactose, fructose, ribose and xylose) than non-pregnant women and the incidence of pregnant women displaying glycosuria increases during gestation. The glycosuria is caused by greater amounts of glucose entering the kidney tubules, due to the increased glomerular filtration rate and also to a decreased ability of the tubules to reabsorb glucose.

Anatomical Changes

The major anatomical change in the urinary tract during pregnancy is dilatation of the ureters, occurring as early as the tenth week. The right side becomes more affected and the dilatation may extend to the renal pelvises. The dilatation is more likely to be due to mechanical compression of the ureters by the dilated ovarian vein plexus or iliac artery than an earlier suggestion that it was due to the smooth muscle relaxing effect of progesterone. Vesicoureteric reflux is more common during pregnancy, being one of the reasons for the increased risk of pyelonephritis.

ALIMENTARY SYSTEM

A change in appetite is one of the commonest things a woman will notice on becoming pregnant. The increase in appetite is more marked in the earlier stages of pregnancy and falls off towards the end. The changes in appetite and food consumption may be under the same regulation as those of thirst, although this is still speculative. The desire for salted and spicy foods may be due to a dulling of the sense of taste in pregnancy, because the threshold for all tastes (salt, sweet, sour and bitter) has been found to be raised in pregnant women when compared to non-pregnant women. Changes in appetite and metabolism that occur during pregnancy lead to increased energy requirements (Fig. 6.3) and changes in plasma lipids (Fig. 6.4).

There is a reduction in gastric secretion during pregnancy which explains why women suffering from peptic ulcers are often much better during their pregnancy. Gastric tone and motility are also reduced and, consequently, passage of food through the stomach is delayed. This process may contribute to the high incidence of nausea and vomiting during pregnancy. Occasionally, the nausea and vomiting is frequent and severe enough to result in

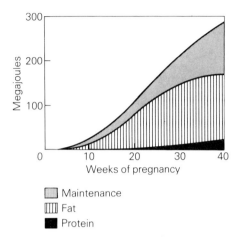

Fig. 6.3 *The energy cost of maintenance of pregnancy. Due to increased food consumption early in pregnancy (800 kJ per day over non-pregnant levels), fat reserves are built up and could be utilised to support pregnancy in the later stages in the absence of food. (Adapted from F.E. Hytten, 1978. In* Scientific Basis of Obstetrics and Gynaecology, *2nd edn. R.R. Macdonald, ed. London: Churchill Livingstone.)*

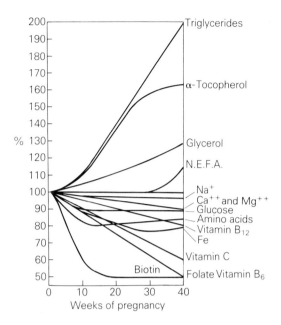

Fig. 6.4 *Changes in plasma nutrients during pregnancy. 100% represents non-pregnant level. Increased levels of triglycerides, glycerol, a-tocopherol and non-esterified fatty acids (NEFA) reflect increased lipid turnover and metabolism during pregnancy. Decreased glucose may reflect the decreased glucose tolerance which is characteristic of pregnancy, but in the majority of cases this is not pathological. (Adapted from F.E. Hytten, 1978. In* Scientific Basis of Obstetrics and Gynaecology, *2nd edn. R.R. Macdonald, ed. London: Churchill Livingstone.)*

hyperemesis gravidarum. This condition is characterised by dehydration, electrolyte imbalance and ketosis, due to a lack of carbohydrate and fluid.

There is evidence to suggest that the small and large intestines also have reduced motility during pregnancy and, as a consequence, transit time through the gut is generally reduced. Absorption is not thought to be affected by pregnancy, except that greater quantities of iron are absorbed in the small intestine and greater quantities of water and sodium are absorbed in the colon.

Alterations in liver function are implied during pregnancy by increasing levels of plasma globulins, renin substrate and serum enzymes and falling concentrations of plasma albumin. Stores of liver glycogen and their mobilisation seem to be unaffected.

The gallbladder empties more slowly during pregnancy with an increase in concentration of bile, although there seems to be no chemical changes in its composition.

ENDOCRINE CHANGES

There is increased secretion of pituitary hormones. TSH levels are raised, causing increased thyroid

activity which, in turn, increases a pregnant woman's basal metabolic rate by 25%. ACTH production increases, causing a greater output of adrenal corticosteroids which, in turn, may account for the improvement of conditions such as rheumatoid arthritis or ulcerative colitis during pregnancy. Increases in melanin stimulating hormone cause the increased skin pigmentation which is characteristic of pregnancy.

Prolactin, important in lactation, is produced in greater amounts, as is oxytocin which rises significantly during the second half of pregnancy and is an important factor in the onset of labour. Oestrogens and progesterones are produced in large quantities by the placenta, the predominant oestrogen being oestriol. Oestrogens, made throughout the placenta, are the main stimulus to uterine growth and development, while progesterone made by the cytotrophoblast has an inhibitory action on the myometrium. Other placental hormones are placental lactogen which alters glucose and insulin metabolism, and may be involved in the initiation of lactation. Chorionic gonadotrophins prolong corpus luteum function in early pregnancy and may be involved with progesterone metabolism in later pregnancy.

DIAGNOSIS OF PREGNANCY

There are many changes which occur during early pregnancy which enable the diagnosis of pregnancy to be made. These can be divided into clinical, biochemical and biophysical in nature.

Clinical

The symptoms of pregnancy begin with a missed menstrual period. The woman who becomes pregnant fails to menstruate at the expected time in the majority of cases, but some bleeding may occur (called an implantation bleed) and this may confuse the issue for both patient and doctor. The failure to menstruate is, of course, due to maintenance of the corpus luteum which continues to produce progesterone, thereby maintaining the endometrium. After pregnancy is established, the secretory endometrium undergoes changes and is known as decidua.

The mother may well complain of nausea, supposedly due to HCG production which affects the vomit centre in the hypothalamus. Her breasts become enlarged and tender due to the influence of progesterone and the rising progesterone levels will also increase the glomerular filtration rate possibly causing the symptom of urinary frequency.

The signs of pregnancy begin with pigmentation due to increased production of melanin stimulating hormone (MSH) from the anterior pituitary. The pigmentation occurs in a number of areas, i.e. facial, in a butterfly distribution over the malar region, known as cloasma; the nipples with associated protruberance of Montgomery's tubercles; the midabdominal line, usually below the umbilicus, known as the linea nigra (black line). The vulva becomes engorged and because of this, the labia majora may have a bluish appearance, as do the vagina and cervix. The uterus becomes enlarged (the size being appropriate to the gestation) and soft, and the body of the uterus and the cervix can

almost be felt separately. The blood supply to the uterus is much increased, and on bimanual examination, the uterine arteries may be felt pulsating. The examination of the ovaries may reveal one or both to be enlarged by the corpus luteum, which by 6 weeks' gestation is often cystic, perhaps 3–5 cm in diameter.

Biochemical

A number of steroid and protein hormones are produced during pregnancy, whose presence is indicative of pregnancy (Table 6.1).

The most widely used diagnostically is HCG which is produced from the time of implantation onwards throughout pregnancy. There is an increasing rate of production until about 10–12 weeks' gestation when it levels off and by 14 weeks has fallen to a maintenance level for the rest of the pregnancy. Detection of the presence of HCG in the blood or urine of the woman confirms the presence of a pregnancy. This involves the detection of HCG by an immunological technique using an antibody to it. In the presence of HCG, the antibody binds to the protein and forms a complex which may be identified by the presence of a marker, e.g. a dye. Another test involves inhibition of agglutination. Latex particles labelled with HCG are mixed with antibody to HCG and urine to be tested. If HCG is absent from urine, there will be an antigen/antibody reaction leading to agglutination (negative test). The presence of HCG in the urine binds with the antibody in the test system, and thereby prevents agglutination of the latex particles. There is a low false negative/positive rate, and a higher degree of sensitivity with monoclonal antibody techniques.

Recent introduction of enzyme colorimetric techniques to the antigen-antibody concept has further improved detection of βHCG to <5/u/ml.

Ultrasound

A gestation sac may be seen in the uterus from $5\frac{1}{2}$ to 6 weeks' gestation with modern ultrasound equipment. The fetal parts may be identified at 7 weeks and the movement of the fetal heart seen using real time ultrasound. Crown-rump length can be measured very accurately from 7 weeks onwards and this gives an accurate estimate of gestation.

Table 6.1
Site and Time of Main Production of Steroid and Protein Hormones formed during Early Pregnancy

Steroid protein hormone	Main site of production	Main increase commences (weeks after conception)
Oestrogens	Placenta Ovary	4
Progesterone	Placenta Ovary	6
Human chorionic gonadotrophin (βsubunit)	Trophoblast	1
Relaxin	Corpus luteum of pregnancy	1–2

ANATOMICAL CHANGES IN THE UTERUS AND ANATOMY OF THE PLACENTA

The uterine vasculature undergoes quite remarkable and unique changes in the first half of pregnancy, specifically to accommodate increasing flows of blood to the placental intervillous space under conditions of low pressure. Maternal blood supply to the placenta is by way of up to 9–14 branches of the uterine artery on both sides of the uterus. These branches give rise to the arcuate arteries, which encircle the uterus in the basal third of the myometrium to form the stratum vasculare. The radial arteries, which come off the arcuate arteries, pass through the remainder of the myometrium and eventually lead to the spiral arteries with their branches, the basal arteries, supplying the superficial myometrium.

The changes in the spiral arteries during pregnancy are brought about by and are an extension of placental growth. The trophoblast of the placenta invades the uterine wall, migrating through the decidua of the placental bed and also within the lumen of the spiral arteries, where they can be seen on histological section to form cytotrophoblastic plugs. The trophoblast cells begin to invade the walls of the spiral arteries, which are gradually replaced by a mixture of trophoblast in a ground substance of fibrinoid. The spiral arteries become inert and widely expanded down to the level of the myometrial-decidual junction. A second migration of trophoblast early in the second trimester extends this 'physiological change' of the spiral arteries deep into the myometrium. Failure of this process is thought to play some part in the pathogenesis of pregnancy induced hypertension and fetal growth retardation.

Placentation

The placenta begins to form as soon as implantation takes place. The outer layer of the blastocyst (trophoblast) invades the endometrium and loses its form to become the syncytiotrophoblast. The outermost layer of this, called the chorion, forms projections or villi, some attached to the endometrium, but mainly lying free in the lacunae, filled with blood.

The maternal blood supply becomes concentrated on the deep surface of the embryo. The trophoblast grows most profusely here, forming the chorion laeve, which, in turn, forms a villous system called the chorion frondosum. The other areas of trophoblast tend to become less active. The chorion frondosum becomes the placenta proper and its formation is completed by Day 70.

There are about 200 projections of trophoblastic cells which branch indefinitely, but there are about 10 main branches called cotyledons and many other smaller cotyledons of less significance.

By about Day 20, fetal blood vessels invade the villous trunks and by Day 23 there is a primitive circulation as these vessels join with the blood vessels in the inner cell mass which becomes the heart.

The intervillous spaces are formed by septae from the maternal surface and these are filled with arterial blood from the uterine arteries, and drained by the uterine veins, bathing the fetal surface in maternal blood. The maternal blood flow through the placenta is estimated to reach 600 ml/min at term, over a surface area of villi of about 11 m^2.

Blood supply

Two umbilical arteries supply one half of the placenta each, although this functional arrangement is not entirely discrete due to an anastomosis of the arteries (Hyrtle's anastomosis) prior to the point of insertion into the placenta. The umbilical arteries divide at the point of insertion to give rise to first order chorionic vessels, which travel along the surface of the placenta, branching up to three more times to give chorionic vessels of the 2nd, 3rd and 4th order. The chorionic veins (1st, 2nd, 3rd and 4th order) sometimes travel in conjunction with the arteries in an inferior position, but can also be seen to meet the artery only at the point at which they descend into the placenta. First order villous vessels (2–3) branch off from chorionic arteries of the 2nd, 3rd and 4th order and descend into villous stems. First order villous arteries subsequently divide to give 4–8 vessels of the 2nd order, which run parallel to the fetal surface of the placenta. The 2nd order vessels then curve in the direction of the basal plate, at which point they are termed villous vessels of the 3rd order. Third order villous vessels pierce the basal plate to return in a retrograde course to the chorionic plate (fetal surface of the placenta).

The capillary network of the placental villi arises from branches of 3rd order villous vessels. The capillaries of a single villous anastomose by way of short connecting parts and quite often show wide, sinusoidal dilatations. At the point of these dilatations, the syncytiotrophoblastic covering of the villous thins and appears almost to fuse with the endothelial lining of the capillary to form the vasculosyncytial membranes.

A placental cotyledon is defined as the villous 'tree', which is supplied by a single villous artery of the 1st order. The intervillous space is loosely divided into 10–38 lobules by foldings of the basal plate (placental septa). Each lobule may contain 1–3 cotyledons, individually supplied by one, or less often two, spiral arteries which are thought to open into the centre of the cotyledons. Drainage of the intervillous space is by way of a complex of venous sinusoids, which may have their openings located around the periphery of each cotyledon. A cotyledon may thus be viewed as a functional unit of the placenta, comprising a fetal part, which is the villous tree, and a maternal part, which is the immediate surrounding portion of the intervillous space and the vessels which supply it. Loss of one of these units due to blockage of a spiral artery, therefore, does not compromise the overall function of the placenta as an organ of exchange.

The widening of the spiral arteries leads to large amounts of blood entering the intervillous space at low pressure which is less than 20 mmHg in the primate placenta and low velocities (0.1–10 mm/s in the primate placenta). The direction of flow is probably from the centre of the cotyledon outwards and by way of thin capillary-like spaces formed by the high density of the branching villi. The low velocities of flow safeguard this loose arrangement of the placental villi and reduces transit time through the placenta, allowing longer times for exchange. Exchange is further facilitated by a gradual reduction in the diameters of the villi and, as a consequence, the closer apposition of the fetal villous capillaries with the syncytiotrophoblastic layer. This development is epitomised by the formation of the vasculosyncytial membranes which decreases the diffusional barrier of the villi (Fig. 6.5).

Clinical aspects

The shape of the placenta is determined at the time of implantation and there are considerable variations, none of which are of any functional significance.

Generally, the cord enters at the midpoint, but it may enter at the placental edge (marginal) or the vessels may divide some distance from the placenta and traverse its surface (velamentous insertion).

As regards implantation, the decidual plate and the chorionic plate are of similar sizes, but if the chorionic plate is reduced, the lateral invasion is reduced and thus is poorly supplied with blood and so villi die. The resulting outer ring of the placenta tends to have its membranes unfolded (circumvallate placenta).

Occasionally, a lobe of placental tissue develops separately from the main placenta (succenturiate lobe) and remains within the uterus after delivery.

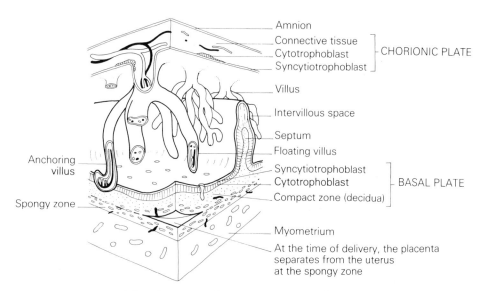

Amnion
Connective tissue
Cytotrophoblast — CHORIONIC PLATE
Syncytiotrophoblast
Villus
Intervillous space
Septum
Floating villus
Anchoring villus
Syncytiotrophoblast
Cytotrophoblast — BASAL PLATE
Compact zone (decidua)
Spongy zone
Myometrium
At the time of delivery, the placenta
separates from the uterus
at the spongy zone

Fig. 6.5 *Structure of the placenta. Villous tissue consists of an outer continuous layer of multinucleate syncytiotrophoblast with an inner layer of mononucleate germinative cytotrophoblast cells. The cytotrophoblast cells are less prevalent in the later stages of pregnancy, but will reform syncytiotrophoblast damaged by hypoxia. (Adapted from H. Tuchmann-Duplessis, G. David and P. Haegel, 1972.* Illustrated Human Embryology, Vol 1. Embryogenesis. *Paris: Masson et Cie Editeurs.)*

In rare instances, invasion of the uterus is so deep that there is a morbid attachment of the placenta (accreta) onto the myometrium, into the myometrial cells (increta) or through the serosal surface (percreta). This condition may well necessitate hysterectomy.

THE BREASTS

The breast is made up of numerous lobules, which are collections of hollow spheres called alveoli that are the secretory units of mammary gland. Each alveolus consists of secretory cells surrounded by contractile myopithelial cells. Small ducts connect the alveoli to a lactiferous sinus from which 10–15 ducts extend to the openings in the surface of the nipple.

During early pregnancy, the breasts receive an increased blood flow and hypertrophy. The increase in size, under the regulation of steroid hormones and human placental lactogen, is due to the full development of lobules with the alveoli and ducts becoming dilated. The cells of the alveoli differentiate, so that by the fourth month of pregnancy they are capable of producing milk. Colostrum, a concentrated yellow fatty substance, is usually secreted in small quantities during the last few weeks of pregnancy.

Further information on the anatomical and physiological changes of the breast and on lactation is to be found in Chapters 12 and 16.

POSTURE AND PELVIC CHANGES

The changing centre of gravity of the pregnant woman leads to increasing lordosis. The effect of raised levels of oestrogen, progesterone, and possibly the effect of relaxin causes laxity of ligaments throughout the body. Slight movement in otherwise very firm joints, such as the sacroiliac joints and the pubic symphysis can cause discomfort on movement which in extreme cases can be severe. Laxity of the pelvic ligaments allows for maximum pelvic capacity during labour and delivery.

FURTHER READING

Chard T., Lilford R. eds. (1986). *Basic Sciences for Obstetrics and Gynaecology*, 2nd edn. London: Springer Verlag.

Hytten F.E., Chamberlain G.V.P. (1980). *Clinical Physiology in Obstetrics*. Oxford: Blackwell Scientific Publications.

Panigel M. (1986). Anatomy and morphology of human placenta. In *Clinics in Obstetrics and Gynaecology*, 2nd edn., T. Chard, ed. London: Saunders.

7

Antenatal Care and Prenatal Diagnosis of Abnormalities

Antenatal care is a form of preventive medicine by which risk factors are recognised and specific intervention instioned when necessary. Structured access to medical attention is provided for this purpose. This also allows common symptoms of pregnancy to be dealt with promptly and provides an ideal opportunity for population screening measures, such as cervical cytology, and testing for rubella immunity. Above all, perhaps, antenatal care fulfils a psychological role in which the woman prepares for childbirth and motherhood. This chapter is mainly concerned with the most ostensible aim: recognition of factors which may harm the mother or her baby. A detailed knowledge of the conditions involved encompasses most of obstetrics and forms the subject matter of much of this book. Here, we are concerned with the methods by which antenatal care is implemented, rather than the conditions themselves.

THE BOOKING VISIT

This is important as at this time the medical risk factors are ascertained (Table 7.1). It consists of three components: the history, examination and special investigations.

Timing of the Booking Visit

Traditionally, women have been asked to book by 16–18 weeks of gestation. This is the ideal time for maternal alpha fetoprotein screening, assessment of gestational age by ultrasound and amniocentesis.

Early booking is desirable, as some obstetric interventions are required at an earlier gestational age (chorion villus biopsy at 8–12 weeks, cervical encirclage at 12–14 weeks). There is also a move towards preconception counselling. In this way, rubella immunity can be confirmed and patients on some potentially teratogenic drugs, such as coumarin, may be changed to alternative treatment such as heparin. It has been shown that among juvenile diabetics optimal control reduces the incidence of congenital abnormality, and it is suggested that periconceptual vitamins, especially folate, may reduce the risk of neural tube defects. Preconceptual counselling also enables couples to be screened for carrier status to certain diseases such as Tay-Sachs and to discuss issues that may be worrying them.

Booking History

The booking history may be divided into identification factors, the psycho-social history, the menstrual/contraceptive history, past obstetric history, maternal conditions, factors suggesting an increased risk of congenital abnormalities and miscellaneous.

Identification details

Some of the information recorded under this section, which includes the patient's name and address, and that of her general practitioner and next of kin, is also of medical importance. Thus a history that the patient is unmarried or that she and her husband/partner are unemployed is associated with a higher perinatal mortality and calls for more rigorous assessment of fetal well-being in later pregnancy.

Social history

A general assessment of the patient's social circum-

Table 7.1

Some Medical Disorders that Constitute Risk Factors

Risk factor	Action
1. Oral anticoagulants for deep vein thrombosis or prosthetic heart valve	Consider changing to heparin in first and third trimesters
2. TB contact	Chest x-ray
3. Recurrent cystitis	Serial midstream urine examination
4. Idiopathic thrombocytopenic purpura	Observe baby for coagulation disorder
5. Endocrine disorder	Check fetus and baby for neonatal thyrotoxicosis
6. Myasthenia gravis	Observe newborn for myasthenia (transient)
7. Steroid therapy within 6 months	Cover labour with steroids
8. Poliomyelitis with persistent deformity or congenital defect of spine or pelvis	Pelvimetry in third trimester
9. Allergies	Avoid allergenic drugs
10. Hyperprolactinaemia	Serial visual fields; Repeat x-ray after delivery
11. Hyperprolactinaemia with adenoma	The above, plus bromocryptine after delivery Monitor dose of anticonvulsant required
12. Epilepsy	Special instructions for breast feeding

stances is appropriate. This should include details of whether she is married or single, supported or unsupported, and what is her attitude and that of her partner's to the pregnancy. Details of her occupation and housing should be recorded as this may influence the antenatal period. Her partner's occupation is also noted. Where relevant, advice about availability and eligibility for the various social services and benefits is of value. Consumption of alcohol should be stopped or restricted to 1 or 2 units/day, while cigarette smoking should also be stopped or restricted to less than five per day. Any current drug medication should be recorded in detail.

Menstrual and contraceptive history

One of the most difficult, but nevertheless important, items to acquire accurately at the booking clinic is an estimate of the patient's gestational age. This calculation requires the following data:

1. The date of the last menstrual period
2. The degree of certainty of the above
3. The regularity of the menstrual cycle
4. The average length of the menstrual cycle
5. Whether the last menstrual period was abnormal

6. If it was abnormal, date of pervious menstrual period
7. Whether this menstrual period was normal
8. Presence of bleeding in the first 3 months after the apparent last menstrual period
9. Date of ovulation induction, if applicable
10. Date of stopping an ovulation inhibitor
11. Whether a withdrawal bleed followed the stopping of an ovulation inhibitor.

In some cases, no relevant menstrual history can be obtained. These include pregnancy after a previous confinement with no intervening menstruation, pregnancy after a long period of amenorrhoea and even pregnancy before the first period.

It is important to ascertain, while obtaining the contraceptive history, whether an intrauterine device was in use at the time of conception. Such a device should be removed if possible and, if the patient is less than 10 weeks pregnant, an ectopic gestation should be excluded.

Previous obstetric history

This is the most important source of risk factors for the current pregnancy. A history of a previous unexplained stillbirth or severe growth retardation is an indication for more careful monitoring of fetal wellbeing in the third trimester by one or more of the methods discussed in Chapter 10. A history of recurrent midtrimester abortion in the absence of fetal growth retardation or infection may call for cervical encirclage. This is described on p. 58. A history of previous caesarean section should lead to further questions about the type of caesarean section and the indication, as it is on these factors that a decision to perform elective surgery or encourage a trial of labour will depend. If necessary, this information must be obtained by writing to the hospital where the previous confinement took place. A history of postpartum haemorrhage, retained placenta or third degree tear should be sought, as this is an indication for the obstetrician to attend the subsequent delivery. A history of a baby weighing over 4.5 kg suggests gestational diabetes and is an indication for a glucose tolerance test in centres where this is not routine.

Past medical history

Most patients volunteer any history of previous illnesses, but this is one area where direct questioning is of value to achieve completeness and save time. Current medication should be clearly recorded and specific medical conditions enquired about, e.g. diabetes mellitus, epilepsy, anaemia, chest disease, tuberculosis, hypertension, rheumatic fever, cardiac disease — congenital or acquired — renal disease, venereal disease, rubella and previous blood transfusion. Conditions such as heart disease and diabetes mellitus have extremely wide implications for subsequent management of the pregnancy and a history of these should be sought by specific questions. A history of chronic hypertension or renal disease increases the chance of subsequent pre-eclampsia and calls for more frequent assessment in the second half of pregnancy. Other maternal conditions with specific obstetric implications are listed in Table 7.1. Previous surgical procedures may be relevant to the current pregnancy, especially gynaecological operations such as dilatation and curettage, cervical cone biopsy and pelvic-floor repair. Any previous psychiatric disorder should be recorded. Allergies, especially to previous drug treatment, require clear annotation.

Additional gynaecological history

The following features in the gynaecological history

may prove relevant to the present pregnancy in greater or lesser degree:

Postcoital bleeding
Intermenstrual bleeding
Vaginal discharge; colour, consistency, odour, blood-stained, irritative
Previous or current contraception; pregnancy occurring with an intrauterine contraceptive device *in situ*; continued use of an oral contraceptive in the early weeks of an unrecognised pregnancy
Primary or secondary infertility and the details of any treatment
Previous abortions, spontaneous and therapeutic, including the period of gestation attained and any subsequent complications, such as vaginal bleeding and pelvic infection
Date and result of last cervical smear.

Other questions

The patient should be asked about her present complaints. Some of these, such as backache, are indications for general advice, i.e. the use of a firm mattress, while others, such as heartburn, require specific medication. Heartburn in pregnancy is due to oesophagitis resulting from regurgitation of stomach contents due to a relatively incompetent cardiac sphincter and increased pressure on the stomach from the gravid uterus. These contents are usually acid and respond to alkalis and often elevation of the head of the bed to reduce reflux. Occasionally, there is incompetence of the pyloric sphincter resulting in biliary reflux causing gastritis and sometimes oesophagitis. These rare cases respond to ingestion of dilute hydrochloric acid.

A history of insulin-dependent diabetes in the patient's parents should be sought, as a glucose tolerance test is then indicated if this is not the routine policy of the clinic. Some questionnaires include a family history of twins, but as this does not significantly increase the chance of multiple pregnancy, a possibility which should always be considered, this question is unnecessary. Similarly, a history of consanguinity should not be sought, as nothing can be done to pre-empt the increased risk of an autosomal recessive disease.

Factors pertaining to genetic risk

Risk of chromosomal trisomy rises with maternal

age and is an indication to offer amniocentesis or chorion biopsy if the patient is aged 37 or more. Certain racial groups are at increased risk of specific diseases; for example, Negroes of West African stock should be screened for sickle trait, Ashkenazy Jews for Tay-Sachs disease and people of Mediterranean and eastern origin for haemoglobinopathies. In all of these cases, prenatal diagnosis is available if both parents are found to be carriers. A history of recent rubella contact, especially in an unimmunised person, is an indication for serial specific IgM estimations. Patients with previous 'multifactorial' conditions, such as neural tube defects, congenital heart disease and cleft lip/palate, have a higher incidence of recurrence which calls for specific diagnostic methods. In addition, couples should be asked about any known inherited diseases, such as haemophilia or muscular dystrophy, in their family.

Examination of the Obstetric Patient

The patient is weighed and her height and development recorded, including any abnormal gait or deformity. The heart and lungs are examined and blood pressure is recorded. The breasts are examined for any discreet mass or inverted nipples. Pelvic examination should take place at this first visit so that a cervical smear may be performed. This will also confirm that the pregnancy is the appropriate size for gestational age and allow other pelvic pathology such as fibroids and ovarian cysts to be detected.

During the second trimester, the uterus becomes palpable on abdominal examination. The position of the uterine fundus within the abdominal cavity is used to estimate the duration of pregnancy, but is misleading in the presence of fibroids, hydramnios or multiple pregnancy. Traditionally, the umbilicus is taken as a reference point (Fig. 7.1), but its position varies from one patient to another and it is not always midway between the xiphisternum and symphysis pubis. However, such an estimate does reflect the progression of pregnancy and its accuracy and reproducibility is enhanced by measuring fundal height from the symphysis pubis in centimetres.

Palpation

Abdominal palpation. The woman lies supine, arms by her side, with her head and shoulders

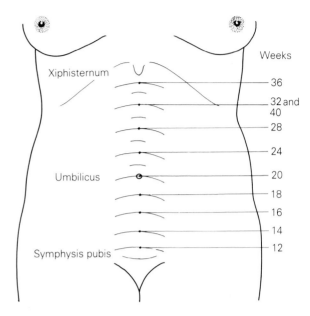

Fig. 7.1   *Fundal position and gestation.*

slightly raised. The examiner stands on the right side and gently palpates the abdomen in a routine sequence.

Fundal palpation (Fig. 7.2). The uterine fundus may be located by applying light pressure either with the ulnar border of the left hand or by the parted fingers of the left hand placed flat in the region of the uterine fundus. The height of the fundus above the symphysis pubis can thus be determined. Both hands are then applied to each side of the fundus and the polarity of the fetus (breech or head) ascertained.

Lateral palpation. (Fig. 7.3). The hands are then gently moved along the contour of the uterus. The lie of the fetus is thus determined. When the presentation is cephalic and in the usual lateral or anterolateral position, the fetal spine is identified as a continuous firmness on one side, and the limbs as irregular shapes on the other side, giving a softer impression to the examining hand. Fetal movements are often felt at this stage. When the fetus has adopted a posterior position, the findings are slightly different. The fetal spine lies over the maternal spine giving a characteristic flattening below the mother's umbilicus and, if not obviously visible, may be realised by placing the hand flat

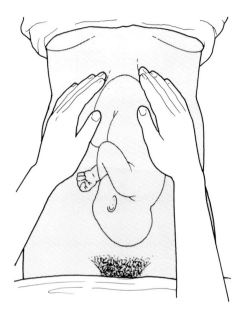

Fig. 7.2 *Abdominal palpation. Step 1 — fundal palpation.*

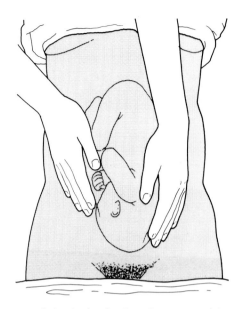

Fig. 7.4 *Abdominal palpation. Step 3 — pelvic palpation.*

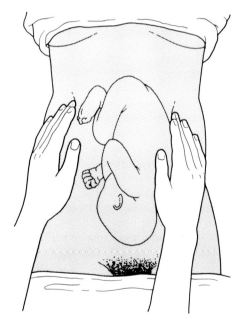

Fig. 7.3 *Abdominal palpation. Step 2 — lateral palpation.*

across the abdomen below the umbilicus. Fetal limbs are usually palpable on both sides of the midline.

Pelvic palpation. The examiner now faces the patient's feet, placing his/her hands on either side of the lower portion of the uterus (Fig. 7.4). Gentle pressure is applied with the distal phalanges of the fingers and the presenting part identified. The presenting part is usually the fetal head and is identifiable by its hard, rounded character. If unengaged, it will be easily ballotable. Engagement has occurred when the widest diameter of the presenting part has passed through the pelvic brim. As the fingers of each hand are moved towards the pelvis, the impression will be of the head becoming wider until the pubic rami are touched. However, when the head is unengaged, the impression will be of the head becoming wider and then narrower again as the fingers are advanced towards the pelvic brim. If the head is deeply engaged, it may be completely impalpable. Vaginal examination will confirm a cephalic presentation.

The Pawlik grip. This stage of the palpation is not always required, but should be left to last as it is the most uncomfortable part (Fig. 7.5). The examiner faces the woman and, spreading the fingers and thumb of the right hand, places it suprapubically. With gentle fundal pressure from above, the fingers and thumb are approximated across the presenting

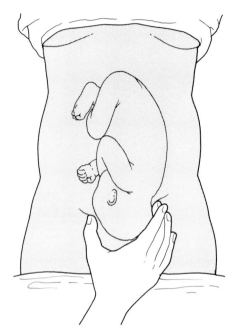

Fig. 7.5   *The Pawlik manoeuvre.*

part and its mobility either above or within the pelvic brim is assessed.

To complete the examination of the fetus, the fetal heart is auscultated with a Pinard fetal heart stethoscope. Its presence, rate and rhythm are noted.

At this stage, the examiner should have a clear impression of (1) the height of the fundus (interpreted as gestational age equivalent); (2) the lie of the fetus; (3) the position of the fetus; (4) the presentation; (5) whether the presenting part is engaged or unengaged; and (6) the rate and character of the fetal heart.

Special Investigations

The blood group is determined and an antibody screen carried out. The latter is performed irrespective of the patient's Rhesus group in case antibodies against other red blood cell antigens are present. A base line haemoglobin estimation is performed and Negro patients and those of Mediterranean origin are screened for haemoglobinopathies by electrophoresis. The serological test for syphilis is carried out and rubella titre investigated, so that vaccination can be offered in the puerperium if the patient is not immune. In many clinics, the serum is examined for alpha-fetoprotein as a screening test for neural tube defects and this is most reliable between the 16th and 18th week. Some clinics screen all patients for the hepatitis β surface antigen. If this is present and the patient has the e antigen (or lacks anti e antibodies), she may infect staff. Precautions are needed at delivery or when taking blood samples. Such patients are also likely to transmit the virus to the fetus at birth, and some authorities recommend immediate vaccination of the newborn to prevent a chronic infection and later hepatoma. Another investigation, which is routinely offered in many clinics, is a modified glucose tolerance test in which only fasting and 1 h glucose estimations are made.

A routine ultrasound scan is commonly carried out in early pregnancy; optimally at the 18th week of gestation. Some patients may decline this investigation on the basis of unconfirmed reports of harmful effects. Animal and human studies on the effects of *diagnostic* sonar have been reassuring and doses a hundred times greater than those in current use are required to produce any biological effect. Most patients, therefore, consider the following concrete advantages to outweigh any hypothetical disadvantage:

1. It forms an accurate assessment of gestational age. Thirty per cent of patients have one of the menstrual ambiguities mentioned on p. 34. Even among those patients who are sure of their last menstrual period, ultrasound has been shown in some series to provide a more reliable indication of the due birthdate. Furthermore, randomised trials have shown that the induction rate for presumed postmaturity may be reduced by means of early ultrasound dating.
2. The maternal alpha-fetoprotein estimation is a more specific index of spina bifida when the gestational age is calculated on the basis of the biparietal diameter.
3. It provides a firm and objective baseline against which further growth assessment may be judged. (This is a by-product of the first advantage.)
4. Twins, one-sixth of whom would otherwise remain undiagnosed by the start of labour, will be detected (Fig. 7.6).

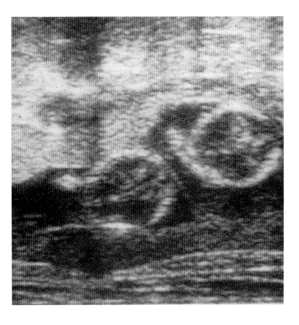

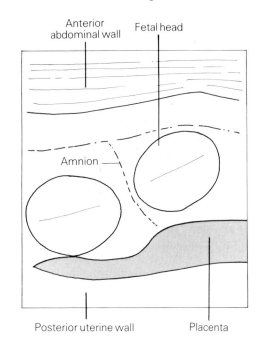

Fig. 7.6   *Detection of twin fetal heads by ultrasound.*

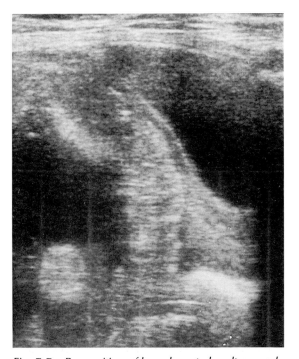

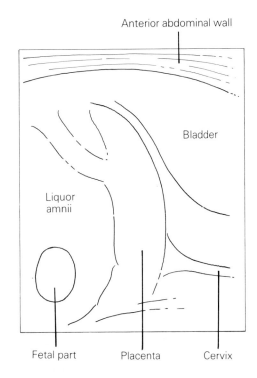

Fig. 7.7   *Recognition of low placenta by ultrasound.*

5. A large number of congenital abnormalities, the proportion of which will be determined by the expertise of the individual ultrasonographer, may be observed. All cases of anencephaly, 80% of spina bifida and the majority of patients with severe dwarfism, renal and intestinal obstruction will be recognised. More subtle anomalies, such as congenital heart disease, diaphragmatic hernia, mild hydrocephalus and fetal tumours should also be detected.

6. Recognition of the low placenta (Fig. 7.7); 5–10% of the scans at 18 weeks will demonstrate a low-lying placenta and, in 5% of these, placenta praevia can be confirmed by a subsequent scan in the third trimester. This information may warrant hospital admission in order to pre-empt a severe haemorrhage in the case of a major degree of placenta praevia. In addition, subsequent management of antepartum haemorrhage is easier if a low placenta has been diagnosed or excluded by an early scan.

7. A psychological benefit has been claimed, and there is no doubt that most mothers and fathers enjoy the experience of seeing their unborn child on the ultrasound screen.

It is only fair to point out that this technology also has some disadvantages (apart from the hypothetical dangers of high frequency sound waves), in that the discovery of self-correcting conditions, such as minor dilatation of the renal tract and small cysts of the choroid plexus, will engender unnecessary anxiety.

SUBSEQUENT ANTENATAL VISITS

A guide to subsequent antenatal visits and the important factors to be considered at these times is shown in Fig 7.8. At every subsequent visit, the mother's weight and blood pressure are measured, and the urine checked for protein and glucose. Weight gain should average about 10 kg during pregnancy. Excessive weight gain may contribute to the onset of pregnancy-induced hypertension and calls for dietary advice.

Blood pressure should be considered abnormal if, in a previously normotensive patient, it reaches 140/90 mmHG or if there is a rise in systolic and diastolic pressure of 20 mmHg or more between visits.

Proteinuria in an ordinary specimen of urine usually represents contamination of the urine by vaginal discharge. If present in an MSU, it is either due to infection, chronic renal disease or, occasionally, orthostasis. In the presence of hypertension occurring during pregnancy, it indicates renal and placental pathology which warrant urgent admission.

Glycosuria can indicate gestational diabetes, or merely the lowered renal threshold for tubular reabsorption of glucose, the latter being more common. Oral glucose tolerance test should be carried out to make the diagnosis.

On each visit the fetal size is assessed and the distance from the symphysis pubis to the uterine fundus may be recorded. From the 32nd week onwards, the presentation of the fetus is also recorded. After the 36th week, it is customary to determine whether the fetal head is engaged or will engage in the pelvis.

The amount of liquor should also be determined from the 32nd week onward and a general impression obtained of fetal size, so that any suspicion of inadequate fetal growth can be confirmed by ultrasonic measurements. From 24 weeks onward, the mother should be asked about fetal movements as any sudden diminution warrants further investigation.

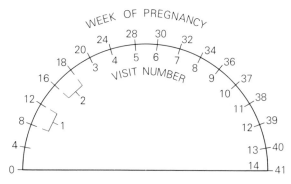

Fig. 7.8 *Summary of special points of antenatal care to be considered at the following visits: (1) History, physical examination, cervical smear, blood group, rhesus factor and antibodies, Hb, VDRL, rubella immune status, chorion villous biopsy if appropriate. (2) Ultrasound, serum AFP, amniocentesis if appropriate. (3) GTT if at risk for gestational diabetes. (5) Rhesus antibodies, Hb. (7) Ultrasonicplacentography if placenta thought to be low lying at 16–18 weeks. (8) Rhesus antibodies; repeat GTT if at risk for gestational diabetes. (9) Hb. (10) Lateral pelvimetry if breech presentation. (14) Induction of labour at 42 weeks.*

The haemoglobin concentration is re-estimated at 30 and 36 weeks, and antibody titres are obtained at this time from Rhesus negative mothers and those with other pre-existing antibodies. It is becoming increasingly common to offer Rhesus negative mothers an anti D γ globulin injection at 28 and 34 weeks. This reduces the chance of sensitisation prior to delivery which otherwise occurs in 1% of mothers.

The number of times that such antenatal examinations should be carried out varies according to the patient's history. Where there are no specific risk factors, the patient should be seen every 4 weeks until 28 weeks, fortnightly until the 36 week, and thereafter every week until the onset of labour. Many patients and general practitioners prefer a policy of shared care, and this is usually carried out on an agreed basis between the hospital and referring general practitioners. A 'shared care' card facilitates information exchange in such circumstances.

Engagement of the Fetal Head

In primigravida, the head may be engaged by 38 complete weeks. Some of the causes of non-engagement are shown in Table 7.2, but cephalopelvic disproportion must be actively excluded. In multigravida, the head may not become engaged until the onset of labour, but cephalopelvic disproportion should, nevertheless, be excluded even though the pelvis has already been tested by a previous delivery.

Table 7.2

Causes of Non-Engagement of the Presenting Part

---

1. Full bladder or rectum
2. Mistaken dates
3. Occipitoposterior position
4. Cephalopelvic disproportion
5. Hydramnios
6. Multiple pregnancy
7. Placenta praevia
8. Pelvic tumours
9. Fetal malpresentation, e.g. brow, face
10. Short umbilical cord
11. Fetal abnormality, e.g. hydrocephalus
12. High assimilation pelvis

Three methods of assessing the capacity of the pelvis to allow the presenting part to engage will be considered.

Abdominal palpation

The mother is placed supine (*see* p. 78), and gentle pressure is applied to the fundus with the left hand to push the fetal head towards the pelvis. The right hand is placed flat across the suprapubic region with the ring finger overlying the symphysis pubis. The fetal head is gently pressed backwards and will normally enter the pelvis easily. Should there be doubt, the assessment may be aided by asking the mother to sit up partially by supporting herself on the elbows and placing the forearms by the side of her chest. By raising the upper portion of her body in this manner, the rise in intra-abdominal pressure assists descent of the head.

Combined abdomino-vaginal palpation

This is the Munro-Kerr method and is depicted in Fig. 7.9. The left hand, placed suprapubically, pushes the head downwards and backwards into the pelvis to meet the fingers in the vagina at the level of the ischial spines. The thumb of the right hand may be used to assess the degree of any

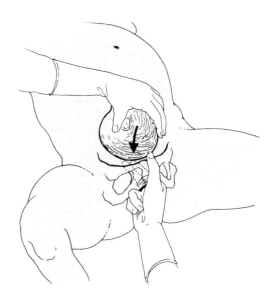

Fig. 7.9 *Estimating the relative size of the fetal head and the maternal pelvis by the Munro-Kerr 'head fitting' test.*

overlap. This method also allows an assessment of the bony pelvis and will detect any soft tissue pelvic tumour. Placenta praevia as a reason for non-engagement of the presenting part must be excluded before this manoeuvre is performed.

Vaginal examination

Pelvic assessment by vaginal examination is employed to predict the possibility of cephalopelvic disproportion. The sacrum is gently palpated and its anterior surface should be concave with the coccyx following the line of the curve. The fingers are then moved to the lateral borders of the sacrum, in turn, and placed on the sacrospinous ligament allowing assessment of the greater sciatic notch, which should accept two fingers' breadth with ease. The sacrospinous ligaments are attached anteriorly to the ischial spines which should lack prominence and, therefore, not encroach into the pelvic cavity. The pelvic outlet is now assured. The subpubic angle should easily accept two fingers' breadths, but must be assessed gently. The transverse diameter of the outlet is reflected by the distance between the ischial tuberosities and normally four knuckles of the hand will fit between them.

Such manoeuvres provide an impression of pelvic capacity which can prove useful. The student is well advised to practise the examination on a pelvic model, when the technique of the assessment will be better appreciated.

GENERAL ADVICE TO THE PATIENT IN PREGNANCY

Counselling is an essential part of the antenatal care, and helps the mother to prepare for childbirth and cope with some of the common symptoms of pregnancy. It is axiomatic, therefore, that a relaxed atmosphere should be created, although this ideal is sometimes compromised by the tempo of busy antenatal clinics. It is important that each patient should be given a booklet in which the policies of the hospital and general practice are laid out, and explanations of the events of pregnancy and labour can be found. This booklet should also explain the purpose and possible hazards of various investigations which the woman may be offered. Specific

issues which may be discussed include the following.

Diet

The pregnant woman requires extra energy to supply the needs of the growing fetus and to keep pace with her own increased metabolic rate and weight gain (Fig. 7.10 and Table 7.3). The average person requires 2500 calories a day and this is not greatly increased from her daily non-pregnancy food consumption. The total increased calorie requirement of pregnancy is relatively small and a balanced diet should be able to supply all the extra

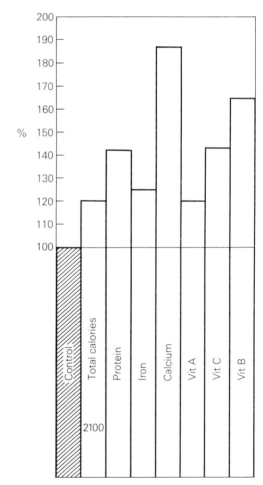

Fig. 7.10 *Approximate increases in daily requirements of important dietary constituents during pregnancy expressed as a percentage above non-pregnant needs.*

Table 7.3

Daily Dietary Requirements for Non-Pregnant, Pregnant and Lactating Women

Nutrients	Normal	Pregnant	Lactating
Calories	2100	2500	3000
Protein (mg)	60	85	100
Calcium (mg)	0.8	1.5	2.0
Iron (mg)	12	15	15
Vitamin A (i.u.)	5000	6000	8000
Thiamin (mg)	1.1	1.8	2.0
Riboflavine (mg)	1.5	2.5	3.0
Nicotinic acid (mg)	11	18	20
Vitamin C (mg)	70	100	150

protein and fat required, together with most of the minerals such as zinc, a deficiency of which may be associated with congenital abnormalities, and calcium. The question of iron supplements is more controversial and, again, may be unnecessary provided the mother is not vegetarian. If the mother is not given iron, her iron stores will inevitably decline during pregnancy. This is not a cause for concern provided she was not anaemic to start with and did not become pregnant with already depleted iron stores. Iron supplements combined with folic acid should be given in the case of multiple pregnancy. Folic acid without iron should be the treatment for otherwise uncomplicated haemoglobinopathies. Doses of iron and folic acid vary considerably from one preparation to another. The average requirements for prophylaxis are 50–100 mg elemental iron and 350–500 µg folic acid per day. Intolerance to iron is very variable, usually causing diarrhoea or constipation.

Rest and Exercise

It has been shown by Doppler studies that violent exercise causes increased femoral artery flow at the expense of the uterine supply and competitive running is, therefore, unadvisable. Furthermore, body temperature rises during strenuous exercise, especially in fit people and, as the fetus is unable to control its own heat loss, any extreme form of physical exertion is contraindicated during pregnancy. It is, nevertheless, important for a sense of wellbeing and in preparation for labour that gentle exercise is taken. Swimming, cycling and walking are all beneficial during pregnancy.

Sexual Activity

The bulk of evidence seems to indicate that coitus is not harmful during pregnancy. Nevertheless, most obstetricians would counsel patients with repeated abortions against having sex during the critical period of up to 14 weeks.

Preparation for Lactation

No single measure would cut down on mortality throughout the world as much as the widespread resumption of breast feeding. The best preparation for this is to ensure that the mother is aware of the normal course of events following delivery and is mentally prepared for breast feeding. Inverted nipples usually correct themselves spontaneously during pregnancy and can be made to protrude by means of gentle manipulation, or occasionally by the use of a nipple shield.

General Education and Instruction

This varies from specific instruction on items such as the preparation of the baby's clothes and the advantages of breast feeding to a discussion of what to expect during labour and the provision of breathing exercises to help cope with pain. Analgesia should be discussed in order to give the mother a deeper appreciation of the options open to her. These discussions should include the husband, who should be encouraged to be present during the labour which is, after all, a family event. It is also important that the patient should have a tour of the labour ward, so that this is not a frightening or strange place when the big day arrives. A number of patients will have specific requests about issues such as birth position which will be discussed later in this book.

THE ISSUE OF HOME BIRTH

Many women will wish to discuss this possibility with their doctors and it is, therefore, important to have an appreciation of this issue. Arguments for and against home births often evolve around overall perinatal mortality associated with hospital and domiciliary confinement. This is inappropriate; the overall perinatal mortality of home births is slightly higher than that of the country as a whole, but it is quite fairly pointed out by proponents of this method that these figures include many premature and precipitate labours and a number of unbooked deliveries among high risk patients. The perinatal mortality which is defined as stillbirths and neonatal deaths occurring during the first 7 days of life among low risk patients especially selected for home birth is 4 per 1000 births. This, however, cannot be compared with the perinatal death rate in hospital, as many patients booked for home births will be transferred to a hospital as an emergency, and fetal deaths among these patients will appear in hospital statistics which, of course, also include all other high risk patients. The 0.4% perinatal mortality quoted above, therefore, constitutes the intrapartum and early neonatal death rate. The proportion of this accounted for by intrapartum asphyxia is not known, but it is unlikely to compare favourably with intrapartum death rates quoted by hospitals of 0.1–0.2%. It seems reasonable to conclude, therefore, that women electing to have a home birth, because of the emotional warmth and comfort of their own surroundings, do so at the cost of a small increase in the risk of fetal death. Perhaps of greater importance, however, is the observation that such losses represent only the tip of the iceberg and permanent damage is a more likely and, in a sense, more serious sequel of unrecognised intrapartum hypoxia. A compromise for women wishing to be at home during childbirth is to deliver the baby in hospital, and return home, if all is well, within 6–12 hours.

PRENATAL DIAGNOSIS OF FETAL ABNORMALITIES

The detection and prevention of congenital disorders is the most rapidly expanding area in obstetric practice. The relative importance of this topic has become greater as perinatal mortality due to all causes has diminished to levels of around 10/1000 births. Single gene defects alone occur this frequently (Table 7.4). Structural congenital abnormalities are now three or four times as common as perinatal loss from other causes. With a birth prevalence of 2/1000, serious chromosomal abnormalities are as common as intrapartum death and have more serious long-term consequences. In developed countries, 30% of stillbirths, 20% of neonatal deaths and 30% of all paediatric admissions are the result of congenital disorders. This section will deal with the prenatal diagnosis rather than the genetics of these disorders. The two subjects are, however, intimately connected, as indica-

---

Table 7.4

Contribution of Different Categories of Congenital Abnormality to Overall Incidence

Category of defect	Incidence per thousand	
	Detectable abnormality	*'Serious' abnormality* i.e. with permanent life-threatening implications
Chromosomal	5 (includes balanced translocations and sex chromosome abnormalities)	2
Single gene defects	10	10
Structural abnormalities*	30–40 (includes talipes and congenital dislocation of hip)	10–20 (includes congenital heart disease)
Congenital infection	4–8	1–2

* A small proportion of structural abnormalities are the result of chromosomal, single gene or infective causes. Thus, duodenal atresia is sometimes caused by Down's syndrome; many forms of dwarfism have autosomal inheritance; and microcephaly may have an autosomal recessive or infective basis. Most structural abnormalities, however, are caused by a combination of many genes and environmental agents. We call these conditions multifactional or polygenetic and they include the majority of organ defects such as congenital heart disease, neural tube defects, cleft-lip and palate and gastrointestinal and renal anomalies.

tions for many diagnostic tests depend on the risks of inheritance. The genetics of single gene defects and structural abnormalities are, therefore, summarised in Table 7.5. However, no attempt to provide a comprehensive account of genetics is made.

The fetus is not amenable to traditional methods of physical examination, and prenatal diagnosis, therefore, involves the use of specific technology. Detection of abnormalities is dependent on one of three basic methods:

1. **Imaging techniques.** In practice, ultrasound is much the most important, although conventional radiology still has a place, and nuclear magnetic resonance may be useful in the future.
2. **Measurement of fetal products in maternal blood.** In practice, this involves measurement of the fetal protein, alpha-fetoprotein, but techniques to harvest minute numbers of fetal cells from the maternal circulation have exciting implications for the future.
3. **Analysis of fetal tissue or fluids.** Prenatal

Table 7.5

Mechanisms of Genetic Inheritance

Type of inheritance	Recurrence risk	Other features	Examples
Autosomal dominant	1:2 if present in a parent	May be new mutation (with very low recurrence risk) if no family history. The more lethal the condition, the more frequently is it caused by new mutation. Penetrance also varies for some conditions.	Achondroplasia Huntington's chorea Tuberose sclerosis Neurofibromatosis Von Willebrand's disease Congenital spherocytosis Multiple endocrine adenomatosis
Autosomal recessive	1:4	Includes most inborn errors of metabolism. Prenatal diagnosis frequently available.	Cystic fibrosis Thalassaemia Tay Sach's disease Phenylketonuria
Sex-linked recessive	1:2 males affected 1:2 females carriers (the female is an obligatory carrier if she is the daughter of an affected man)	The probability that a female is a carrier can often be increased or decreased by specific testing, e.g. creatinine phosphokinase for Duchenne dystrophy and factor VIII for Haemophilia.	Haemophilia Christmas disease Duchenne and Becker dystrophies Lesch-Nyhan syndrome Ornithine carbamyl transferase deficiency
'Polygenetic' (multifactorial)	1:20 where the condition is common to 1:100 where it is rare	A number of genes and environmental agents (usually unidentified combine to produce the abnormality. Concurrence rate in identical twins is 50%	This group includes most of the major structural abnormalities such as congenital heart disease, intestinal atresia, cleft lip and palate. Sometimes, however, these are caused by single gene defects, e.g. the Meckel syndrome (*see text*) or as part of a chromosomal abnormality, or as a result of infection or drugs

diagnosis has great potential in reducing the total of suffering and the economic consequences of congenital disease. The incidence of the world's most common and one of the most serious autosomal recessive disorders, beta-thalassaemia, has been reduced by 70% in Sardinia by means of fetal tissue sampling and gene probe diagnosis. Similarly, the incidence of Tay Sachs disease has been reduced by an even greater amount in the state of New York, where a specific enzyme assay is carried out on pregnancies at risk. It must be mentioned, however, that prevention of congenital disorders is dependent upon selective termination of affected fetuses. An essential component of genetic counselling is that it should be as non-directive as possible. Couples should be provided with the facts they require to make their own informed decision. Thus, counselling serves largely as an educational function in which the couple assess the risks of various courses of action in the light of their own values. Many counselling sessions may be required for patients to absorb the information which they have been given, and it is often helpful to write a letter following the consultation in which the essential points are enumerated. This allows prospective parents to consider the situation more carefully.

Ultrasound Diagnosis of Congenital Abnormalities

Anomalies are detected by one of three means:

1. Direct visualisation of the abnormality, e.g. the absence of the fetal head in anencephaly;
2. Demonstration of abnormal growth of a particular fetal part, e.g. slow growth of the limbs in achrondroplasia;
3. A recognition of the effect of the abnormality on adjoining structures, e.g. dilatation of renal tract in cases of urethral atresia.

In Table 7.6 indications for detailed, high resolution ultrasound scan are listed. Where these indications apply before the time of fetal viability, the woman will have the option of selective termination of pregnancy if a serious anomaly is discovered. Some of the indications, however, apply after the time of fetal viability. This information may still be of use in clinical management. For instance, mothers may be spared the risk of caesarean section for fetal distress where it is known that the fetus has an unequivocally lethal congenital anomaly. In other cases, the paediatric surgical team can be placed on standby before the delivery.

Ninety per cent of congenital anomalies will arise in patients who do not have any of these specific risk factors. Routine antenatal screening of all women between 16 and 20 weeks' gestation is, therefore,

Table 7.6
Indications for High Resolution Ultrasound

Indications in mid-pregnancy (i.e. 16–20 weeks' gestation)	Previous child with structural anomaly (recurrence risk 1–5% unless part of a single gene defect)
	Parent with a structural anomaly
	Raised maternal alpha-fetoprotein
	Maternal diabetes (four times increased incidence)
	Exposure to potential teratogens
	Suspicious findings on routine ultrasound
Indications which usually apply after fetal viability (i.e. >24 weeks' gestation)	Breech presentation (four times increased incidence)
	Oligohydramnios
	Polyhydramnios
	Severe symmetrical growth retardation

Table 7.7

Some Important Conditions which can be Diagnosed by Ultrasound

	Disorder	Comments
Central nervous system	Anencephaly	Ultrasound diagnosis effectively 100% reliable
	Spina bifida	80% accompanied by mild hydrocephalus
	Hydrocephalus	Presents with increased size of cerebral ventricles; head enlarges much later
	Encephalocele	Prognosis poor if brain tissue herniates
Gastrointestinal	Oesophageal atresia	Polyhydramnios and persistent absence of stomach vesicle on scan
	Diaphragmatic hernia	Stomach vesicle adjacent to heart; may be intermittent
	Duodenal atresia	Double vesicle
	Jejunal atresia	Multiple peristaltic vesicles
	Cystic fibrosis	Speckled reflections of inspisated meconium commonly seen
	Large bowel obstruction	Dilated bowel loops
	Omphalocele	Central abdominal defect covered with peritoneum; frequently associated with other anomalies and associated with chromosomal defects
	Gastroschisis	Smaller eccentric abdominal defect; bowel free in amniotic cavity; not associated with other anomalies or trisomies, but more difficult to treat surgically
Urinary system	Renal agenesis	Oligohydramnios; absent kidneys
	Hydronephrosis	Dilated renal pelvis and calyses; has good prognosis especially if unilateral
	Urethral obstruction	Dilated bladder and ureters; prognosis poor if obstruction complete, i.e. accompanied by severe and early oligohydramnios; intermittent obstruction may be caused by urethral valves which has a better prognosis and may be treated by *in-utero* drainage after exclusion of aneuploidy (especially trisomy 13)
Skeletal abnormalities	Osteogenesis imperfecta	The lethal form may usually be diagnosed by the middle of pregnancy
	Lethal hypophosphatasia	Less echogenic skeleton
	Achondroplasia	Non-lethal heterozygous form cannot be diagnosed until late in the second trimester
	Many other forms of dwarfism	
Cleft lip and palate		Specific search required for detection
Heart		Most lethal abnormalities can be diagnosed by experts in high risk patients; many defects will be overlooked on routine scanning

required to detect the majority of congenital abnormalities. In leading units, the great majority of structural anomalies may be diagnosed in this way.

The ability of routine ultrasound to detect anomalies is lower in the average hospital service where vigilance and expertise are not as great. Thus, while

97% of cases of spina bifida may be detected in centres of ultrasonic excellence, detection rates of 60–80% are more usual. Some common conditions which may be diagnosed by ultrasound are shown in Table 7.7. It can be seen from this Table that anomalies which can be identified by direct visualisation can usually be diagnosed earlier in pregnancy than those which rely on an effect on surrounding structures or the demonstration of differential growth rates. A further important principle of anomaly scanning is that congenital anomalies frequently affect more than one system. The detection of one abnormality should, therefore, always lead to very careful examination of other organ systems. Furthermore, certain non-lethal anomalies are frequently associated with chromosomal aneuploides, and karyotyping should be obtained in these cases to provide a more accurate prognosis. Some anatomical variants are of no clinical importance; thus small choroid cysts always disappear and many cases of pelvi-ureteric junction obstruction resolve spontaneously.

It is very important to provide couples with sensitive and comprehensive counselling following the discovery of a congenital abnormality. A member of the team of obstetrics should be available to speak to the couple as soon as any suspicious observation is made, and this should be followed up by more detailed counselling which may involve the Paediatrician or Paediatric Surgeon who will be responsible for the baby's care after delivery. It is important to seek parental permission for a postmortem examination following termination of pregnancy, stillbirth or neonatal death due to congenital abnormality. Definitive diagnosis is made in this way, thereby providing information for subsequent genetic counselling. Thus, the finding of polycystic disease and encephalocele suggests the diagnosis of *Meckel* syndrome. This is an autosomal recessive condition with a much higher recurrence rate than the 1–5% usually associated with structural abnormalities. Similarly, isolated hydrocephalus is usually a 'polygenetic' abnormality (*see* Table 7.5, p. 87) with a 2 or 3% recurrence rate but, when caused by aqueduct stenosis, it may be inherited as a sex-linked condition. A chromosome culture should also be obtained from congenitally abnormal neonates or abortuses as many of the conditions listed in Table 7.6 are the result of chromosomal abnormalities, and this knowledge will affect counselling and prenatal diagnosis in future pregnancies.

Alpha-fetoprotein Estimations

Alpha-fetoprotein (AFP) is the main fetal serum protein produced during the first half of pregnancy. It leaks across exposed membranes in conditions such as open spina bifida and anencephaly. The birth prevalence of these conditions varies from 2 to 6 per thousand in the UK. It is most common along the west coast of the country. It has been suggested that the recurrence risk (1 in 20 or 25 after one affected child) can be considerably reduced by periconceptual vitamins, but this has not been proven by completely randomised trials.

Anencephaly is best detected by ultrasound. Spina bifida can be accurately diagnosed in this way by careful high-resolution ultrasound. Where this is not available, centres rely on maternal serum alpha-fetoprotein screening, which is less critically dependent on individual expertise.

The recurrence risk for these conditions is around 4% and amniocentesis is frequently carried out on women with a previously affected child, especially if high resolution ultrasound scanning is not available or difficult for technical reasons (unfavourable fetal position, obesity). Acetyl cholinesterase, which is liberated from exposed neural tissue in open neural tube defects, is also measured in amniotic fluid under these circumstances.

Fewer than 5% of pregnancies associated with open neural tube defects occur in women who have already had an affected offspring. The finding that maternal serum alpha-fetoprotein (MSAFP) levels are higher in affected pregnancies has led to the use of this estimation as a screening test. As can be seen from Fig. 7.11, this test does not provide perfect discrimination between affected and normal fetuses. Nevertheless, the sensitivity is reasonably good in that 90% of anencephalics and 80% of open neural tube defects will be detected at the usual cut-off point (2.5 multiples of the median). The predictive value of the test is, however, not high in that only about one-tenth (the exact figure depending on the prevalence of neural tube defects) of patients with a high MSAFP level will be confirmed to have a neural tube defect. Thus, high levels should be followed up by more specific tests: ultrasound and/ or liquor AFP or cholinesterase.

The optimum time for screening is 16–18 completed weeks of gestation and an accurate knowledge of gestational age is, therefore, essential. AFP levels in fetal blood and amniotic fluid decrease progressively during the second trimester. The

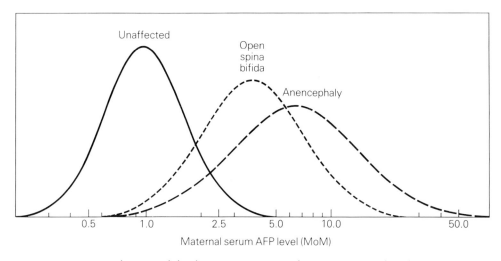

Fig. 7.11 *Maternal serum alpha-fetoprotein in normal pregnancies and in those with open neural tube defects. It can be seen that there is a degree of overlap in values obtained from normal and affected pregnancies, especially those with spina bifida. Thus, although MSAFP is quite sensitive (detecting 80% of spina bifida fetuses) it is not specific.*

concentration of AFP in maternal serum, however, increases progressively over this period due to greater leakage across the placenta. As a result, when the pregnancy is thought to be less advanced than it really is, the MSAFP concentration would appear to be relatively high and is more likely to be interpreted as positive. Similarly, if a pregnancy is thought to be more advanced than it really is, a genuinely high level might not be regarded as positive.

High levels of maternal serum AFP are also caused by other congenital anomalies in which fetal serum proteins are able to leak into amniotic fluid in large amounts. Thus congenital nephrotic syndrome, and abdominal wall defects such as omphalocele and gastroschisis are also associated with raised MSAFP levels. Omphalocele is a large midline abdominal wall defect with the bowel covered by peritoneum, which can be associated with other congenital abnormalities. Gastroschisis is a lateral abdominal wall defect with no peritoneal covering for the bowel, and unassociated with other abnormalities. Recovery of bowel function does not always take place. Other causes of false positive results are multiple pregnancy, threatened abortion and intrauterine death. It should be stressed, however, that most false positive results simply represent the upper end of a normal range. Low maternal serum AFP in conjunction with maternal age may increase the detection rate of Down's syndrome.

Antenatal Diagnosis on Fetal Tissues and Fluids

Clinical practice depends on a knowledge of three main methods of obtaining fetal tissue: amniocentesis, fetoscopy and chorion villus biopsy, along with the three predominant laboratory techniques — chromosome analysis, enzyme assay and gene probe technology.

Techniques for obtaining fetal tissue

Amniocentesis. This is still the most widely practised technique for chromosome analysis, enzyme assay and gene probe diagnosis. It is also used for biochemical tests in the detection of neural tube defects and, in later pregnancy, for assessment of rhesus isoimmunisation and the prediction of fetal lung maturity. When indicated for prenatal diagnosis, the procedure is best carried out at 15–16 weeks' gestation. Before this time, the number of cells available for culture and analysis is much lower and the procedure is technically more difficult. Culturing of amniotic fluid cells takes approximately 3 weeks. The procedure allows termination of pregnancy, where necessary, to be carried out before 20 weeks.

In order to avoid placental and fetal injury, amniocentesis should be performed immediately after ultrasound examination or, ideally, under continuous ultrasound control. Twenty ml of fluid are aspirated, but the first ml should be aspirated into a separate syringe and discarded in case any maternal cells have contaminated this portion of the specimen. The chance of causing an abortion ranges between 0.3% and 2% in different studies. The most widely quoted procedure-related abortion rate is 1%, although recent authors have reduced this to 0.5%.

Fetoscopy. The most frequent indication for this technique is to obtain fetal blood. This may be used to diagnose congenital infections and haematological disorders, such as haemoglobinopathies, coagulation defects and the severe combined immunodeficiency syndrome. Fetal blood is also used to obtain a rapid karyotype after the detection of a congenital abnormality on detailed scan. Carriers of haemophilia and Christmas disease normally undergo amniocentesis in order to ascertain the gender of their fetus and, if this is a male, fetoscopy is offered. It should be noted that the indications for fetal blood sampling are dwindling rapidly, as chorion villus biopsy and gene probe diagnosis play an increasing role.

Tissue biopsy may also be obtained under fetoscopic guidance. Skin biopsies have been used for the diagnosis of a number of lethal bullous conditions. Fetal liver biopsy may be used to detect deficiency of enzymes not expressed in normal amniotic fluid cells. These include deficiencies of the urea cycle enzymes. Fetoscopy is feasible after 18 weeks' gestation and causes fetal loss in approximately 3% of cases. In addition, there is an increased premature delivery rate and some patients develop a persistent leak of liquor. Recently, a technique has been developed in which fetal blood may be obtained under direct ultrasound guidance from umbilical vessels without the need for fetoscopy. This method is already superseding fetoscopy for many of the remaining indications for fetal blood sampling.

Chorionic villus biopsy. This technique has received considerable recent attention because it is carried out much earlier in pregnancy than amniocentesis (9–11 weeks versus 16–18 weeks). Villus tissue is amenable to direct analysis without the need for culture. Thus termination of pregnancy, when required, can be carried out in the first trimester which has a much lower mortality and morbidity, and is emotionally less distressing.

The tissue obtained by this technique may be used for chromosome analysis, enzyme assay and gene probe technology. All these techniques may be carried out on direct preparations or on cultured chorionic villus cells.

Until recently, all chorionic villus sampling was carried out by a transcervical route. Over 10 000 cases have now been reported to a central registry in Philadelphia and the procedure seems to cause abortion in about 2–3% of cases. Furthermore, there is a slight risk of maternal septicaemia. These considerations have led to the recent development of a transabdominal ultrasound-directed technique.

Laboratory procedures

These are carried out on fetal tissue obtained from one of the above methods and consist of:

1. Chromosomal analysis
2. Enzyme analysis
3. Haematological tests
4. Recombinant DNA technology.

Chromosomal analysis. A large number of chromosomal anomalies are described, but much the most important of these are the aneuploidies (abnormalities in chromosome number).

Polyploidy. Duplication of the entire chromosome set usually leads to abortion in the first trimester. Those few fetuses which survive will die soon after birth with multiple congenital abnormalities. The most important abnormalities of chromosome number are the trisomies and monosomies, involving an extra or deficient chromosome respectively. Only five trisomies, of which chromosomes 21, 18 and 13 are the most important, and one monosomy, XO (Turner's syndrome), survive to term. The most common of these at birth is trisomy 21 (Down's syndrome). The incidence of trisomies increases with advancing maternal age; paternal age has been excluded as a predisposing factor. Down's syndrome has an overall birth incidence of 1 : 1000. The incidence at amniocentesis rises from 1 : 300 at the age of 35, to 1 : 100 at 40 and 1 : 20 at the age of 45. Thereafter, the incidence declines; older mothers abort abnormal embryos more successfully, especially after the age of 45. The incidence of Turner's syndrome does not show the increasing trend noted for trisomies with maternal age. The single X chromosome found in this condition is contributed by the mother and the non-disjunction, therefore, takes place in the father. The incidence of Turner's syndrome declines slightly with advancing maternal age, again reflecting the enhanced ability of the older mother to abort abnormal embryos.

The other important risk factor for trisomies is a previously affected child. In this situation, the overall recurrence risk is 1.5%. If the previous baby had Down's syndrome, more than half the recurrences will also be of chromosome 21. Low serum alpha-fetoprotein measurements are also associated with an increased incidence of Down's syndrome and it is possible that, in future, the combination of this result and maternal age will be used to define a high-risk population.

Implications of the above findings are that mothers with a previous history of trisomy or mothers over a certain age should be offered prenatal diagnosis. The age at which this offer should be made routinely depends on individual perception of the relative risk of procedure-related abortion and an affected child. Thus, if the birth of a Down's syndrome child is regarded as being as unacceptable as fetal loss in the middle of pregnancy, then the age at which amniocentesis should be offered routinely is 40. If a Down's syndrome baby is regarded as being three times more traumatic than an abortion, then amniocentesis should be offered to all patients at the age of 35 and above (these figures are based on the widely quoted 1% procedure-related abortion rate of amniocentesis). In most developed countries, it is customary to offer the procedure to mothers over this age. For some women, or couples, however, the possibility of a Down's syndrome child is ten or more times worse than that of a late abortion. Such patients will frequently request amniocentesis irrespective of their age and place a considerable extra load on existing resources.

About 97% of cases of Down's syndrome and the other trisomies arise from non-disjunction during the meiotic division of the oocyte. A small number, however, result from a balanced translocation in a parent. The risk of recurrence in these cases is high, affecting a third of established pregnancies and around 10% of infants. The latter discrepancy is caused by frequent abortion of affected embryos. Patients who are known to carry such translocations usually ask for prenatal diagnosis.

Abnormalities of the sex chromosomes sometimes appear as an unexpected finding after genetic amniocentesis. Turner's syndrome (XO) produces severe phenotypic abnormalities and sterility, but no mental retardation, while the Triple X syndrome produces mental retardation in a phenotypically normal female. Another abnormality of the sex chromosomes associated with impaired brain development is the Fragile X syndrome. In this condition, the X chromosome is abnormally prone to breakage when culture is carried out in the presence of an antimetabolite. This syndrome is inherited as a sex-linked recessive and is the most common congenital cause of male mental retardation after Down's syndrome.

Trisomies and monosomies can be diagnosed on both cultured cells and on direct chorionic villus preparations. The detection of more subtle anomalies of chromosomes such as inversion and small deletions requires detailed banding and these are best obtained from cultured cells.

Enzyme defects. Many of the inborn errors of metabolism can be diagnosed by incubation of fetal tissue with a specific substrate. In addition, a small number of conditions may be diagnosed by the measurement of an accumulating metabolite in amniotic fluid supernate. This type of diagnosis is applicable in two circumstances: parents who have already had an affected child or those known to be carriers of conditions such as Tay Sachs on the basis of population screening.

An exciting recent discovery is that altered levels of intestinal alkaline phosphatase in amniotic fluid after 18 weeks' gestation provide reasonable diagnostic discrimination where parents are known carriers of cystic fibrosis. A negative test result reduces the chance that the fetus is affected from the 1 in 4 genetic risk for an autosomal recessive condition to 1 in 60. This is an important development because cystic fibrosis is the most common single gene defect in Caucasians; with an incidence of more than 1 : 2000 the gene frequency is 1 in 22. Nevertheless, this will probably be surplanted by even more accurate gene-probe diagnosis in the future (*see below*).

Haematological tests on fetal blood. Haemophilia A and Christmas disease may be diagnosed by assay for factors VIII and IX respectively. These are present in much lower quantities than in adult plasma, but are nevertheless detectable.

Fortunately 10% of fetal haemoglobin at 20 weeks' gestation is haemoglobin A, and beta thalassaemia may, therefore, be diagnosed by specific assay for the beta globin chains. Again, these techniques are being replaced by gene-probe technology.

Use of recombinant DNA technology. Recombinant DNA (deoxyribonucleic acid) technology is providing a valuable tool to detect defects at a molecular level in genes. While genes are normally expressed in the appropriate tissue, they are also present in all other cells of the body, even though they are not expressed. For example, while a globin gene is only expressed in fetal haemopoietic tissue and is thereby inaccessible, its presence and structure can be detected in other cells such as skin fibroblasts, which are readily obtained and cultured. Fluorescent activated cell sorting (FACS) is a technique which uses the fact that DNA has an affinity for a fluorescent dye, ethidium bromide. Chromosomal size is reflected in the amount of fluorescence present. The labelled chromosomes can then be sorted using laser beams so that a flow type with peaks of fluorescence for each chromosome can be obtained and then separated from each other. A chromosome specific library can then be built up.

Having separated chromosomes, gene mapping must take place. Each chromosome has a specific binding pattern demonstrated by special stains such as Giemsa. Each arm of the chromosome is divided into regions and each region into bands. A typical example is shown in Fig. 7.12. The site of a gene will be so localised.

Techniques for isolating genes or sequences of nucleotide bases include the Southern and Western blotting techniques and the use of gene probes. The principles of blotting techniques are as follows:

Restriction endonucleases are a range of enzymes produced largely from bacteria, which act on DNA at sequence specific sites to break it, usually into segments of four to six sequences in length. Appropriate restriction endonuclease acts on extracted DNA and the resultant fragments separated by electrophoresis on agarose gel. The DNA so isolated is denatured by placing the gel in sodium chloride/sodium hydroxide mixture, rinsed and then neutralised. A filter of nitrocellulose is placed on top of the gel, which binds the denatured DNA fragments to it as the buffer containing these fragments is drawn through the gel. The filter can be fixed and DNA hybridised subsequently with a P^{32} recombinant cDNA probe at a later date. Autoradiography

will demonstrate the specific site on the gel of the DNA in question.

Gene probes may be synthesised from constituent nucleotides if these are already known. An alternative is to make a recombinant DNA (cDNA) probe from messenger RNA (mRNA) using the enzyme reverse transcriptase. The basis of this technique is to isolate the appropriate mRNA, expose this to reverse transcriptase and thereby produce a single stranded DNA copy. Alkali destroys the mRNA part of the mRNA-DNA hybrid leaving the cDNA strand intact. P^{32} is then incorporated into the DNA using a process whereby DNA-ase enzyme produces small nicks along the DNA strand. Deoxynucleotide triphosphates labelled with P^{32} are incorporated into the DNA molecule at these nicks by means of the action of DNA polymerase.

The effectiveness of the DNA probe depends to a large extent on the purity of the protein and mRNA concerned. If there are a number of mRNAs involved, then the specificity of the gene probe generated from these will be correspondingly reduced. If the gene is copied frequently within the

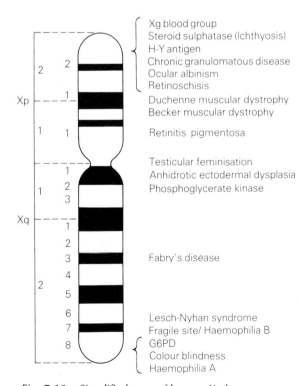

Fig. 7.12   *Simplified map of human X chromosome.*

cell (polymorphism), this process of amplification may be accompanied by mutations. Again, the specificity of the DNA in question will be diminished in these copied and mutated sequences, making the gene probe less effective.

About 15 or 20 mg of chorionic tissue is required to extract sufficient DNA (approximately 20 µg) to perform gene probe diagnosis.

Gene probe methodology has been most widely used for the diagnosis of haemoglobinopathies. However, gene probes are available for a number of other conditions such as Duchenne muscular dystrophy, Haemophilia A, Christmas disease, Huntington's chorea, ornithine carbamyl transferase deficiency and many others. The first and easiest type of gene probe analysis occurs when the gene is completely deleted (as in alpha thalassaemia) or the aberrant mutation removes a cutting site for the endonuclease (sickle cell anaemia). For most conditions, however, this kind of diagnosis is not possible and linkage studies to the presence or absence of various endonuclease cutting sites (restriction fragment length polymorphisms) in the DNA between genes are required. In order to conduct this kind of analysis, more detailed family studies are required including, in most cases, analysis of DNA from an affected family member or many known carriers. This is the case in many forms of beta thalassaemia.

FURTHER READING

Emery A.E.G. (1984). *An Introduction to Recombinant DNA*. Chichester: John Wiley.

Golbus M.S., Pollycove R. (1984). Diagnosis of congenital disorders. In *Maternal-Fetal Medicine*. Creasy R.K., Resnik R., eds., pp. 93–114. Philadelphia: Saunders.

8

Medical Disorders and Pregnancy

The principle of management of pregnant women with medical disorders is to achieve the most effective control of the medical disorder, and then to deal with subsequent problems along standard obstetrical lines. The principle is best applied if the patient is seen before she conceives. This enables review of the medical disorder, readjustment of treatment, appraisal of risks, and achievement of the understanding and cooperation of the patient. She can then start her pregnancy with the best possible prognosis. In order that preconception review can become routine in patients with medical disorders, it is still necessary to convince physicians that almost any woman between 12 and 48 years of age may become pregnant, regardless of her apparent circumstances.

HYPERTENSION IN PREGNANCY

Arterial blood pressure is a continuously distributed variable in the general population. The difference between normal blood pressure and hypertension is an arbitrary level. It is generally accepted that a blood pressure above 140/90 mmHg is abnormal in women of reproductive age.

Measurement of blood pressure

When taking blood pressure in a pregnant woman, the patient's position should be consistent. Semi-prone with lateral tilt is best, but the sitting position is convenient. The first phase of the Korotkoff sounds defines the systolic pressure. In pregnancy, the diastolic pressure is best recorded when the Korotkoff sound becomes muffled (fourth phase), and errors then tend to cause an overestimation.

Hypertension Occurring Before Pregnancy

Hypertension can be classified into primary or essential hypertension where there is no apparent precipitating factor, and secondary hypertension, which is much less common, and where there is some identifiable cause. Malignant hypertension occurs in a minority of patients with essential hypertension and is characterised by the rapid development of severe hypertension and the presence of papilloedema.

Essential hypertension tends to occur in older parous and obese women, often with a family history of hypertension. The blood pressure is usually raised in the first half of pregnancy, but may be masked by the physiological decline in the blood pressure during the middle trimester. Patients with intermittent hypertension in early pregnancy have an approximately fivefold increased risk of developing significant hypertension in the third trimester.

Causes of secondary hypertension are:

1. Renal disorders, whether ischaemic, infective, congenital or an infiltration such as amyloid;
2. Endocrine disorders such as thyrotoxicosis, Cushing's syndrome, Conn's syndrome or phaeochromocytoma;
3. Congenital heart disease such as coarctation of the aorta or aortic regurgitation;
4. Collagen disorders such as systemic lupus erythematosus.

The approach to secondary hypertension is to obtain the best therapeutic control possible of the underlying condition, and then to treat any residual hypertension.

Diagnosis of hypertension antedating pregnancy

If the blood pressure is 140/90 mmHg or higher in the first 24 weeks of pregnancy, chronic hypertension can be inferred, and this is most likely to be due to essential hypertension, although the possibility of secondary hypertension must be borne in mind. In the latter half of pregnancy, diagnosis can be a problem because pre-eclamptic symptoms may superimpose on pre-existing hypertension.

Physical signs. The displacement of the apex beat to the left and its prominence may indicate left ventricular hypertrophy, suggesting long-standing hypertension. Renal enlargement such as occurs in polycystic disease, or a renal systolic bruit, as in renal artery stenosis, suggests hypertension secondary to renal causes. Examination of the optic fundi may show arteriolar tortuosity, silver wiring and arteriovenous nipping in long-standing hypertension. In most women who develop pre-eclampsia, there is no abnormality in the optic fundi. Palpation of femoral arteries may reveal a diminished or absent pulse in coarctation of the aorta.

Investigations. In pregnancy, levels of plasma urea above 5 mmol/l and plasma creatinine above 100 μmol/l suggest an underlying renal problem.

Measurement of creatinine clearance will establish any degree of renal failure.

Platelet counts tend to fall to 100 000/mm^3 (100 × 10^9/l) or less with severe hypertension associated with placental insufficiency and intrauterine growth retardation. Occasionally, severe exacerbations are associated with coagulopathy and should be investigated appropriately.

In essential hypertension, plasma uric acid is usually below 0.35 mmol/l. It rises in pre-eclampsia. In the absence of urinary tract infection (bacterial count of >10^5/mm^3), proteinuria of 0.5 g/l or more in a 24 h urine collection is significant. Progressive rise of proteinuria to more than 4–5 g/day suggests severe pre-eclampsia and may indicate serious renal impairment.

Urinary vanillyl-mandelic acid is raised in phaeochromocytoma. This condition is rare, but can have fatal consequences to mother and baby. It should be remembered that in pregnancy phaeochromocytoma presents more commonly with sustained than with unstable hypertension, and the most common misdiagnoses are diabetes mellitus and Cushing's syndrome.

Management of chronic hypertension

Patients who are on antihypertensive treatment should be encouraged to seek advice before becoming pregnant. Commonly used antihypertensive agents are not teratogenic, but revision of an antihypertensive regimen may be appropriate. Theoretically, the usual combination of a β-blocking drug and a diuretic is not ideal for pregnancy, as both components would be expected to impair utero-placental blood flow. On the other hand, a patient whose blood pressure is well controlled by a modest dose of a β-blocker alone may be expected to do well if the drug is continued in pregnancy. It is the sudden introduction of large doses of these drugs during pregnancy to control severe hypertension, which has been associated with fetal loss. Methyldopa is well established as an extremely safe basic drug for treatment of hypertension in pregnancy, and transfer to this agent should be considered, particularly in women who have had a perinatal loss on the other agents. Side effects of postural hypertension or depression are uncommon in pregnancy. The safety for the fetus of the newer antihypertensive drugs, captopril, nifedipine or clonidine, has not been established. Reserpine and ganglion-blockers convey a risk to the fetus; the maternal side-effects of the increased doses of hydralazine, which may be needed, often render this agent unsuitable for long-term use in pregnancy.

Close control of hypertension is best instituted with well divided doses. Should it not be possible to secure overnight control with methyldopa alone, a β-blocker such as atenolol, the safety of which in pregnancy is reasonably established, may be added.

Rest, the elimination of obesity and controlled weight gain in pregnancy are of value in managing chronic hypertension in pregnancy. Finally, low dose aspirin (75 mg/day) treatment during pregnancy should be considered for patients with a history of intrauterine growth retardation.

Patients who present during the first 20 weeks of pregnancy with a blood pressure of more than 150/90 mmHg need admission for observation and investigation. If the blood pressure settles to completely normal, management without antihypertensive drugs is reasonable until such time as the blood pressure rises again. Some obstetricians feel that these patients should be treated from the start, even though doses required in the middle trimester may be small, to protect the placental bed circulation from irreversible structural damage. Other obstetricians prefer to wait until the need for treatment becomes obvious.

The object of treatment is to control hypertension, thereby protecting the mother against cerebral haemorrhage, kidney damage, eclampsia and placental abruption as well as maintaining uteroplacental circulation to prevent placental infarction. In general, achievement of a maternal blood pressure consistently at or below 140/90 mmHg is good.

Control to levels below 120/80 may impair uteroplacental perfusion.

Oral antihypertensive agents

Methyldopa. The metabolite α-methylnoradrenaline acts by decreasing sympathetic outflow from the central nervous system, with a reduction in arteriolar resistance, but with little or no effect on heart rate or cardiac output. Initially, an oral dose of 250 mg twice or three times daily is given and adjusted at intervals of not less than two days. If 2 g/day proves inadequate to control hypertension, the addition of small doses of a β-blocker or oral hydralazine should be considered.

β-Adrenergic blocking agents. Propranolol was the first of these to be used in pregnancy and was held responsible for fetal bradycardia, neonatal hypoglycaemia and perinatal losses. In fact, modest doses are reasonably safe and in severe hypertension the fetus is at risk anyway. The risks may have been increased by attempts to secure rapid control of acute situations with propranolol. In general, β-blockers take two or more days of consistent administration before their effects are stabilised.

Both atenolol (50–100 mg daily) and oxprenolol (40–120 mg twice daily) have been used with safety in pregnancy, either alone or in combination with methyldopa.

Labetalol (100–400 mg twice daily) is said to act by peripheral vasodilation without change in cardiac output or uteroplacental blood flow. It has been used without harm in cases of mild hypertension in pregnancy. When it is used intravenously in acute situations to control severe hypertension, some patients do not respond to the first dose, and some to a subsequent administration.

Prazosin is primarily an α-blocker but, in severe hypertension in pregnancy, addition of other drugs is nearly always necessary. The dose is 0.5 mg thrice daily, increased at weekly intervals up to a maximum of 20 mg/day. It may be of value in treating primarily systolic hypertension coming on early in pregnancy.

Hydralazine is a vasodilator and reduces blood pressure by decreasing peripheral resistance. It tends to improve renal, uteroplacental and cerebral blood flow. Oral hydralazine combined with

another antihypertensive drug is particularly useful in controlling blood pressure. The dose is 25–50 mg by mouth every 6 h. Its use is safe in pregnancy, although prolonged use may cause skin rashes and headaches. The parenteral dose is considerably lower (10–15 mg i.m.).

Adrenergic neurone blockers. Bethanidine, guanethidine and debrisoquine are not commonly used, as their effects in pregnancy are not well understood. They convey a risk of impairing autonomic responses which may be needed in emergency obstetric situations.

Diuretics are not recommended as components of antihypertensive regimens in pregnancy except in emergency situations, such as heart failure.

HEART DISEASE IN PREGNANCY

Pregnancy imposes an extra haemodynamic burden on the cardiovascular system. Although the incidence of organic heart disease in pregnancy is less than 1%, symptoms of breathlessness and haemodynamic murmurs may occur in a majority of women with normal hearts.

Preconception counselling is of importance. Cardiac status can be fully assessed, risks discussed with the patient and future cooperation secured. Anaemia can be corrected and drug treatment modified. Cardiac surgery can make the difference between a risk to the mother's life and an uncomplicated pregnancy; with severe aortic valve lesions, operation may permit a successful pregnancy.

Physiological changes in pregnancy

Plasma volume increases throughout pregnancy and, by term, it is 40–50% above that in the non-pregnant state. Cardiac output is increased by about 40% by the end of the second trimester, and during the last trimester it may remain the same or increase slightly. In the first half of pregnancy, increase in cardiac output is achieved by an increase in stroke volume, while in the last trimester it is due to an increase in heart rate with a slight fall in stroke volume.

With the onset of labour, cardiac output increases further by 10–20%, especially in the lateral position, and reaches a peak immediately after delivery with values as high as 80% greater than before labour began. This peak increase is reduced by caudal and spinal anaesthesia, and to a greater extent by epidural anaesthesia.

Incidence of heart disease in pregnancy

There has been a steady decline in the incidence of rheumatic disease and an apparent increase in the incidence of congenital heart disease in pregnancy. The most important rheumatic lesion is mitral stenosis, accounting for 90% of cases with mitral regurgitation and aortic regurgitation; aortic stenosis accounts for the rest. The common lesions with congenital heart disease are atrial septal defect, patent ductus arteriosus, ventricular septal defect, pulmonary stenosis, aortic stenosis, Fallot's tetralogy, and coarctation of the aorta.

Maternal mortality is highest in conditions where there is pulmonary hypertension, such as Eisenmenger's syndrome. Maternal mortality is low in rheumatic heart disease. Perinatal mortality in patients with rheumatic heart disease in pregnancy is comparable to that in normal patients, although babies tend to be lighter. With cyanotic congenital heart disease, babies are usually growth retarded, and perinatal mortality may be as high as 40–50%.

Diagnosis during pregnancy

Some cases of heart disease are not diagnosed until the patient has become pregnant. Some symptoms and signs of normal pregnancy may mimic heart disease. Complaints of breathlessness, palpitations, syncope and ankle swelling are all consistent with a normal heart in pregnancy; chest pain and haemoptysis suggest heart disease. Again, increased pulse volume, forceful apex beat, ectopic beats, a systolic ejection murmur, an internal mammary murmur at the second left intercostal space and peripheral oedema may be simple consequences of pregnancy; an apex beat more than 2 cm lateral to the midclavicular line, a raised jugular venous pressure, a diastolic, pansystolic or late systolic murmur, ejection clicks, and signs such as cyanosis, finger clubbing or splinter haemorrhages, all suggest heart disease.

Investigations

Chest x-ray. Significant cardiac enlargement may

be detected, although this investigation is unhelpful in the diagnosis of minor degrees of heart disease.

Electrocardiography is more helpful in diagnosis of arrhythmias than in demonstration of an anatomical abnormality.

Echocardiography. The majority of structural cardiac abnormalities may be demonstrated and this is becoming the investigation of choice.

Antenatal care

At each visit, pregnant cardiac patients should be seen if possible by both an obstetrician and a cardiologist so that the nature and severity of their heart disease can be assessed. Assessments include a decision as to whether the pregnancy should continue and if there is a need for cardiac surgery.

Congenital mitral valve prolapse is now recognised as benign in pregnancy. There are no haemodynamic problems and outcome is good. At the other extreme, primary pulmonary hypertension and Eisenmenger's syndrome (p. 101) are definite indications for early termination of pregnancy as there is a maternal mortality rate of about 30%; the abortion itself conveys a marked risk to life. The indication for closed mitral valve surgery is usually deteriorating pulmonary oedema not responding to medical treatment. The patients do well during pregnancy unless a life threatening situation arises, for example with an aortic valve defect. It is difficult to establish and maintain a by-pass circulation adequate to sustain the fetus, which usually succumbs, unless caesarean section precedes the heart surgery.

The aim of antenatal care is to reduce the risk of heart failure.

1. Obesity and excessive weight gain during pregnancy should be avoided.
2. Dental treatment with antibiotic cover should be advised early in pregnancy to prevent any dental sepsis and reduce the risk of subacute bacterial endocarditis.
3. Anaemia should be prevented with iron and folic acid supplements.
4. Upper respiratory tract infections may be an indication for hospital admission. At each visit, the patients should be examined to detect arrhythmias and raised jugular venous pres-

sure and for evidence of pulmonary oedema at the lung bases.

5. Over-exertion and stress should be avoided.

Hospital admission for bed rest

Between the 28th and 32nd week of pregnancy the load on the heart has usually reached its height, and any patient with deterioration will benefit from hospital rest for the remainder of the pregnancy. The mistake is to consider that the strain on the heart diminishes after 32 weeks; the risk of failure remains or increases throughout the third trimester. The development of pre-eclampsia indicates urgent hospital admission and control of hypertension, not only because of the increased burden on the heart, but also because of fluid retention.

All patients with signs of heart failure must be treated in hospital.

Treatment of Heart Failure in Pregnancy

The principles of management are similar to those of heart failure developing at any other time.

Increase the oxygen supply. Supplemental oxygen may be given by face mask or nasal cannula. Anaemia may be corrected by iron supplements. If the haematocrit is less than 30%, transfusion of packed red blood cells may be given after initiating a diuresis with a modest dose of frusemide.

Decrease peripheral circulatory demand. Bed rest is important, especially after meals. Any infection must be treated and fever must be suppressed as pyrexia increases cardiac workload. Drugs and food additives which increase cardiac output, such as sympathomimetics like ritodrine, terbutaline, salbutamol, and theophylline compounds and caffeine should be avoided as should psychological stress and anxiety.

Augmentation of myocardial contractility. Digoxin is used to control the heart rate in atrial fibrillation and to increase the force of myocardial contraction. Digoxin crosses the placenta, but there is no associated fetal toxicity or reported teratogenicity. Myocardial depressants such as alcohol, or large doses of β-sympatholytics should be avoided.

Reduction of intravascular volume. Treatment is with diuretics such as oral thiazides or frusemide. Hypokalaemia should be avoided. Excess salt intake should be restricted and intravenous overload avoided.

Decrease in left ventricular afterload is achieved by controlling hypertension. Methyldopa is the best drug available, but moderate doses of β-blockers are acceptable.

Anticoagulation

Treatment with anticoagulants is necessary in patients with atrial fibrillation or pulmonary hypertension from congenital heart disease. In the acute situation, intravenous heparin may be necessary but, subsequently, subcutaneous heparin is adequate. There is a small risk of alopecia and of demineralisation of bone with prolonged heparin treatment and x-ray bone density in a hand, and serum calcium and phosphate, should be checked each month or two after 3 months. Patients with artificial plastic heart valves must be fully anticoagulated. There are small risks of abortion with heparin in the first trimester, of warfarin embryopathy at 6–9 weeks after conception, and of warfarin fetal central nervous system damage in the second and third trimesters. Heparin may be used during the first trimester to avoid possible teratogenicity. The best regimen for anticoagulation is then an oral anticoagulant throughout most of pregnancy, with a change to heparin for the last 2–3 weeks. Oral anticoagulants cross the placenta and so there are risks of fetal haemorrhage during labour. Heparin is safe as the large molecule does not cross the placenta.

Management in Labour

The patient who has no obstetric complication is best allowed to go into spontaneous labour. Nevertheless, induction should not be withheld if there is an obstetric indication.

During labour a sitting or semireclining position is most comfortable. Aortocaval compression should be avoided. Respiratory support, frusemide, digoxin and aminophylline should be readily available.

Dyspnoea may be avoided by administration of

oxygen and, if analgesia is required in the second stage, nitrous oxide and oxygen can be used. Breathlessness may be due to anxiety and the discomfort of labour, so effective analgesia must be provided, either with narcotic analgesics or with epidural anaesthesia, provided hypotension is avoided and there is neither a cardiac outflow obstructive lesion nor anticoagulation. Strict fluid balance is very important, as patients with heart disease cannot cope with an increase in intravascular volume and easily develop pulmonary oedema.

It is wise to keep the second stage of labour short to reduce maternal effort. If the patient is likely to deliver herself, an episiotomy may reduce the effort in delivery. If forceps are to be applied, it is better to wait for the fetal head to descend to the pelvic floor provided that the patient is not seriously distressed.

There has been debate as to the use of oxytocic drugs in the third stage of labour, but a postpartum haemorrhage is a disaster. Oxytocin is generally safer than ergometrine and is the drug of choice. In patients with heart failure, an oxytocin infusion may be given with intravenous frusemide.

There should be no reluctance to deliver cardiac patients by caesarean section for the usual obstetric indications.

Antibiotic prophylaxis

The basis of antibiotic cover in labour is to prevent the development of subacute bacterial endocarditis. Women with valvular disease, particularly those with artificial heart valves and those with septal defects, should be given antibiotic prophylaxis. Amoxycillin 500 mg and gentamicin 80 mg i.m., 8 hourly, is a suitable regimen.

Management of the puerperium

The first 12 hours after delivery are the most critical, as venous return is increased. Signs of pulmonary congestion and oedema must be carefully sought. If oral anticoagulants have been used antenatally, these should be recommended; warfarin is not contraindicated with breast feeding, but phenindione does pass into breast milk. If there are no signs of heart failure, the patient is not restricted to bed and graduated activity is allowed before she returns home. Domestic assistance may be required when the patient is at home.

Specific Heart Conditions in Pregnancy

Mitral stenosis

Pregnant women with mitral stenosis are particularly prone to develop pulmonary oedema but, with good conservative management, mitral valvotomy is only rarely needed in pregnancy. Patients considered for closed valvotomy should have no significant mitral regurgitation in conjunction with mitral stenosis. The mitral valve should not be calcified and there should be no other significant valve involvement. Echocardiography is valuable to discover the severity of the lesion and assess the state of the valve cusps.

Artificial heart valves

Patients who have had a successful isolated mitral or aortic valve replacement do not usually have haemodynamic problems in pregnancy. Patients with biological heart valves usually do not require anticoagulation.

Cyanotic heart disease

The incidence of premature delivery and intrauterine death is increased because of the development of severe placental insufficiency. When ultrasound measurements show that the fetus has failed to grow, there should be no hesitation about delivering the baby, if necessary by caesarean section, especially after 34 weeks.

Eisenmenger's syndrome is a severe form of cyanotic heart disease. It consists of pulmonary hypertension with a raised pulmonary vascular resistance together with a congenital cardiovascular lesion that allows shunting from the right to the left side of the heart. Pregnancy should be avoided in this condition and early termination of pregnancy is recommended if it does occur. The risk is high in the puerperium and in those with pre-eclampsia. Fetal loss has been quoted as high as 80%.

VENOUS THROMBOEMBOLISM AND PREGNANCY

Deep vein thrombosis is a relatively common complication of pregnancy and the puerperium. It is important because it predisposes to pulmonary embolism which is an important cause of maternal mortality. Pregnancy increases the risk of thromboembolism by five to six times compared to non-pregnant women who are not on oral contraceptives. The incidence of deep vein thrombosis is about 0.5% and that of pulmonary embolism about 0.3% of all pregnancies.

Aetiology

Clotting factors. In pregnancy there are increases in clotting factors VII, VIII and X, together with an increased fibrinogen level and decreased fibrinolytic activity. This can be presumed to occur in preparation for haemostatic efficiency at the time of delivery. There is thus an increased tendency to thrombosis.

Venous stasis. The pregnant uterus compresses the inferior vena cava and reduces venous return from the legs. There is also a reduced venous tone. Restriction of activity and prolonged bed rest promote venous stasis.

Operative procedures. The incidence of fatal pulmonary embolism is about ten times greater after caesarean section than after vaginal delivery. Difficult forceps deliveries and prolonged labour also increase the risk of thromboembolism. Surgical procedures during pregnancy and tubal ligation in the puerperium cause an increased risk of thromboembolism.

Age and parity. The risk of fatal pulmonary embolism is greater with a fourth or subsequent parity and in women over 30 years of age.

Obesity. Excessively obese women are especially at risk.

Other factors. There is an association with the use of oestrogen to suppress lactation and thromboembolism. Women with blood group O are less likely to develop thromboembolic disease in pregnancy; women with sickle cell anaemia are at risk of developing pulmonary embolism. Women who are severely anaemic in the puerperium are thought to be at increased risk of thrombosis.

Diagnosis of Pulmonary Embolism

In the first place the diagnosis of pulmonary embolism is clinical. A major embolism presents with a sudden onset of chest pain, usually pleural in character, dyspnoea, cough, hypotension, cyanosis and collapse. There may be haemoptysis, a parasternal heave, a raised jugular venous pressure and a third heart sound. Blood P_{O_2} is usually reduced and P_{CO_2} is sometimes low. In many cases, pain may be absent or minimal and the main symptom is dyspnoea. Pulmonary embolism should be considered in all cases of unexplained dyspnoea in pregnancy. The most important differential diagnoses are myocardial infarction, pulmonary atelectasis, aspiration, or viral or bacterial pneumonia. To this extent an e.c.g. and a chest x-ray may be of some value. Definitive diagnosis of pulmonary embolism is made by ventilation perfusion isotope scanning. In late pregnancy or in relation to a confinement, the additional important differential diagnosis is amniotic fluid infusion, which is nearly always related to a clinical event such as rupture of the membranes, abruptio placentae, violent uterine contractions, rupture of the uterus, or delivery, and the most prominent clinical sign is dyspnoea. The other important early diagnostic features of a major amniotic fluid embolism are a normal chest x-ray soon after the initial episode, diffuse floccular shadows all over the lung fields 2–4 h later and a prompt response to intravenous heparin (given in the absence of acute bleeding). Subsequently, the consequences of a consumption coagulopathy will make the diagnosis clear.

Diagnosis of Deep Vein Thrombosis

Symptoms and signs are calf pain and tenderness, with a positive Homan's sign; unilateral oedema, a difference of 2 cm or more between identical sites on the legs is significant; increase in warmth of the leg.

Many patients who have an acutely tender swollen calf do not necessarily have deep vein thrombosis. Thus an objective technique should be used whenever diagnosis is in doubt.

Objective tests

Tests that are safe in pregnancy and reasonably effective are:

1. *Doppler ultrasound* examination of flow in the femoral vein. The sound of blood flow may be absent if the vein is completely obstructed, or altered compared with the opposite side if there is a partial obstruction.
2. *Isotope venography.* Albumin macroaggregates labelled with technetium ($^{99}Tc^m$) concentrate around the thrombus to form a 'hot spot'. An accuracy of 85–98% may be obtained.
3. *Limb impedance plethysmography* is accurate in only about 50% of cases.

Treatment of Pulmonary Embolism

Management of massive pulmonary embolism includes routine cardiac arrest procedures, 10 000–20 000 units of heparin as an intravenous bolus, with continued cardiac massage followed by full intensive care. Pulmonary embolectomy or streptokinase may be indicated if severe hypotension persists and pulmonary peripheral perfusion is reduced by 75%.

Early phase of management

Heparin is effective in arresting active thrombosis and does not cross the placenta. It is best given as a continuous infusion of 40 000 units of heparin in saline per day. Intravenous heparin should be given initially for 48 h, but may be continued for 7 days in severe cases. Bleeding is the most important complication, and stopping a heparin infusion for a few hours will usually allow haemostasis to recover. In urgent situations, protamine sulphate will rapidly reverse the action of heparin.

Thrombolytic drugs, like streptokinase and urokinase, are rarely used in pregnancy due to the hazards of bleeding from the placental site.

Thrombectomy may be indicated in major iliofemoral deep vein thrombosis.

Later management

Coumarin derivatives such as warfarin are the most commonly used oral anticoagulants in pregnancy. They are competitive inhibitors of vitamin K. Warfarin is ideal for chronic treatment in the non-pregnant patient but, as it crosses the placenta, it can cause fetal abnormalities in the second half of the first trimester and, occasionally, central nervous system abnormalities in the fetus if given in the second or third trimester. The main abnormalities are saddle nose, nasal hypoplasia, frontal bossing and short stature with stippled epiphyses. Intracerebral bleeding in the fetus, especially if premature, many occur causing mental retardation and blindness. For these reasons, it has been recommended that, if there is a real need to continue full anticoagulation after the initial treatment with heparin, although there is some risk of abortion, this drug should be continued for the first trimester and, if necessary, followed by warfarin between 13 and 36 weeks of pregnancy, reverting to heparin in the last few weeks of pregnancy.

Long-term treatment with subcutaneous, self-administered heparin is the method of choice in pregnancy. Between 5000 and 10 000 units of heparin 12-hourly given in 0.2–0.4 ml into the lateral aspect of the subcutaneous abdominal wall fat is usually adequate. Ideally, heparin levels should be checked frequently; peak levels should not exceed 0.4 iu/ml. After delivery, treatment with subcutaneous heparin or warfarin should be continued for 5–6 weeks. Demineralisation of bone or alopecia may result from long-term heparin therapy.

If thromboembolism occurs in the puerperium, anticoagulant treatment should be continued for a total of 6 weeks.

Prophylaxis for Venous Thromboembolism

When a woman has had thromboembolism in the previous pregnancy, she will be at increased risk during the present pregnancy and in the puerperium, though the risk of recurrence is now recognised as small. Prophylactic measures are:

1. Elastic stockings worn regularly;
2. Calf muscle exercises;
3. Anticoagulants — heparin subcutaneously.

Prophylaxis may be given for 6 weeks after delivery.

Superficial Vein Thrombosis, Thrombophlebitis

A superficial vein cannulated for transfusion or varicose veins in the leg are usually affected. There is pain and swelling along an inflamed and tender superficial vein. In such cases, the thrombus is firmly attached to the vein wall, so there is little risk of pulmonary embolism. In the calves, there is often an undetected deep extension of the thrombosis and a period of anticoagulation is wise.

Pelvic thrombophlebitis may occur following caesarean section, and treatment involves antibiotics and a short course of heparin.

HAEMATOLOGICAL DISORDERS

Physiological Changes in Pregnancy

The increases in plasma volume and red cell mass are described in Chapter 6.

As the expansion of plasma volume is greater than that of red cell mass, the red cell count, haematocrit and haemoglobin concentrations tend to fall during pregnancy. Nevertheless, total circulating haemoglobin is higher than before pregnancy.

Iron Deficiency Anaemia

In pregnancy, nutritional iron deficiency anaemia is the most common haematological problem. It is found in between 20 and 30% of pregnancies, being more common with lower social grade, multiparity, previous history of menorrhagia and in women whose nutrition is poor. Chronic infection, particularly urinary tract infection, is an important cause. The World Health Organization has suggested that, in pregnancy, the minimum acceptable haemoglobin concentration is 11.0 g/dl.

Iron metabolism

Iron is required mainly for the expanding red cell mass and for the fetus and placenta. The requirement for pregnancy is about 4 mg of iron per day. A normal daily diet contains 10–20 mg, but of this only 1–2 mg may be absorbed. Approximately 120 mg of iron is conserved by amenorrhoea, so an extra 800–1300 mg of iron are required during pregnancy.

Diagnosis

Iron deficiency is most often diagnosed from the results of a peripheral blood count. When iron stores are depleted, there is a reduction in serum iron; this is followed by a reduction in haemoglobin concentration (Table 8.1).

Marrow biopsy. Marrow aspiration is rarely indicated in pregnancy. If required, a sample obtained from the iliac crest or the sternum is reliable in assessing iron stores in pregnancy.

Prophylaxis and treatment

The World Health Organization recommends that supplements of 30–60 mg of elemental iron per day be given to pregnant women with normal iron stores, and 120–240 mg to women with low stores. Supplementation with a daily dose of 100 mg elemental iron from about 16 weeks of pregnancy until delivery will maintain the stores and prevent iron deficiency anaemia. Side-effects of oral administration of iron, such as nausea, epigastric pain, diarrhoea and constipation occur in about 20% of women. Most preparations used commonly in pregnancy now contain small amounts of folic acid.

The risks of folate deficiency occur (a) in women with an inadequate diet; (b) when absorption is defective, in malabsorption syndromes, patients taking anticonvulsant drugs and in the grand multipara; (c) when demand is increased, namely in the anaemic patient who is responding to iron treatment, patients with haemolytic anaemia, patients with malaria, in multiple pregnancy and in patients who have an antepartum haemorrhage.

Megaloblastic Anaemia

Megaloblastic anaemia should be suspected when the expected response to adequate iron treatment is not achieved. Sometimes, after an initial haemopoietic response to iron, no further increase in haemoglobin occurs until folic acid supplements are given.

Diagnosis

In megaloblastic anaemia, haemoglobin concentration is usually below 10.0 g/dl and films of the buffy coat layer show hypersegmented neutrophils, Howell-Jolly nuclear inclusion bodies, nucleated red cells, orthochromatic macrocytes and giant polymorphs. Early diagnosis can be made from marrow biopsy. Serum and red cell folate are decreased. It is important to exclude vitamin B_{12}

Table 8.1

Diagnosis for Iron Deficient Anaemia in Pregnancy

		Normal range	Iron deficiency
Red cell indices			
Mean Corpuscular Volume (MCV)	$= \dfrac{\text{Packed Cell Volume (PVC)}}{\text{Red Cell Count (RBC)}}$	75–99 fl	Decreased
Mean Corpuscular Haemoglobin (MCH)	$= \dfrac{\text{Haemoglobin concentration (Hb)}}{\text{Red Cell Count (RBC)}}$	27–31 pg	Decreased
Mean Corpuscular Haemoglobin Concentration (MCHC)	$= \dfrac{\text{Haemoglobin concentration (Hb)}}{\text{Packed Cell Volume (PVC)}}$	32–36 g/dl	Decreased
Biochemistry			
Serum iron		13–27 µmol/l	<9 µmol/l
Total iron binding capacity		45–72 µmol/l	>98.5 µmol/l
Ferritin		10–150 µg/l	<10 µg/l

deficiency in patients from the Indian subcontinent and in vegetarians.

In the puerperium, folate levels are often low, sometimes being depleted by the haemopoietic response to blood loss at delivery. Lactation increases the demand on folate while, on the other hand, the diminished folic acid absorption of pregnancy and the requirements of the fetus have been relieved. If megaloblastic anaemia has been undiagnosed and untreated in late pregnancy, it may persist and need management in the puerperium. Megaloblastic anaemia arising *de novo* in the puerperium is rare, and the response of puerperal anaemia to iron treatment alone is as good as if folic acid supplements were given as well.

Prophylaxis and treatment

For prophylaxis in pregnancy, folic acid 300–500 µg is given daily, usually in the form of iron-folic acid preparations. Prophylaxis is particularly important in multiple pregnancies, in patients with malabsorption syndromes, those taking anticonvulsants or sulphasalazine, during treatment with co-trimoxazole or antimalarial drugs, and in patients with haemolytic anaemia (who do not need iron). In all these groups, folic acid, 5 mg daily, is an appropriate dose.

For the treatment of folic acid deficiency, 5 mg orally, three times daily, should be prescribed.

Reticulocytosis usually occurs about 5 days after initiation of treatment.

In malabsorption states, i.m. injections of folic acid, 3 mg each week, may be needed and, by implication, should be accompanied with mixed parenteral B vitamins.

Vitamin B₁₂ deficiency

Vitamin B_{12} deficiency

Megaloblastic anaemia of pregnancy is rare and is due to inadequate diet, malabsorption syndrome and, rarely, true pernicious anaemia.

When macrocytic anaemia and low serum vitamin B_{12} levels are found, hydroxycobalamin should be given i.m., 1 mg every 2 months.

Haemolytic Anaemias

Red cell survival span is shortened either by an intrinsic red cell abnormality or by an extrinsic factor. Reticulocyte counts are usually increased. Iron treatment is only indicated if serum iron levels are low, and then it should be oral, as otherwise there is a risk of iron overload.

Intrinsic red cell defects

Hereditary spherocytosis and elliptocytosis. This condition is diagnosed by appearances of a blood film. Inheritance is dominant, hence the baby should be investigated when parents are affected. Treatment is usually with folic acid and, if necessary, by blood transfusion.

Haemoglobinopathies. These are inherited defects in haemoglobin resulting from impaired globin synthesis.

β-chain haemoglobin variants such as HbS and HbC are common in black Africans and white Mediterranean women. Clinical manifestations occur mainly in the homozygous patient. If the sickle cell test is positive, electrophoresis is performed. In homozygous sickle cell disease, the patients are particularly prone to infection; thrombotic episodes or bone crises may be precipitated by infection and dehydration. Fetal loss is increased in pregnant women with sickle cell disease, but not in the heterozygous form. Many cases do not need treatment other than folic acid and, if a patient has already had a successful pregnancy without haemolytic crises, it is a mistake to submit her to intensive treatment. In patients who do need treatment, repeated blood transfusions may be required to maintain HbA levels at 60–70%.

During labour, hypoxia, acidosis and hypotension must be avoided and prophylactic antibiotics should be given. It may be considered that the best way of achieving this is caesarean section under general anaesthesia, but this is unreasonable in a woman who has previously had a normal confinement without complications.

Thalassaemia. Homozygous α-thalassaemia is incompatible with life and the fetus becomes hydropic *in utero* or shortly after birth. Patients with homozygous β-thalassaemia (Cooley's anaemia) often die in childhood. If they do survive and conceive, pregnancy does not seem to affect the disease process adversely. Heterozygous thalassaemia patients are usually healthy apart from mild anaemia, and normal pregnancy is possible.

Antenatal diagnosis of the status of the fetus is important if both parents carry the trait. Fetal blood sampling can be performed by fetoscopy and legal abortion may be indicated. Methods of DNA analysis on chorion biopsies, which convey less risk than fetoscopy, are being developed.

In maternal thalassaemia in pregnancy, the red cells have a reduced haemoglobin content, and anaemia may be severe. There is a large decrease in MCV and MCH values, but the MCHC is within the normal range. In pregnancy, the haemoglobin

concentration should be maintained above 8 g/dl, and routine treatment is with folic acid, 5 mg orally, three times a day. Blood transfusion may be necessary. Iron supplementation is contraindicated unless there is iron deficiency.

Glucose-6-phosphate dehydrogenase deficiency has a sex-linked inheritance. Oxidation of haemoglobin leads to formation of methaemoglobin, and drugs like sulphonamides, salicylates, nitrofurantoin, nalidixic acid, antimalarials and vitamin K may precipitate a haemolytic crisis. If these drugs are being given to the mother in late pregnancy, transplacental passage may lead to haemolytic problems in the newborn.

Extrinsic haemolytic anaemias

Autoimmune haemolytic disease can be divided into warm antibody and cold antibody types. About 50% of patients with warm antibody haemolytic anaemia have demonstrable underlying disorders, such as systemic lupus erythematosus and lymphoma. The blood shows polychromasia with spherocytes and a reticulocytosis and Coombs' test is positive. Treatment is with corticosteroids. The cold antibody type is associated with infections, particularly with *Mycoplasma pneumoniae*. Red cells undergo autoagglutination at 4°C, which is dispersed at 37°C. The direct Coombs' test is positive. Treatment is not usually required. Many drugs can, rarely, cause haemolysis.

Coagulation Disorders

Idiopathic thrombocytopenic purpura

This autoimmune disorder tends to occur in women during the childbearing years. With careful management, prognosis for mother and baby is fairly good.

When patients are in remission at the onset of pregnancy, two-thirds of them will have uneventful pregnancies. A short course of steroids (prednisolone 10 mg/day) started a day or two before labour is anticipated and continued with parenteral hydrocortisone during the confinement may prevent neonatal thrombocytopenia. The latter condition is usually self-limiting over the first few weeks of life, if it does occur. Patients not in remission at the start of pregnancy, those having recurrences during pregnancy, and those where the disease develops during pregnancy need full doses of steroids (prednisolone 20–40 mg/day, increased to 60–100 mg/day before a planned delivery).

The objective should be a planned vaginal delivery, avoiding episiotomy, with good control of the third stage, including i.v. ergometrine, controlled cord traction, and immediate manual removal of the placenta if the cord breaks.

Von Willebrand's disease

This is the most common clinically significant abnormality of blood coagulation in women. It is characterised by a prolonged bleeding time, decreased levels of factor VIII and defective platelet function.

In general, factor VIII levels of more than 30% do not require treatment in pregnancy. Levels of 60% or more are associated with safe vaginal delivery, 100% levels are recommended for caesarean section. One transfusion of fresh frozen plasma daily will maintain levels of factor VIII, three units of fresh frozen plasma or six units of cryoprecipitate produce a maximal level.

Disseminated intravascular coagulation

This term is used to indicate a range of consumption coagulopathies associated with prolonged retention of a dead fetus, severe pre-eclampsia, abruptio placentae, amniotic fluid infusion, Gram negative sepsis and prolonged shock of any aetiology. The features of the full syndrome are a coagulopathy, a low platelet count and the presence of fragmented red cells in the peripheral blood. Fibrin degradation products in the plasma are elevated, but the use of this as a diagnostic feature is limited, as all the associated conditions can also have this effect. With abruptio placentae the predominant characteristic is hypofibrinogenaemia. Sometimes, there is considerable activation of fibrinolytic enzymes.

In the serious acute situation with bleeding, management is with fresh blood, fresh frozen plasma and cryoprecipitate with central venous pressure monitoring; and sometimes platelet infusions. The definitive manoeuvre is to deliver the baby, when improvement will ensue. Even if there is evidence of fibrinolysis, antifibrinolytic agents are best avoided, as renal infarction and other ischaemic organ damage can occur. Sepsis must be treated vigorously with broad spectrum antibiotics and the patient managed by maintenance of cardiovascular, respiratory and renal systems in an intensive care situation.

In less acute situations where there is no active bleeding, heparin infusions are of value and may protect the kidney from deposition of fibrin and red cell fragments in the glomeruli. Response is monitored by platelet counts and fibrin degradation product levels. Dipyridamole infusions, low dose oral aspirin and prostacyclin infusions have also been used.

DISEASES OF THE RESPIRATORY SYSTEM

The respiratory system adapts to the physiological stress of pregnancy more easily than does the cardiovascular system. Nevertheless, as many as 70% of previously normal women experience dyspnoea at some time during pregnancy, this being most common at term.

Physiological Changes in Pregnancy

Oxygen consumption rises by an average of 18% from 250 ml/min to about 300 ml/min. About one-third of the increased oxygen consumption is required by the fetus and placenta, the remainder is for maternal metabolism.

Pulmonary function testing in the normal pregnant patient shows an increased minute ventilation due to an increased tidal volume, with no change in respiratory rate. Tidal volume increases by about 40% from 500 to 700 ml. In the second half of pregnancy, functional residual capacity and total lung capacity are reduced, but vital capacity is unchanged.

Ventilation increases twice as much as oxygen consumption and so arterial P_{CO_2} falls, with an equivalent fall in plasma bicarbonate, while arterial P_{O_2} remains fairly constant, viz. the increased progesterone influence in pregnancy affects the respiratory centre, and there is also an increased sensitivity to carbon dioxide, resulting in the increase in ventilation.

Bronchial Asthma

About 1% of pregnancies are complicated by acute asthma, and the risk to the fetus is very small.

Asthma is not generally affected by pregnancy, though a few patients deteriorate symptomatically in every pregnancy. If one parent has asthma, the risk of the child having asthma is doubled compared to the general population. Classically, asthmatics have been divided into two clinical groups, extrinsic and intrinsic.

Extrinsic

Affected individuals are usually younger and have had their disease since childhood. Their attacks are often seasonal, precipitated by allergens and accompanied by a history of hayfever or atopic dermatitis.

Intrinsic

Intrinsic asthma is an adult onset illness without an atopic history and requires long-term treatment. Associated bronchitis is common.

Treatment

The presence of green or yellow purulent sputum is evidence of chest infection, and an appropriate broad spectrum antibiotic should be prescribed. Tetracycline should not be used, because it colours fetal teeth brown.

A rational principle is to use as little as possible of the safest drug required to keep the patient free from symptoms. For occasional attacks, selective β_2-sympathomimetic bronchodilators, salbutamol or terbutaline taken orally or as an aerosol are used. It should be noted that ritodrine is devoid of bronchodilator activity. When there are more frequent attacks, prophylactic treatment is with sodium cromoglycate taken regularly in maximal dose and reducing to the minimum to maintain control. If cromoglycate fails, steroid aerosols like beclomethasone dipropionate or betamethasone valerate may be used. Theophylline or aminophylline may be added to the regimen. If there is no improvement in the patient's condition, corticosteroids in a titrated dose are used to control asthma, beginning, for example, with a high dose of 20–30 mg prednisolone for 2–3 days and reducing progressively until symptoms begin to recur. Once steroid treatment is initiated in pregnancy, it is better to continue a maintenance dose until the pregnancy is over.

Objective measurement of airway obstruction using a peak flowmeter or a spirometer is important in the management of asthma. This is useful to establish the severity and to confirm objectively that treatment is effective.

When the asthmatic goes into labour, treatment with inhaled β-sympathomimetic agents should be used first. The corticosteroid dependent asthmatic should be given hydrocortisone 100 mg i.m., every 8 h to cover the course of labour. Epidural analgesia is preferable to narcotic analgesics but, when general anaesthesia is required, it is not contraindicated.

Respiratory Infections

Influenza

In relation to pregnancy, influenza is associated with a higher fatality rate than in non-pregnant women. In general, the condition is self-limiting and the patient improves with symptomatic treatment, such as bed rest, antipyretics, and increase in fluid intake. The influenza virus can cross the placenta. No definite congenital defects have been attributed to it, but there is some evidence of a slightly increased rate of childhood leukaemia in the offspring (4/1000). Effective vaccination is with a live attenuated virus, and is best delayed until the second trimester, but it is desirable when an epidemic is anticipated.

Bacterial pneumonia

Bacterial pneumonias are commonly due to *Streptococcus pneumoniae*, *Haemophilus influenzae* and the haemolytic streptococcus. Pneumococcal pneumonia classically begins with a shaking chill, pleuritic chest pain, fever, cough and dyspnoea. Chest x-ray evidence of lobar consolidation may help to distinguish it from pulmonary embolism and infarction. A sample of sputum should be sent for culture and antibiotics such as amoxycillin, erythromycin or a cephalosporin prescribed. As premature labour is a definite risk associated with pyrexia, antipyretic measures, such as tepid sponging and paracetamol, should be used in addition to aggressive antibiotic therapy.

Bronchitis and bronchiectasis

Management is as with non-pregnant patients,

except that the use of iodine containing expectorants and tetracyclines is contraindicated.

Pulmonary tuberculosis

Pulmonary tuberculosis in pregnancy is becoming less common. Chest radiography in pregnancy should be performed in those populations at significant risk and in those in contact with the disease.

In general, with treatment, pregnancy has no unfavourable effect upon the course of the disease. There is no good evidence that the outcome of pregnancy is adversely affected by tuberculosis, although transplacental passage of the tubercle bacilli to the fetus has been reported.

Cough, purulent sputum, fever, weight loss and chest pain occur in pulmonary tuberculosis. Diagnosis is usually made from chest x-ray findings and the presence of acid-fast bacilli on examination and culture of the sputum. The Mantoux test becomes positive in 1–3 months after a primary infection. Treatment of the mother should be as if she were not pregnant.

There is a risk of the neonate being infected by the mother with sputum positive active disease, although the risk is minimal a few days after chemotherapy has been initiated. Exposed babies may be protected with isoniazid and immunised with isoniazid-resistant BCG vaccine if the organism is sensitive to isoniazid. There is no need to separate the baby from the mother.

Cystic Fibrosis

This is a common inherited disease with 1 in 20 carrying the gene. Heterozygous people are asymptomatic, but homozygous people are affected, the incidence being 1 in 2300 births. Fertility is markedly impaired, particularly in males. In pregnancy, maternal mortality is the same as the general rate for women with the disease. Pulmonary hypertension and pancreatic insufficiency are adverse prognostic factors. Perinatal mortality is increased, and related to degree of dyspnoea and cyanosis before conception. Maternal weight gain in pregnancy is poor, but the fetus grows normally.

Management in pregnancy includes monitoring of pulmonary function and continued physiotherapy. Any suggestion of infection is treated promptly with hospital admission and antibiotics. Vaginal delivery is preferred; epidural analgesia is useful

and general anaesthesia is avoided if possible. The occurrence of pneumothorax in the second stage of labour may be reduced by elective forceps delivery.

GASTROINTESTINAL DISORDERS

Vomiting and Heartburn

The vomiting centre in the reticular formation of the medulla controls vomiting. Irritation of the mucosa of the upper gastrointestinal tract generates impulses which are relayed by the sympathetic nerves and the vagi to the vomiting centre. Emotionally charged stimuli causing emesis are also conducted to the vomiting centre from the diencephalon and limbic system. Circulating chemical agents may stimulate the chemoreceptor trigger zone in the medulla which can initiate vomiting.

Morning sickness

The term 'morning sickness' is used to describe mild symptoms of nausea and vomiting, often occurring at other times in the day, between 6 and 14 weeks of pregnancy. The incidence is between 50 and 80%. Usually there is some disturbance of appetite, but in general there are no signs of disturbed nutrition. The aetiology of morning sickness is uncertain, but oestrogen has been suggested to be a cause, as has excess human chorionic gonadotrophin. Cultural attitudes and social disturbance during pregnancy may also be associated.

It is important to exclude medical and surgical causes before attributing vomiting to pregnancy alone. Following explanation of the possible aetiology, all that may then be required is to stop any oral iron treatment and to give simple advice on taking small frequent meals containing a lot of carbohydrate. When an antiemetic is indicated, an antihistamine with or without pyridoxine should be selected initially. Promethazine has been widely used for many years.

Hyperemesis gravidarum

Hyperemesis gravidarum is a term applied when the patient develops intractable vomiting with ketosis, acetonuria, alteration of electrolyte imbalance and weight loss of 5% or more. If untreated, renal and liver damage and neurological disturbances may occur. This condition may be associated with hydatidiform mole, multiple pregnancy, and hydramnios.

The immediate management of hyperemesis involves correction of fluid and electrolyte balance, parenteral vitamins, bed rest and sometimes sedation. Phenothiazines and related drugs have antiemetic and sedative properties and are suitable for use parenterally for 1–3 days at a time. Promethazine, 25 mg, promazine, 50 mg, chlorpromazine 25–50 mg, or prochlorperazine, 1 mg, may be given i.m. three times a day. Steroids are occasionally useful in controlling recurrence. In certain cases subsequent care may include psychiatric consultation.

Vomiting in late pregnancy

Vomiting sometimes recurs in the last few weeks of pregnancy in women who have had troublesome vomiting in the early months. Nevertheless, full investigations should be undertaken as it may be due to a serious condition. The vomiting often appears to be due to mechanical factors, such as gastro-oesophageal reflux, but the possibility of other conditions, such as urinary tract infections, pre-eclampsia, acute hydramnios, gastroenteritis and appendicitis, cholecystitis, pancreatitis or intestinal obstruction must also be considered.

Heartburn and hiatus hernia

Heartburn often accompanies nausea and vomiting and is especially common in late pregnancy. It is due to regurgitation of gastric contents into the oesophagus. The reflux of bile is even more irritant than reflux of gastric acid. The reduced tone in the muscle of the lower oesophagus is probably responsible for regurgitation. Other factors such as increased intragastric pressure, pyloric sphincter incompetence and hormone influences may be related.

In the first trimester, it is best to confine treatment to simple dietary measures, upright posture and simple antacids. Magnesium trisilicate mixture is adequate for most purposes. Magnesium hydroxide mixture may be used in patients who have a tendency to constipation.

In late pregnancy, preparations containing local anaesthetics such as oxethazaine, gastric antispasmodics such as belladonna alkaloids and their synthetic analogues or a gastric motility stimulant such as metoclopramide, may all be given to alleviate symptoms.

Hiatus hernia is a well recognised cause of heartburn. It appears to be more common in women with advancing age and multiparity. About 10–20% of women in late pregnancy have been shown to have some degree of hiatus hernia. Severe heartburn with pain radiating to the neck is made worse by lying down, stooping or straining. Rarely haematemesis may occur.

Ptyalism

Ptyalism, which is excessive salivation and compulsive expectoration is a rare complication of early pregnancy of neuropsychiatric origin. It sometimes results in mild hypokalaemia, but without systemic effects. The condition is self-limiting and specific treatment is seldom required.

Peptic Ulceration

The incidence of peptic ulceration during pregnancy is low. In nearly 23 000 deliveries, only 12 patients were admitted for ulcer-like symptoms and of these only 6 were thought to be active. Most women with a history of peptic ulceration seem to improve during pregnancy, probably due to reduction in gastric secretion of acid. Perforation is very rare in pregnancy. In the third trimester, acidity in the stomach may be increased with delayed gastric motility. This may explain the occasional complication of peptic ulceration occurring in pregnancy. Quiescent ulcers may suddenly become active in the puerperium, presenting with haemorrhage.

Management in pregnancy follows general principles in peptic ulcer treatment. Mucosal barrier strengtheners, such as carbenoxolone, have side-effects of salt and water retention, hypokalaemia and, occasionally, raised blood pressure. Their use in pregnancy has been limited. Histamine H_2 receptor antagonists, cimetidine and ranitidine, may be used in late pregnancy for the treatment of peptic ulceration.

As a general rule the pregnant woman with severe gastric haemorrhage or perforation should be treated as if the patient is not pregnant. Hesitation to operate on a pregnant patient with perforated ulcer and peritonitis yields a high mortality.

Acute Appendicitis

Acute appendicitis is seen with equal frequency in the first two trimesters of pregnancy and only slightly less often in the third trimester.

Pregnancy confuses the clinical picture of acute appendicitis. The base of the appendix is pushed upwards and outwards by the enlarging uterus, causing the appendiceal inflammatory reaction to occur progressively higher and more laterally in the abdomen. The diagnosis becomes much more difficult and peritoneal involvement occurs much more readily in late pregnancy.

The normal leucocytosis of pregnancy (up to 15 000/mm^3) makes this guide unreliable. Urinary tract symptoms and abnormalities of urine analysis are common during pregnancy and make the differentiation between appendicitis and urinary tract infection difficult. Other causes like cholecystitis, renal colic, or torsion of an ovarian cyst should be considered.

The mortality of appendicitis in pregnancy is the result of delay. Where real doubt exists, it is far better to perform a laparotomy.

Appendicectomy performed during pregnancy for an appendix that is found to be normal carries only minimal risk for mother and fetus. Antibiotics should be used in all cases to reduce the chance of infection.

Intestinal Obstruction

The most common cause is strangulation by bands of adhesions from previous operations, which become stretched by the enlarging uterus. Vomiting secondary to bowel obstruction occurring in early pregnancy may be mistaken for morning sickness and the pain of obstruction late in pregnancy may be similar to that of labour pains. The presence of surgical abdominal scars, localised tenderness, a peristaltic rush and air-fluid levels in an upright x-ray film may help to diagnose intestinal obstruction. Volvulus may occur.

Adequate replacement of fluid and electrolytes should be achieved before surgery. The obstruction must be identified and relieved; necrotic bowel requires resection; obstruction of the colon requires colostomy. If the pregnancy is close to term, a caesarean section may be necessary to give access to the intestinal obstruction.

Non-specific Inflammatory Intestinal Disorders

This group of intestinal disorders include ulcerative colitis, Crohn's disease and non-specific colitis. They occur almost equally between females and males and usually manifest before the age of 30 years. The incidence in developed countries is between 40 and 100 per 100 000 population and is probably lower in developing countries. Ulcerative colitis is more common than Crohn's disease, but this difference is becoming less marked.

Well-managed inflammatory bowel disease has a good fetal outcome in 70–90% of cases where the disease presents before pregnancy and even if a relapse occurs in pregnancy. There appears to be no overall increase in the incidence of congenital defects.

Between 40 and 50% of affected women have a clinical relapse during pregnancy. Relapse may occur at any time during pregnancy, but is more likely during the first trimester and early in the puerperium.

Management. Patients should be encouraged to embark on a pregnancy when their disease is clinically quiescent, and when taking a minimum number of drugs. When they are seen before conception, any anaemia should be treated and folic acid and B vitamin supplements should be prescribed to continue in pregnancy. Management during pregnancy should involve monthly monitoring with blood counts and estimations of serum iron, folic acid, calcium, phosphate and, in severe cases, magnesium. Hospital rest is a primary measure in treatment of exacerbations.

Ulcerative colitis

Medical treatment suppresses disease activity, but never cures. Mild attacks can be treated with sulphasalazine and topical steroids.

Sulphasalazine is considered safe for use throughout pregnancy and also in breast feeding mothers. It impairs absorption of folic acid and supplements of 5–10 mg/day will be required in pregnancy. There is a small risk of neonatal jaundice.

Local applications of corticosteroids in the form of prednisolone enemas are preferable in mild cases when the disease is confined to the distal rectum. Patients with severe bowel symptoms, and those who fail to respond to topical steroids, need bed rest, an adequate diet, correction of fluid and electrolyte deficits, especially potassium, the correction of anaemia and treatment with systemic steroids.

Oral broad-spectrum antibiotics aggravate ulcerative colitis and should be avoided. The value of intravenous antibiotics in severe attacks is not well established.

Crohn's disease

Simple measures should be tried before any treatment. Fluid stools can often be controlled by codeine phosphate and bulk-forming agents are helpful in colonic disease. Patients should be allowed a full diet with adequate protein. Diarrhoea usually responds to a low milk diet. Supplementation with folic acid is advisable and vitamin B_{12} is essential in patients with ileal disease or after ileal resection.

Sulphasalazine may improve symptoms in patients with modestly active disease. Broad-spectrum antibiotics are indicated in patients with intra-abdominal or perianal sepsis. Corticosteroids are indicated in acutely ill patients or for persistent disabling disease which has failed to respond to simpler measures. Azathioprine may be used to maintain a steroid induced remission. The clinical response often requires a latent period of several weeks.

Indications for surgery in ulcerative colitis and Crohn's disease during pregnancy are usually perforation, toxic megacolon and, rarely, intestinal obstruction.

Patients who have been on corticosteroids should have hydrocortisone 100 mg i.m. every 8 h to cover general anaesthesia, a surgical procedure or labour.

Constipation

There is a tendency to constipation during pregnancy. This may be due to increased sodium and water absorption in the colon, general hypotonia of the intestine, caused by increased progesterone activity on smooth muscle, and it is sometimes aggravated by iron supplements given in pregnancy. Simple measures include advice on a diet containing a high fibre content, bran and adequate fluids. Cellulose-containing foodstuffs and hydro-

philic stool bulking agents should be the initial treatment. If these fail, magnesium hydroxide mixture, senna, or bisacodyl may be used. Purgatives such as liquid paraffin should be avoided for they impair absorption of fat-soluble vitamins A, D and K.

Diseases of the Liver

Liver diseases can be caused by conditions which are associated with and peculiar to pregnancy or conditions which are unrelated to pregnancy.

Conditions peculiar to pregnancy

Hyperemesis gravidarum. In severe cases of hyperemesis gravidarum, jaundice may occur. If so, then the odds are strong that the diagnosis of viral or toxic hepatitis or, rarely, fatty degeneration, has been missed.

Pre-eclampsia and eclampsia. Liver dysfunction has been detected in about 18% of pre-eclamptic and eclamptic patients and is due to ischaemia. The right upper quadrant pain sometimes present in pre-eclampsia is traditionally due to hepatic oedema and haemorrhage, with distension of Glisson's capsule. Subcapsular haemorrhage is now uncommon and if haemorrhage into the liver occurs, it is usually parenchymal. Pruritus does not usually occur. The level of serum transaminase, usually slightly raised (50–300 iu/l), is a sensitive guide to hepatocellular involvement. Bilirubin elevations are usually mild and reflect both hepatic dysfunction and intravascular haemolysis.

Acute fatty liver. This is a rare, but serious, complication of unknown aetiology, characterised by the accumulation of microvesicular fat in the hepatic parenchyma. Patients usually present in the third trimester of pregnancy or in the puerperium with abdominal pain, nausea, vomiting and varying degrees of jaundice. Pruritus is rare. The course of acute fatty liver of pregnancy is characterised by the rapid progression to acute hepatic failure, with coagulation disturbances and encephalopathy. In contrast to hepatitis, the disease has a short prodromal period, abdominal pain is a predominant feature, and serum transaminase and alkaline phosphatase levels are only moderately elevated. Complications include hypoglycaemia, gastrointestinal bleeding, renal failure and metabolic acidosis. Remission of the disease is frequently observed after the pregnancy; vaginal delivery is preferred.

Intrahepatic cholestasis of pregnancy. This condition, which is related to excess oestrogen influence, is due to an exaggeration of the difficulty in transport of bilirubin into the biliary canaliculi in pregnancy. The predominant symptom is pruritus due to accumulation of bile acid in the skin and jaundice is usually mild. Right upper quadrant abdominal pain is rarely present and the general health of the patient is usually unaffected. Liver enzymes, and particularly alkaline phosphatase, are elevated. Extrahepatic causes of cholestasis and drug toxicity must be excluded.

Antipruritic drugs, such as antihistamines, are only partly effective; potentially hepatotoxic agents must be avoided. Cholestyramine has been used to alleviate pruritus, but it is not very effective. Regular vitamin K injections should be given to the mother for 2 weeks before labour is anticipated to prevent fetal haemorrhage. Fetal outcome is generally good.

Patients with a history of intrahepatic cholestasis of pregnancy should avoid the oral contraceptive pill.

Conditions incidental to pregnancy

Acute viral hepatitis. This is due either to hepatitis A (infective hepatitis) or to hepatitis B (serum hepatitis).

In hepatitis A, the infective agent is found only in faeces and transmission is by the oral-faecal route. The onset is usually abrupt with gastrointestinal symptoms, low-grade fever and general influenza-like manifestations. Recent infection is confirmed by a rising titre of anti-HA IgM. Hepatitis A usually resolves within 2–3 weeks and chronic hepatitis is not observed.

In hepatitis B, the infective agent can be detected in the blood. Transmission is parenteral with a high incidence in drug addicts. Maternal-fetal transmission also occurs. The disease has a long incubation period with a prodrome of arthralgia and urticaria. In the acute period, hepatitis B antigen (HB_sAg) is present in the serum. This may be followed by HB_eAg in serum. When the 'e' or core antigen is present, there is a high incidence of neonatal hepatitis B infection.

Hepatitis B carriage. The incidence of symptomless carriers of hepatitis B surface antigen among antenatal patients varies greatly from country to country. It is highest in Africa and South-East Asia. The incidence in Europe is about 0.5%, with most of the carriers coming from the higher incidence areas. Carriers of the 'e' antigen (mainly patients of Far East extraction) are by far the most infectious and are likely to transmit the infection to their babies. Hepatitis B antibody positive patients are usually immune and not infectious. The disease is blood-borne, and so it is desirable that medical and nursing staff should be immunised against the disease, but precautions should also be taken to prevent cross-infection. The babies of 'e' antigen positive mothers should be immunised with antihepatitis B immunoglobulin or a new vaccine genetically engineered from yeast. The vaccine should also be given to staff when there is a possibility of infection.

Acute pancreatitis. Although rare, acute pancreatitis in pregnancy has a maternal mortality of 20%. There is no causal relationship between pancreatitis and pregnancy. Biliary tract disease is a prominent cause. In pregnancy, it has been suggested that the actions of progesterone may promote bile reflux into the pancreatic duct, and that hyperlipaemia, which occurs normally in pregnancy, may cause pancreatitis. About half the cases of pancreatitis occur during the third trimester.

CENTRAL NERVOUS SYSTEM DISORDERS

Epilepsy

The prevalence rates for epilepsy vary from about 5% of the population who will suffer a non-febrile epileptic seizure during their lifetime, to about 0.5% with chronic epilepsy. The risk of an epileptic adult having a child with epilepsy is small, about 1 in 30; but still 5 times that of the general population. The risk is greatest among those with an electroencephalographic pattern showing symmetrical three cycles per second spikes and slow wave discharges.

In pregnancy, it has been estimated that one-third of epileptics will suffer an increase in seizures, one-third a decrease and in one-third there will be no significant change. Factors responsible for the increased frequency of seizures may be a fall in the plasma concentrations of the anticonvulsant drugs. This can be due to decreased drug absorption, increased hepatic metabolism and impaired patient compliance.

Some patients develop seizures for the first time during pregnancy or the puerperium. Care should be taken to distinguish petit mal in particular from syncope in early pregnancy. A small number of patients suffer seizures only during pregnancy or the puerperium. It should be remembered that some cerebral tumours increase in size during pregnancy, and the development of seizures may be the first sign of this condition.

Clinical differentiation between epilepsy and eclampsia may be difficult. In eclampsia, there is usually a history of signs and symptoms of pre-eclampsia such as hypertension and proteinuria, and there may have been severe headache, visual disturbances, epigastric pain and vomiting.

In epilepsy, blood pressure is unchanged, and proteinuria and oliguria are not features.

Management

This should begin in a preconception clinic. The decision whether to treat in pregnancy is generally made on the same grounds as for non-pregnant patients. The risks of uncontrolled seizures to the fetus are greater than the risks of exposure to anticonvulsant drugs. If a woman having treatment for epilepsy is planning a pregnancy, it is best if she can be controlled on a single drug with monitoring of free plasma levels. Nevertheless, if a patient is on combination therapy to control seizures and is found to be pregnant, it may be best to continue on the same drug regimen. Sudden withdrawal or change of drug therapy may lead to status epilepticus.

In general, the choice of drugs in pregnancy should be governed by the same considerations as in the non-pregnant patient. Phenobarbitone may be best if epileptics can be managed on a barbiturate alone. If anticonvulsants are to be used in pregnancy, folic acid supplements (5 mg/day) should be started well before conception, as there is evidence that the teratogenicity of phenytoin is related to its effect on folate absorption and metabolism. Rarely, the frequency of fits increases with folic acid, so there should be ample time to adjust anticonvulsant dose. Folic acid supplements also prevent develop-

ment of megaloblastic anaemia. Prophylactic vitamin K tablets should be started 2 weeks before delivery is anticipated; 5 mg of phytomenadione i.m. should be given to the mother at the onset of labour and 0.5–1 mg i.m. to the newborn to reduce the risk of neonatal haemorrhage when phenytoin or barbiturates have been used at the end of pregnancy.

There is a two- to threefold increase in the incidence of congenital malformations in the off-spring of epileptic mothers treated with anticonvulsants, but not given folic acid, but it must be made clear to the potential mother that there is a 95% chance that she will have a normal baby.

Breast feeding is not contraindicated when mothers are on anticonvulsant drugs.

Cerebrovascular Disease

Arterial occlusive disease

Ischaemic stroke presents with the sudden onset of deficits in the central nervous system function such as hemiplegia, hemianopia, aphasia and apraxia. The incidence of an arterial occlusion in pregnancy and the puerperium has been assessed at 1 per 20 000 live births, with a mortality rate about three times that in non-pregnant women. Middle cerebral artery occlusion is the most common finding in pregnancy and internal carotid artery occlusion in the puerperium. The differential diagnosis in late pregnancy is cerebral vascular spasm.

Cerebral phlebothrombosis

Aseptic cerebral venous thrombosis usually presents in the second or third week after delivery. It presents with severe headaches, usually culminating in generalised and focal seizures, which are followed by weakness, aphasia and other deficits in cerebral cortical function. If the patient survives the initial episode, long-term prognosis is good, but a progression of symptoms is a poor prognostic sign.

Subarachnoid haemorrhage

In normal pregnancy, the incidence of spontaneous subarachnoid haemorrhage is not increased. A majority of cases are due to ruptured berry aneurysms on the circle of Willis, and less frequently due to arteriovenous malformations which have a tendency to rupture during labour. Patients often have hypertension, and may complain of a sudden onset of severe headache, neck stiffness and nausea. The finding of heavily and uniformly blood-stained cerebrospinal fluid at lumbar puncture confirms the diagnosis.

About a third of the patients die within 24 h. In those who survive, initial treatment is sedation and bed rest. Delivery is by caesarean section or, in selected cases, vaginal delivery with full epidural anaesthesia to prevent bearing down. Diagnosis of cerebral vascular lesions involves cerebral angiography and computerised axial tomography (CAT) or nuclear magnetic resonance (NMR) scans.

Chorea Gravidarum

Jerky purposeless movements associated with limb hypotonia acquired during pregnancy usually begin after the first trimester and cease within 2 or 3 months after childbirth. There is a strong link with a history of rheumatic fever. These movements are absent during sleep. Severe chorea can lead to rhabdomyolysis, myoglobinuria and hyperthermia. Treatment is with chlorpromazine or haloperidol.

Brain Tumours

Brain tumours sometimes increase in size during the second half of pregnancy and temporarily remit after childbirth. Their neurosurgical treatment is frequently postponed until several weeks postpartum, when the tumour is less vascular. Exceptions include pituitary tumours, acoustic neuromas, metastatic chorioncarcinoma, and tumours such as supratentorial malignant gliomas and posterior fossa tumours which require prompt surgical intervention.

Prolactinoma

Hyperprolactinaemia may be due to prolactin-secreting pituitary adenomas. These may be a macroadenoma (greater than 10 mm in diameter) or a microadenoma (less than 10 mm diameter). Most women with hyperprolactinaemia are infertile until treated with bromocriptine to induce ovulation.

During pregnancy, the growth of pituitary adenomata is accelerated by the influence of oestrogen and may impair vision by pressure on the optic chiasma. It is not possible to predict which tumours will enlarge to cause symptoms. Nevertheless, women known to have macroadenomas who wish to become pregnant should have their tumours treated before starting a pregnancy. This can be with bromocriptine, radiation (yttrium implants) or neurosurgery. During pregnancy, visual fields and acuity should be determined monthly, and more frequently if any visual failure is observed. If there is deterioration, treatment with bromocriptine may be reinstituted and is safe for use in pregnancy. Progressive visual field defects at 38 weeks of pregnancy may be an indication for early delivery as visual defects improve afterwards.

Retinal Detachment

There is a case for delivering patients with a history of retinal detachment by caesarean section; alternatively, epidural anaesthesia and complete avoidance of bearing down in the second stage by means of a forceps delivery can be used.

Otosclerosis

A condition which is often progressive in women of reproductive age. Terminating a pregnancy will not affect its course.

Multiple Sclerosis

This is a condition susceptible to remission and exacerbation. Sometimes these changes occur in relation to a pregnancy. There is no case for legal abortion in a woman with multiple sclerosis who wants a baby.

Neuropathies

Bell's palsy

Bell's palsy is said to be associated with pregnancy. Usually, there is an isolated paralysis of the seventh cranial nerve, without apparent inciting cause. The palsy commonly occurs in the third trimester. Generally, the condition improves during the puerperium. Steroids (prednisolone, 40–60 mg daily) have been used for treatment starting within one week of the onset of symptoms. Electrodiagnostic techniques are valuable in assessment. Patients with conduction block have a good prognosis.

Carpal tunnel syndrome

This is one of the most common neurological causes of pain in the hand. It is thought to be due to compression of the median nerve in the carpal tunnel by oedema of its wall during pregnancy. The pain and tingling tend to occur at night and to wake the patient. The hand feels numb and swollen as well as painful. These symptoms usually disappear when the patient starts to move the hand and fingers. In the fully developed case, there is atrophy of the median-supplied thenar muscles and sensory loss of appropriate distribution. The condition usually responds well to elevation of the arm, splinting of the wrists and treatment with oral diuretics, but occasionally surgical relief of the compression may be indicated.

Meralgia paraesthetica

In this condition there is entrapment of the lateral cutaneous nerve of the thigh under and sometimes through the lateral end of the inguinal ligament. This causes numbness and tingling on the anterolateral surface of the thigh. This condition appears to be more common in pregnancy due to lumbar lordosis. Pain may be precipitated by standing and relieved by recumbency. Weight gain should be restricted by dietary control. Treatment is with analgesics and sometimes infiltration of the nerve with local anaesthetic may be necessary. Surgical decompression is rarely required.

Foot drop

Paralysis of a lower limb of the mother after labour, or maternal obstetric palsy, has been considered to result from injury to the lumbosacral plexus by the fetal head or obstetric forceps. The most common form is unilateral foot drop. Generally, there is improvement within a few weeks. When paralysis is noted, lumbar disc protrusion must be considered. The presence of pain is associated with disc protrusion; pain with plexus injury rarely persists. Peroneal palsy, due to compression of the nerve around the neck of the fibula when the patient is placed in the lithotomy position, may also cause foot drop.

RENAL AND URINARY TRACT DISORDERS

Urinary Tract Infection

In pregnancy, the combined effects of increased progesterone secretion and pressure from the gravid uterus on the urinary tract cause a tendency to urinary stasis and ureteric dilatation and reflux. The result is an increased incidence of urinary tract infection. This can present as asymptomatic bacteriuria or as an overt infection.

Asymptomatic bacteriuria (>100 000 colonies/ml)

This occurs in 4–7% of pregnant women and a proportion of these patients may develop acute pyelonephritis later in pregnancy. *E. coli* is the organism responsible in most cases, but streptococci and proteus are not uncommon. By treating bacteriuria, the incidence of acute infection may be reduced to one-tenth, but the associated incidence of prematurity, pre-eclampsia and anaemia is unchanged.

With bacteriuria, blood urea or creatinine should be estimated to check renal function.

The aim of treatment is to maintain a sterile urine in pregnancy with a short course of appropriate antibiotics. Usually a 5-day course of amoxycillin or a soluble sulphonamide is the appropriate primary treatment. Sulphonamides are best avoided during the last 2–3 weeks of pregnancy because of the chance of neonatal jaundice if the patient goes into labour. If co-trimoxazole is used, then folic acid supplements, 5 mg daily, should be given by mouth. Alternative drugs useful with resistant infections, include cephalosporins, nitrofurantoin and metronidazole. Tetracyclines are contraindicated during pregnancy.

Where bacteriuria has recurred following initial treatment, a full urological assessment should be carried out 3 months after delivery to exclude any renal tract abnormality.

Acute urinary tract infection

Acute pyelonephritis is not confined to the woman with pre-existing bacteriuria; the incidence is about 2%. It is more common for the right kidney to be most affected, perhaps due to the dextro-rotation of the uterus in pregnancy. *E. coli* is the most common infective organism, but *Streptococcus faecalis*, *Staphylococci*, *Proteus*, *Klebsiella*, *Pseudomonas* and other Gram-negative bacteria can also be responsible.

In pregnancy, it is relatively uncommon to find a patient with the full clinical features of pyelonephritis, marked pyrexia, loin pain, severe renal angle tenderness, rigors and severe dysuria. More frequently, the patient has a slightly elevated temperature with vague symptoms of increased frequency, dysuria, backache, malaise and vomiting. There may be minimal loin tenderness and the diagnosis is made only from examination of the urine. Acute pyelonephritis must be distinguished with care from acute appendicitis.

Hospital admission is indicated in the severe case. Immediate antibiotic therapy, rehydration with intravenous fluids, analgesia to relieve pain, and tepid sponging to reduce pyrexia should be prescribed. The risks to the fetus from severe pyrexia are premature labour or intrauterine death. Antibiotic treatment should be continued for 10–14 days, when a further specimen of urine should be examined.

It is desirable to perform midstream urine cultures at subsequent antenatal visits. After a recurrence, prophylactic treatment with amoxycillin or a cephalosporin for the remainder of the pregnancy should be considered. Renal tuberculosis is now rare, but should not be forgotten when there is a sterile pyuria.

Haematuria in Pregnancy

Haematuria in pregnancy is usually related to a contaminated specimen of urine, urinary tract infection or calculus. Nephrolithiasis causes diagnostic problems, because of the difficulty of distinguishing ureteric colic from obstetric causes of abdominal pain. There may be a predisposition to haematuria by the engorgement of veins in the renal pyramids. Haematuria may also be present after a difficult vaginal delivery, especially if the bladder is catheterised. Rupture of a caesarean section scar involving the bladder must be considered in the differential diagnosis.

Other causes of haematuria include renal tuberculosis, renal neoplasm, polycystic kidneys, hydronephrosis, bladder papilloma, viral urinary infection and acute and chronic nephritis.

Acute Renal Failure

Prerenal causes of reduced renal function include renal hypoperfusion due to hypotension associated with acute haemorrhage, including placental abruption, or due to reduced plasma volume, as in the severest forms of hyperemesis, pre-eclampsia or septic shock.

Intrinsic renal causes of renal failure include acute tubular necrosis and cortical necrosis. The distinction is not absolute — a proportion of glomeruli are often damaged in association with tubular necrosis. Complete cortical necrosis is now rare in obstetrics. These conditions may be due to prolonged renal hypoperfusion, disseminated intravascular coagulation, particularly associated with pre-eclampsia, amniotic fluid embolus or sepsis.

Postrenal causes of renal failure include ureteric or bladder outlet obstruction due to calculi, tumours or surgical trauma.

Diagnosis

The cause for the sudden decline in renal function should be sought, as early diagnosis is important. Acute onset of oliguria after haemorrhage, septicaemia or a hypotensive episode during operation suggests acute tubular nephropathy. When the cause is not obvious, obstruction of the urinary tract should be considered. Catheterisation will exclude bladder outlet obstruction. Ultrasound scanning of kidneys and ureters is particularly helpful. Plain abdominal films may reveal radio-opaque calculi. Differentiation of prerenal from intrinsic acute renal failure may be a problem. Comparison of electrolyte, urea and creatinine concentrations in the urine and plasma may be useful, but are not always accurate due to the effects of therapeutic manoeuvres such as salt and fluid repletion and administration of diuretics. Response to plasma volume expansion or frusemide are more helpful in assessing intrinsic renal damage.

Differences between prerenal and intrinsic renal failure are shown in Table 8.2.

Management

The management of acute renal failure in association with obstetrical and gynaecological problems is the same as for any other precipitating factor.

Pregnancy and Chronic Renal Disease

Fertility and the ability to maintain a pregnancy depend on adequate renal function. Estimation of creatinine clearance gives a good guide to renal function. Adverse prognosis for mother and fetus is directly related to whether there is proteinuria alone, when the outlook is good; or in addition hypertension or nitrogen retention.

The incidence of intrauterine growth retardation, prematurity and perinatal mortality is increased in mothers with chronic renal disease.

Well over 1000 patients with renal transplants have now had successful pregnancies, taking steroids and azathioprine. A number taking cyclosporin have now succeeded. The prognosis is best if the transplant has been working well for 2 years, there is no hypertension, there have been no episodes of rejection and graft function is adequate and stable. The transplant seldom interferes with vaginal delivery, and if caesarean section is conducted, it is usually on obstetric grounds.

Very few pregnancies occur in women on chronic renal dialysis. Abortion is common, but there have been some successful pregnancies.

DIABETES MELLITUS

Since the recognition of the importance of good diabetic control during pregnancy, there has been a dramatic improvement in maternal and fetal mortality and morbidity in these patients. The decline in perinatal mortality correlates with lower mean maternal blood glucose levels, and maternal and fetal mortality rates approaching those in non-diabetic pregnancies have been reported in recent studies. Fetal malformation now accounts for at least 50% of deaths among babies of diabetic mothers. It must be recognised that these defects have their origin in the first trimester, and that they are related to lack of scrupulous control in the earliest weeks of pregnancy. It is, therefore, vital that diabetic patients be seen before they conceive and that optimal control, assessed by blood sugar and haemoglobin A_1 measurements, be obtained before they embark on a pregnancy.

The incidence of diabetes is between 1 and 3% of the obstetric population, but much effort is involved in achieving success in this group of pregnant mothers. It is important for the patient to understand the need for the strict control of her diabetes, to comply with frequent hospital visits and to accept admission readily.

Terminology

Clinical diabetes. The glucose tolerance test is abnormal and the patient presents with symptoms or complications of diabetes.

Gestational diabetes. Glucose tolerance is abnormal in pregnancy and reverts to normal after delivery.

Potential diabetes. Certain features (Table 8.3) increase the likelihood of abnormal glucose tolerance in pregnancy.

Latent, chemical, borderline and asymptomatic diabetes are terms often used synonymously and with confusion. They are generally applied to asymptomatic individuals with an impaired glucose tolerance.

Table 8.2
Differences between Prerenal and Intrinsic Renal Failure

	Prerenal	Intrinsic
Urine osmolality (m osm/kg)	>500	<400
Urine/plasma osmolal ratio	>1.5	<1.1
Urine sodium (mmol/l)	<20	>40
Urine/plasma urea ratio	>10	<10
Urine/plasma creatinine ratio	>10	<10

Diagnostic criteria

A fasting blood sugar of greater than 7.8 mmol/l suggests diabetes mellitus.

The pregnant woman given a 50 g oral glucose tolerance test who has a 1 h glucose level of greater than 7.2 mmol/l needs a full glucose tolerance test. When she is given a 100 g oral glucose test, she has gestational diabetes if two or more of the following values are exceeded:

Fasting	5.8 mmol/l
1 hour	10.6 mmol/l
2 hours	9.2 mmol/l
3 hours	8.1 mmol/l

Classification

The White classification of diabetes in pregnancy (Table 8.4) is of prognostic value as fetal mortality increases with duration of diabetes and presence of diabetic complications.

Effect of Pregnancy on Diabetes

There is no deterioration of glucose tolerance in pregnancy in normal women. The increased demand for insulin during pregnancy is probably related to increased metabolic rate, but the precise mechanism is far from clear. The hormone changes of pregnancy may be an important factor. The placental hormones, in particular oestrogen, progesterone, human chorionic gonadotrophin and placental lactogen, play an important role. Increased destruction of maternal insulin by placental insulinase has also been suggested as a causative factor.

The *instability* of diabetes in pregnancy is probably related to dietary changes, erratic absorption, a lowered vomiting threshold and infections.

Effect of Diabetes on Pregnancy

Fertility

When diabetes is well controlled and uncomplicated, there is no significant effect on fertility. Diabetics with severe nephropathy tend to be infertile.

Fetal development

There is an increased incidence (4–12%) of congenital, often multiple, malformations among the babies of diabetic mothers. There is an increase in major congenital abnormalities in the offspring of diabetic mothers with elevated glycosylated haemoglobin (HbA_1) in early pregnancy, indicating less than adequate control of the diabetes.

There is no evidence that there is an increased incidence of fetal malformations in women with potential or gestational diabetes or if the father is diabetic. There seems to be no increase in dysmorphic fetal abnormalities in women normally taking oral hypoglycaemic drugs.

Although fetal hyperinsulinism is unlikely to be a major contributory factor in malformation, it may cause 'unexplained' deaths in the latter stages of pregnancy and perinatal complications from a macrosomic fetus. Inadequate production of surfactant, resulting in respiratory distress syndrome, used to be a more common complication of diabetic pregnancy than it seems to be now.

Infection

Common conditions such as vaginal thrush and urinary tract infections are more frequent among diabetics and require prompt treatment.

Table 8.3

Risk Factors indicating Potential Diabetics

Family history of diabetes in first degree relatives

Past or present glycosuria

Obstetric history of recurrent miscarriages, unexplained perinatal deaths, fetal malformations, large babies (>4.5 kg.), or hydramnios

Maternal obesity (>20% ideal weight), increased age, or parity >5

Table 8.4

White's Classification

A Chemical diabetes or impaired glucose tolerance only
B Maturity onset diabetes (age over 20 years at onset), duration less than 10 years
C1 Onset at age 10–19 years
C2 Duration 10–19 years
D1 Onset under 10 years of age
D2 Over 20 years' duration
D3 Benign retinopathy
D4 Calcified leg vessels
D5 Hypertension
E Calcification of pelvic arteries
F Nephropathy
G Recurrent fetal loss
H Cardiomyopathy
R Proliferative retinopathy
T Renal transplant

Pre-eclampsia

This occurs two to ten times more commonly in diabetic than in non-diabetic pregnancies. It is particularly associated with diabetic nephropathy and the presence of hydramnios.

Hydramnios

Excessive accumulation of amniotic fluid occurs in up to 1% of normal pregnancies, but in poorly controlled diabetic pregnancies the incidence may be as high as 30%. It is associated with fetal macrosomia. Hydramnios can provoke premature labour and pre-eclampsia, thus adding risks for the fetus. In well controlled diabetics, the presence of hydramnios may suggest gastrointestinal or neuro-skeletal defects in the fetus.

Management

Before conception

Abnormal metabolic conditions for the fetus during organogenesis are a major cause of fetal malformation. One of the main aims of preconception management is to achieve normal diurnal blood glucose levels.

Ideally, the patient should be instructed in self-monitoring of her blood glucose levels, using finger prick blood sample applied to a glucose oxidase impregnated strip, and read off by a portable reflectance meter. During pregnancy, urine glucose testing is generally unsuitable for monitoring diabetic control.

Estimations of HbA_1 are now thought to be good indicators of the quality of diabetic control over the preceding 4–6 weeks. The normal (non-diabetic) range of HbA_1 is between 4 and 7% of the total haemoglobin. HbA_1 contains three subfractions, HbA_{1a}, HbA_{1b} and HbA_{1c}. The level of the last is closely related to that of total HbA_1. Serial estimations are useful for month to month monitoring of diabetic control before conception and during pregnancy.

Diabetics on oral hypoglycaemic drugs are best changed over to twice daily doses of combined short and intermediate acting insulin.

Antenatal

The preprandial blood glucose levels should be maintained between 4 and 7 mmol/l and postprandial levels at 8 mmol/l without hypoglycaemic episodes. HbA_1 should be maintained within the normal range.

Gestational diabetics. In most instances, gestational diabetes will respond to a diet regimen alone. In the obese woman, calorie restriction to 1000–1200 kcal is advised. Failure to achieve optimal diabetic control is an indication for insulin.

Insulin dependent diabetics. In pregnancy, if insulin is required to control blood glucose, it should be given at least twice a day, as a combination of medium and short-acting insulin.

Poorly controlled diabetics, with either frequent hyperglycaemia or severe hypoglycaemia, unresponsive to outpatient treatment, should be admitted to hospital. The problem may be poor motivation from, or lack of understanding by, the patient. If control remains poor, continuous insulin infusions may be considered. An assessment of fetal status can be made during the admission.

Diabetics do not frequently go into preterm labour; if they do, the best course may well be to allow them to deliver. If β-sympathomimetics or steroids are used, close monitoring of blood glucose is desirable.

Ultrasound monitoring of fetal biparietal diameters and abdominal girths is desirable not only to detect possible fetal growth retardation, but also macrosomia. The latter may indicate early delivery or caesarean section to avoid the risk of shoulder arrest during vaginal delivery.

Admission and delivery

The optimal time for delivery in a diabetic pregnancy remains a dilemma. The fear of sudden intrauterine death originally led to a policy of preterm delivery by elective caesarean section at 36 weeks of pregnancy in diabetic mothers. This resulted in some neonatal morbidity and mortality from respiratory distress syndrome. It is now clear that well controlled diabetics with normal fetal growth can be allowed to proceed to term and deliver vaginally without added risk to the fetus.

A bad obstetric history, pre-eclampsia, nephropathy, hydramnios, and fetal dysmaturity or macrosomia are indications for admission and early delivery. Delivery of the baby is indicated if hypertension becomes severe or the fetus is compromised by severe growth retardation or intrauterine anoxia. If delivery is planned before 38 weeks, it is important to assess fetal lung maturity by amniocentesis and estimation of both the amniotic fluid lecithin : sphingomyelin ratio and the phosphatidyl-glycerol content. Dexamethasone or betamethasone may be used to accelerate fetal lung maturity.

Planned vaginal delivery at term is preferred, but management of patients who begin labour spontaneously is similar. Elective caesarean section is indicated between 38 and 39 weeks if there are predictable risks to the mother or the fetus, such as suspected disproportion, malpresentation or previous caesarean section.

During labour, it is essential to maintain normoglycaemia, 4–7 mmol/l. Maternal hyperglycaemia causes fetal hyperinsulinism, which can result in hypoglycaemia in the newborn.

The diabetic controlled by diet alone requires no special management during labour except monitoring of blood sugar. Insulin dependent diabetics require control using intravenous dextrose and insulin only.

Postpartum

The gestational diabetic controlled on insulin during pregnancy should have her insulin stopped in the puerperium. Preprandial blood glucose esti-

mations should continue into the puerperium. After 6 weeks, a 75 g oral glucose tolerance test is performed. If the result is impaired, she is referred to a physician for follow-up.

In the insulin-dependent diabetic, the maternal insulin requirements fall within hours of delivery and the patient is then at risk from hypoglycaemia. Frequent blood sugar estimations and close observation are necessary.

Perinatal complications

Fetal endogenous hyperinsulinism causes hypoglycaemia and may compromise the newborn, especially if macrosomia is present. The baby may have fits, apnoea, hypotonia, hypothermia, hypomagnesaemia, hypocalcaemia and hyperbilirubinaemia. For these reasons, it should be delivered and cared for in a unit with neonatal special care facilities.

THYROID DISORDERS

Thyrotoxicosis or hypothyroidism complicating pregnancy are relatively uncommon. In thyrotoxicosis of moderate severity, partial thyroidectomy can be considered before pregnancy, minimising the need for drugs. Goitres of significant size can be removed before they enlarge dangerously in pregnancy.

Physiological Changes in Pregnancy

The increased vascularity of the thyroid gland, increased renal excretion of iodide, increase in thyroxine binding globulin concentration and the production of placental thyroid stimulators contribute to enlargement of the thyroid gland in pregnancy. Despite this and the increase in basal metabolic rate, the normal pregnant woman is euthyroid.

Thyroxine is the main hormone detectable in the fetus. By term, the concentration of thyroxine is just less than the maternal level.

Thyroxine (T_4) and tri-iodothyronine (T_3) undergo metabolic change in the placenta and only small amounts cross to the fetus. Iodine and antithyroid drugs such as propylthiouracil and the imidazole derivatives cross the placenta readily.

Hyperthyroidism

The incidence of thyrotoxicosis complicating pregnancy is 0.2–0.5%. It is uncommon for untreated severe thyrotoxic patients to become pregnant, as they tend to have anovulatory cycles. In untreated cases of lesser severity, there is an increased incidence of spontaneous abortion and perinatal mortality. Premature delivery is also increased. With treatment, the perinatal outcome improves dramatically. In the majority of patients, the disease has been diagnosed before pregnancy and they are under treatment.

The normal pregnant woman exhibits many signs and symptoms of hyperthyroidism, but the presence of goitre with bruit, exopthalmos, myopathy, sleeping pulse greater than 90/min, as well as specific signs such as brisk deep tendon reflexes and pretibial myxoedema all suggest Graves' disease. Due to changes in protein binding, the most important diagnostic and monitoring test in pregnancy is the free thyroxine index.

Medical treatment in pregnancy is usually with propylthiouracil or carbimazole or its active metabolite, methimazole. Both iodine and radioactive iodine (^{131}I) are contraindicated, as they can cause fetal goitre. Propanolol is particularly associated with fetal growth retardation and should be avoided except parenterally for control of the acute situation of a thyroid crisis. Excellent results have been obtained in America with partial thyroidectomy in the second trimester.

Intrauterine growth retardation is a fairly common complication. Management is along the usual obstetric lines.

In labour, problems specifically related to thyrotoxicosis are unusual if the patient has complied with treatment. Should a thyroid crisis occur, treatment is with intravenous propanolol.

The presence of thyroid-stimulating immunoglobulins in the mother seems to be associated with neonatal thyrotoxicosis. About 1 in 20 babies born to mothers treated with antithyroid drugs are affected by neonatal hypothyroidism or thyrotoxicosis, and investigation of the neonate is essential, for treatment is important, but not usually prolonged. About 1 in 20 babies have a goitre.

Treatment of the mother can often be discontinued 6 months after delivery.

All antithyroid drugs pass into breast milk in significant quantities, although there is some evidence that this is less of a problem with propylthiouracil. Treatment should be with propylthiouracil and the baby monitored for any effect on its thyroid function.

Hypothyroidism

Hypothyroidism is often associated with infertility and a high fetal wastage. Symptoms of cold intolerance, excessive weight gain and skin changes together with a slow pulse rate and delayed tendon jerks should make one suspicious of a positive diagnosis. In most instances, thyroid hormone replacement will have been commenced before pregnancy and should be continued.

The serum free T_4 index level is depressed and thyrotrophin (TSH) level is raised; the latter is only noted in primary hypothyroidism. Estimations of free thyroxine index should help with changes in hormone replacement therapy. The usual dose of *l*-thyroxine is between 100 and 300 µg daily.

Goitre

Endemic goitres due to iodine deficiency may present as large multinodular tumours in some parts of the world. Retrosternal extension may cause pressure effects, such as dyspnoea and dysphagia and impaction in the thoracic inlet in labour is potentially lethal. It is important to exclude both hyper- and hypothyroidism. In most instances where the cause is iodine deficiency, increased thyroid activity makes the patient euthyroid. Iodine supplements are provided to compensate for fetal demands, especially in the first trimester of pregnancy, to prevent neurological cretinism which does not respond to treatment. When iodine deficiency occurs after the first trimester of pregnancy, the newborn suffers from hypothyroid cretinism and will respond provided the baby is treated promptly.

In developed countries where iodised salt is used, small euthyroid goitres may occur. Enlargement of these goitres may occur during pregnancy. They pose little difficulty to management except when doubt exists regarding thyroid malignancy. Ultrasonography, needle biopsy and a technetium ($^{99}Tc^m$) scan may help with diagnosis, but surgery may be indicated. When a pregnant woman has a simple goitre, small amounts of supplementary iodine in the form of iodised table salt are advised.

RHEUMATIC DISORDERS

Rheumatoid Arthritis

This chronic inflammatory disorder, affecting one or more joints, is more common in women. Pregnancy has a beneficial effect on the disease, perhaps related to increased free cortisol levels, perhaps to changes in immune factors. Most patients develop recurrence of symptoms about 2 months after delivery, and almost all have an exacerbation within a few months.

The risk of spontaneous abortion, fetal growth retardation and perinatal mortality is no greater than in the general population.

Most patients with rheumatoid arthritis need only simple analgesics, usually non-steroidal anti-inflammatory agents such as aspirin and indomethacin, during pregnancy. These drugs are not responsible for congenital abnormalities, but, as prostaglandin synthesis inhibitors, they tend to delay the onset of labour. Whether or not there is a small risk of premature closure of the ductus arteriosus and pulmonary hypertension in the newborn, if preterm delivery is affected, is debatable. Aspirin is irritant to the stomach and should always be crushed and taken with milk. If full doses are continued until the confinement, there is an increased risk of ultrasonically diagnosed intraventricular haemorrhage due to interference with fetal platelet function, particularly of preterm newborn, although there may be no untoward sequelae. Aspirin is best discontinued when delivery is anticipated within a few days. No risks are documented with paracetamol.

Physicians are reluctant to treat rheumatoid arthritis with steroids, but, in pregnancy, there is no special risk provided supplements are given to cover surgical manoeuvres and labour.

Systemic Lupus Erythematosus

Systemic lupus erythematosus is an autoimmune disease often associated with microvascular abnormalities. It usually affects women in their reproductive years and can present with a variety of manifestations, such as polyarthritis, myalgia, skin rash, alopecia, pleurisy, dyspnoea, pericarditis, proteinuria, anaemia, leucopenia and thrombocytopenia. The disease runs a fluctuating course.

Detection of early stages by measurement of anti-DNA or anticardiolipin antibody and complement (C_3) levels has improved management of these patients.

Provided the disease is in remission, the outcome of pregnancy is generally good. This is where preconception counselling can be of major help. The effect of systemic lupus on pregnancy is an increased risk of spontaneous abortion, intrauterine fetal death, premature labour, intrauterine growth retardation and congenital heart block. Babies born to mothers with lupus nephritis and hypertension tend to be growth retarded, and the perinatal mortality rate is high. These patients should defer pregnancy until the disease is quiescent.

The effect of pregnancy on systemic lupus erythematosus is variable; there may be more exacerbations during pregnancy, in particular during the puerperium. Despite this, the maternal mortality and long-term prognosis are not affected. Anti-DNA antibodies are of little value for monitoring the disease during pregnancy; C_3 levels are more helpful in diagnosing exacerbation; symptomatology is the best guide.

The key to success in management is the free use of steroids when patients have been managed on other drugs; transfer to steroids before pregnancy (preferably not more than 10 mg/day of prednisolone) may be considered. When there has been a previous pregnancy loss taking other drugs, or the patient has been on steroids in the previous 2 years, transfer to steroids before or in early pregnancy is desirable. Patients taking steroids are not capable of the normal increased corticosteroid response to pregnancy, and prednisolone, 7 mg/day, should be regarded as a minimum replacement dose. Exacerbations are treated with increased doses, and if hypertension deteriorates beyond control with reasonable doses of hypotensive drugs, the dose of steroids is *increased*. Patients with a history of intrauterine growth retardation in a previous pregnancy should have low dose aspirin (75 mg/day) throughout pregnancy to minimise platelet aggregation. Labour is managed with parenteral hydrocortisone, continued for 24 h after delivery. Puerperal exacerbation is common and may be prevented by increasing doses of prednisolone for a few weeks, followed by gradual reduction.

Patients with systemic lupus erythematosus should be tested for antiphospholipid antibodies, anticardiolipin and the lupus anticoagulant, preferably before they become pregnant. Those with elevated levels are at high risk for pregnancy loss. Some success has been secured with a combination of high dose steroids (up to 50 mg prednisolone/day), sufficient to suppress the antibodies, and low dose aspirin. The use of plasmapheresis to reduce the antibody level in resistant cases is at present experimental. Patients with thrombotic variants of the disease may need anticoagulation with subcutaneous heparin throughout pregnancy.

ACQUIRED IMMUNE DEFICIENCY SYNDROME (AIDS)

Sexual transmission of the human T cell lymphotropic virus causes suppression of the immune system allowing the patient to develop a number of opportunistic infections such as pneumonia or Kaposi's sarcoma, which in almost all cases are ultimately fatal. The disease has spread from the male homosexual population to women, who are at risk when having intercourse with a male who is seropositive or has the disease. The chances of her becoming seropositive as a result of such a relationship are not known, but they are considerably less than for the recipient male homosexual. Currently, 10% of seropositive adults have developed the disease. A number of people have become seropositive from having used infected blood products and a growing number of drug addicts from using infected needles.

Pregnancy partially suppresses cell mediated immunity, and so it is possible that women with HTLV III antibody may have an increased chance of developing AIDS soon after pregnancy.

Perinatal transmission of the infection can take place before, during or after birth, including possibly through breast milk. The rate of perinatal transmission of HTLV III virus from infected pregnant women is not yet known. Small studies indicate a transmission rate varying from 0 to 65%.

Counselling and screening for HTLV III infection, preferably before conception, should be offered to drug addicts, prostitutes, the sexual partners of bisexual men and male drug addicts and to those who come from countries with a high incidence of AIDS in the female population, such as Haiti and central African countries. The sexual partners of men who have required a lot of blood products such as haemophiliacs also require testing.

The time from exposure to sero-conversion is not known, but is probably several months. For this reason, and if exposure is repetitive, testing will need to be done at regular intervals.

HTLV III infected women should be advised to postpone a pregnancy until more is known about perinatal transmission and to assess their own health further. Infected women delivering a child should be advised against breast feeding to reduce the risks of perinatal infection.

An infected patient should be managed throughout pregnancy and labour with strict precautions to minimise the risk of infecting staff. These will be similar to those used for the management of patients with hepatitis B.

FURTHER READING

De Swiet M., ed. (1984). *Medical Disorders in Obstetric Practice*. Oxford: Blackwell Scientific.

Gleicher N., ed. (1985). *Principles of Medical Therapy in Pregnancy*. New York and London: Plenum Press.

Hawkins D.F., ed. (1987). *Drugs and Pregnancy*, 2nd edn. Edinburgh: Churchill Livingstone.

9

Abnormalities of Pregnancy

PREGNANCY INDUCED HYPERTENSION (PIH) OR PRE-ECLAMPSIA

Hypertension developing during pregnancy (>140/90 mmHg) in a previously normotensive woman is often accompanied by excessive fluid retention and less frequently by proteinurea. This triad of clinical signs is still called pre-eclamptic toxaemia. However, the term 'pregnancy induced hypertension' (PIH) with or without proteinuria is clearer and should be used to differentiate this condition from renal causes of hypertension, proteinuria and oedema, such as glomerular nephritis or renal abnormalities associated with other diseases such as the connective tissue disorders.

Pregnancy induced hypertension occurs in about 10% of pregnancies and is more common in women having their first pregnancy with a particular partner. The importance of prompt diagnosis and appropriate management lies in the prevention of rapidly worsening maternal hypertension with the subsequent risk of cerebral haemorrhage, eclamptic fits or placental separation as well as those of fetal hypoxia.

Factors Predisposing to Pregnancy Induced Hypertension

Genetic. A family history of pre-eclampsia or hypertension tends to increase the risk.

Primigravidae. It is at least twice as common in primigravidae as in multigravidae. A history of an early miscarriage may protect against the risk of PIH, but pregnancy by a new partner increases the risk, suggesting that the disease has an immunological basis.

Social and economic. Pregnancy induced hypertension is more likely to occur in poor and underprivileged women. Inappropriate diet may be a factor; failure to attend for antenatal care delays diagnosis and management. Women who smoke tend to have a lower incidence but, should pre-eclampsia develop, fetal outlook is worse.

Medical. Diabetes mellitus and chronic renal disease are predisposing diseases.

Obstetric. Pregnancy induced hypertension is associated with hydatidiform mole, multiple pregnancy, hydramnios, and rhesus isoimmunisation.

Pathological Changes Occurring in Pregnancy Induced Hypertension

Vascular changes

Hypertension is caused by generalised arteriolar constriction with a normal cardiac output. A sudden rise of blood pressure may cause acute arterial damage with loss of vascular autoregulation, and the most common cause of maternal death from this condition is cerebral haemorrhage. Generalised arteriolar constriction also affects the vessels of the placental bed with a reduction of blood flow. Fibrin deposition in these vessels produces irreversible reductions. The consequences of chronically reduced placental blood flow are intrautcrine growth retardation and placental infarction and sometimes abruption. Acute placental infarction may cause sudden hypertension as a result of thromboxane release, and fetal hypoxia if it is severe.

Renal changes

Renal biopsies in patients with PIH and proteinuria have shown a plethora of different varieties of pathological change. The most characteristic is oedema of the endothelial cells of the glomerular capillaries and fibrinoid necrosis in renal glomeruli and tubules. Renal tubular function is first impaired, causing a reduction of uric acid clearance, reflected by a rise in plasma urate. Proteinuria usually indicates renal glomerular involvement. A rise in plasma creatinine or urea indicates increasing renal impairment in the form of reduced glomerular filtration rate and subsequent reduction in urine output. Acute renal failure with tubular or cortical necrosis is more likely when placental abruption has occurred. Oedema is probably due to generalised changes in membrane function, but is associated with renal retention of both sodium and potassium and also to reduced plasma albumin. Although there is extravascular fluid retention, plasma volume is reduced and the haematocrit rises. Rare complications of fluid retention include ascites and pulmonary and laryngeal oedema.

Liver changes

These occur infrequently and only as a result of severe PIH. Sometimes there is necrosis at the periphery of the lobule which may extend to involve the whole lobule. Occasionally, subcapsular haemorrhage is seen. Liver enzymes in the plasma are raised when there is liver impairment. Jaundice occurs rarely.

Coagulation changes

Disseminated intravascular coagulation may occasionally occur in severe cases and tends to be worse if the liver is involved. Platelet count, fibrinogen, and factors V and VIII are reduced, with a rise in fibrin degradation products. Another hallmark of disseminated intravascular coagulopathy which places renal function at risk is the appearance of fragmented red cells in the peripheral circulation. Potential complications of clotting disturbances include haemorrhage and necrosis in the brain, kidneys, liver, adrenal and pituitary glands.

Possible Aetiology of Pregnancy Induced Hypertension

Numerous hypotheses have been put forward to account for this condition.

Abnormal vasospasm involving both uterine and renal circulations

The hypothesis that vasoconstrictor agents are released when there is excessive uterine distension was put forward to account for the fact that PIH is more common in primigravid patients and those with multiple pregnancies. Renal ischaemia due to vasospasm allows the leakage of albumen through the tubules.

Coagulation abnormalities

Coagulation abnormalities have been said to account for the excessive fibrin deposition in the placenta and kidney which lead to placental infarction and glomerular damage characteristically seen in these cases. The increased fibrin deposition is accompanied by increased fibrinolytic activity and consequently there is an increase in circulating fibrin degradation products seen in cases of severe PIH. Placental damage leading to the liberation into the circulation of thromboplastic substances could cause generalised disseminated intravascular coagulation and consequently thrombocytopoenia, and a further rise in fibrin degradation products which are only seen in severe PIH.

Immunological aspects

The immunological barriers between mother and fetus that prevent rejection are not fully understood. Some inability of the mother to protect herself from the paternal antigens expressed in the conceptus has been suggested to explain the higher incidence of PIH among first pregnancies and in cases of hydatidiform mole, as well as explaining the lower incidence of PIH among antigenically similar couples. None of these theories provides an adequate explanation on its own. The likelihood is that the trophoblast plays a key role of some description and that there could be an interplay between immunological aspects, placental biochemistry and control of maternal blood pressure and coagulation factors.

Placental factors

What is the evidence for the placenta, and the trophoblast in particular, playing a key role in pregnancy induced hypertension? (Fig. 9.1). Firstly, trophoblast cells invade the intima and media of maternal spiral arterioles in early preg-

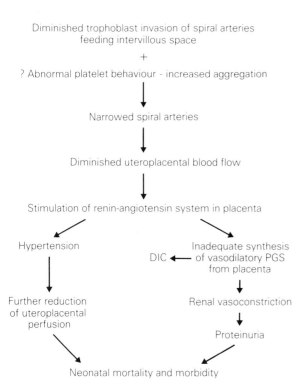

Fig. 9.1 *Possible aetiology of pregnancy induced hypertension.*

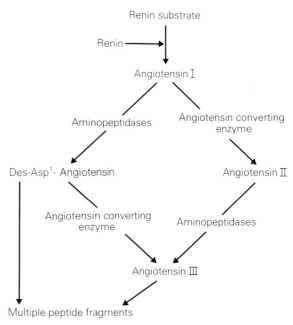

Fig. 9.2 *The renin-angiotensin system.*

nancy. This causes softening and loss of resistance in these vessels allowing for their expansion and so ensuring an adequate flow of maternal blood at low pressure into the intervillous space. A locally produced vasodilator to maintain the low flow and pressure state of the intervillous space should be of benefit. Secondly, the placenta produces renin and angiotensin and is able to carry out, in the same way as the kidney, all the enzymatic conversions within the renin–angiotensin system (Fig. 9.2). The pregnant woman is refractory to angiotensin II infusions, which would cause hypertension in the non-pregnant woman. This suggests that some placental product modulates the pressor effects of angiotensin II.

The placenta and fetal membranes metabolise arachidonic acid to eicosanoids which are the products of the cyclooxygenase and the lipoxygenase enzyme systems (Fig. 9.3). Prostacyclin is a very potent vasodilator and inhibitor of platelet aggregation, while thromboxane A2 has the opposite effect. The placenta has platelet anti-aggregatory activity which could be due to AD Pase or prostacyclin. In cases of PIH, there is a reduction in synthesis of

prostacyclin as determined by low levels of urinary metabolites, reduced levels of $6\text{-}oxo\text{-}PGF_{1\alpha}$ in amniotic fluid and the reduced conversion of C_{14} arachidonic acid to prostacyclin by the umbilical cord. Increased platelet aggregation leading to fibrin deposition and placental infarction would increase local thromboxane production both from platelets and from damaged placental tissue. A local imbalance in these two cyclooxygenase products could then ensue and be important in altering the biochemical balance necessary for maintaining a normal blood pressure.

The roles of lipoxygenase products in reproductive physiology are unknown, but their production in relatively large amounts by placental tissue from early in pregnancy and by fetal membranes suggest that they are of importance. Leukotrienes and monohydroxy fatty acids have both contractile effects on smooth muscle and increase capillary permeability. This could therefore cause vasospasm and an increase in extravascular, and the corresponding reduction in intravascular, fluid volume seen in severe PIH. Deficiencies of essential fatty acids have been demonstrated in PIH which favour increased synthesis of lipoxygenase products which, in turn, will inhibit prostacyclin synthesis. Finally, lipoxygenase products may affect the maternal immune response as leukotriene B_4 (LTB_4) induces

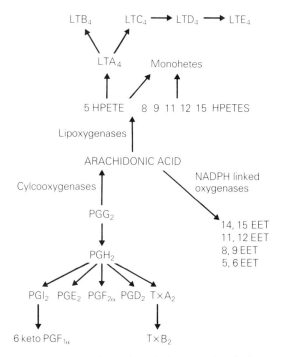

Fig. 9.3   Metabolites of arachidonic acid with the cyclooxygenase and lipoxygenase enzyme pathways. PGG_2, PGH_2 = endoperoxides; PGI_2 = prostacyclin; TXA_2, TXB_2 = thromboxane A_2, B_2; HPETE = hydroperoxyeicosatetraeonic acid; LTA_4, B_4, C_4, D_4, E_4 = leukotriene A_4, B_4, C_4, D_4, E_4; ETT = epoxyeicosatrienoic acid.

active suppressor T cells which down regulate the maternal immune response. An abnormal interplay between the maternal immunological system, alterations of arachidonic acid metabolism and other biochemical factors responsible for control of maternal and fetal vascular homeostasis may be the reasons for PIH.

Abnormal coagulation factors, expressed in severe cases of PIH as disseminated intravascular coagulation, are probably of a secondary nature as a result of placental infarction. These include raised levels of fibrin degradation products and reduced platelet count. There are some suggestions that increases in coagulation factors such as factor VIII may precede the onset of the hypertension.

Diagnosis

Pregnancy induced hypertension is diagnosed when the blood pressure taken in a sitting position

reaches 140/90 mmHg in a previously normotensive woman. The upper limits of normal are between 130/80 and 135/85 mmHg. Pregnancy induced hypertension very rarely occurs before the 20th week of pregnancy except in the case of hydatidiform mole. Usually hypertension is the first sign, but it may be preceded by a sudden retention of fluid manifest by clinically obvious oedema of legs, hands and face or by a sudden weight gain of two or more kilos within a week.

The proteinuria is largely albumen and represents renal ischaemia causing leakage of protein through the glomeruli and tubules. It is usually between 0.5 and 3 g per day. It is a sign of a more severe form of PIH, as renal pathology often reflects the placental pathology. The perinatal mortality rate in these cases is several times higher than in PIH without proteinuria. Proteinuria and/or oedema without hypertension constitutes totally different problems. Fulminating PIH presents with oedema, hypertension, headache, hyperreflexia, irritability and sometimes epigastric pain due to distension of the liver capsule or, rarely, subcapsular haemorrhage.

Management

Management is determined by the need to minimise the possible harmful effects to mother and fetus. Perinatal mortality in severe PIH with proteinuria is increased tenfold. However, this may be partly due to obstetricians' reluctance to perform an elective delivery sufficiently early. Recent experience of delivery between 28 and 32 weeks in cases of severe PIH suggest that the perinatal mortality in these cases can be substantially reduced if the fetus is delivered before significant hypoxia in utero can exert its harmful effects.

If severe PIH occurs suddenly around 26 weeks, with blood pressures of greater than 150/100 mmHg and with proteinuria, the patient must be admitted to hospital immediately and preferably to a centre with neonatal intensive care facilities. Intravenous hypotensive therapy using hydralazine and an anticonvulsant such as diazepam or chlormethiazole given i.v. or phenobarbitone given i.m. is commenced. Methyldopa may be used in addition, for its longer term action.

Fetal weight and liquor volume together with as extensive an assessment of fetal normality as possible are carried out ultrasonically. Cardiotocography is performed twice daily to detect the earliest onset of fetal hypoxia. Renal function is determined by urine output, specific gravity of urine, total protein in grams per 24 hours, plasma creatinine urea and uric acid levels. Fibrin degradation products and platelet count should be carried out. Delivery will be indicated if (1) hypertension is difficult to control without the use of more than one hypotensive drug; (2) there is evidence of rapidly worsening renal function; (3) fetal growth stops and (4) there is evidence of fetal hypoxia. If delivery is anticipated between 28 and 32 weeks, it is our policy to administer corticosteroids to the mother in the form of dexamethasone 12 mg i.m. on two consecutive days, the course finishing at least 24 h before delivery if possible. This therapy reduces the incidence of respiratory distress syndrome and intraventricular haemorrhage in the low birth weight, preterm baby. The mode of delivery depends on the degree of control of maternal blood pressure and whether or not there is fetal distress. Caesarean section will be the preferred mode of delivery in the majority of cases of severe pregnancy induced hypertension to minimise the risks of fetal hypoxia and maternal hypertension.

Moderate (150/100–160/110 mmHg) or mild (less than 150/100 mmHg) cases of PIH will require hospitalisation, bed rest and hypertensive therapy to maintain the blood pressure around 140/90 mmHg, and to improve placental blood flow. Hypotensive drugs suitable for use in pregnancy are described in Chapter 8. It is undesirable to reduce maternal blood pressure excessively, as this will reduce placental perfusion and cause fetal hypoxia. Anticonvulsant therapy is not usually needed unless the blood pressure exceeds 150/100 mmHg or there are signs of increased irritability, visual disturbance, severe headache or epigastric pain. Fetal monitoring should be by ultrasound scan every 2 weeks to assess fetal growth and liquor volume and by daily or twice daily fetal cardiotocography and fetal movement charts. Severe fetal growth retardation is unusual, but milder degrees (10th–3rd centile) are not uncommon. Biochemical monitoring by means of urinary or plasma oestriol estimations or plasma HPL estimations have largely been superseded by biophysical monitoring. The timing of delivery depends on blood pressure control and fetal well-being. Renal function is not significantly impaired in these cases. Delivery will usually be vaginally unless there is fetal distress.

Management in labour

The principles of management in labour and delivery are (1) adequate control of both systolic and diastolic blood pressure, (2) the use of anticonvulsants if required, (3) adequate analgesia and (4) an unstressful delivery by forceps or caesarean section. Continuous fetal monitoring is mandatory. Epidural analgesia is an effective way of providing analgesia and reducing the blood pressure, but coagulation must be normal for it to be used. The use of an anticonvulsant prior to induction of general anaesthesia is desirable.

Management of eclampsia

Eclampsia occurs when a woman with severe pre-eclampsia starts to have convulsions. This constitutes a major emergency as the patient can rapidly suffer from any of the following:

1. Cerebral haemorrhage due to sudden further elevation in her blood pressure.
2. Acute asphyxia due to convulsions or obstruction of her airway by the tongue or inhalation of vomit.
3. Severe fetal hypoxia as a result of the above or from concealed accidental haemorrhage.

If the patient is not in hospital, the Obstetric Flying Squad should be summoned immediately for emergency treatment on the spot and then transfer of the patient to a suitable obstetric unit. Immediate treatment is directed at reducing the blood pressure rapidly, ensuring an airway, and giving anticonvulsant drugs. Thereafter, delivery of the fetus should take place as soon as possible. A number of therapeutic regimens are used for this emergency. Diazepam, magnesium sulphate and chlormethiazone are used as anticonvulsants and should be given intravenously. Hypotensive therapy also needs to be given intravenously, the most commonly used drugs being probably hydralazine, although magnesium sulphate has some hypotensive effects. The drugs must be given in combination and a commonly used effective combination is hydralazine 10 mg and diazepam 10 mg given intravenously, in a period of 30 min.

Delivery of the baby should be by caesarean section once the blood pressure and fits are controlled and provided it is still alive.

Fluid overload should be avoided. Urine output during the first 24 h after an eclamptic fit may be reduced to less than 500 ml, particularly if there has been a caesarean section carried out. This is not a cause for concern but, if urine output continues at less than 500 ml into the second 24 h, an osmotic diuretic such as mannitol may be indicated.

Prophylaxis

On the grounds that enhanced platelet aggregation plays a key role in the pathogenesis of PIH, drugs that suppress this may be of benefit if commenced early in pregnancy and before significant placental or renal damage has taken place. Aspirin in low doses blocks the cyclo-oxygenase enzyme in platelets by acetylation and, as they cannot synthesise new enzyme, they can no longer produce thromboxane A_2 during their lifetime in the circulation. Higher doses of aspirin partially block prostacyclin synthesis by vascular endothelium. Dipyridamole inhibits platelet aggregation and may also be helpful. Recent studies suggest that low dose aspirin (75 mg per day) without dipyridamole from early pregnancy has been beneficial in pregnancies where excessive placental and vascular thromboxane production might be harmful. The possible beneficial effects of new thromboxane synthetase inhibitors require evaluation.

INTRAUTERINE GROWTH RETARDATION (IUGR)

Aetiology

Either the fetus is intrinsically small and, if so, it is often abnormal, or the growth retardation develops at a later stage of pregnancy. The reason for the latter is a reduced flow of maternal blood into the intervillous space and reduced fetal blood flow. What causes the reduction in maternal blood flow in the first place is not clear. When the ratio of the head to abdominal circumference remains constant, growth retardation is defined as being symmetrical. Asymmetrical growth retardation is diagnosed when there is a progressive change in this ratio. Increase in the growth rate of the abdomen is markedly reduced compared with that of the head as a consequence of loss of body fat and liver glycogen.

Asymmetrical intrauterine growth retardation may be associated with severe PIH or severe essential hypertension and is slightly more common in older women and in those who are very active or stressed throughout pregnancy. However, in about one-third of cases there is no obvious associated factor. A reduced blood flow through the uteroplacental circulation, either by fibrin deposition in the cases with severe PIH, or vasospasm in the other instances, leads to the reduced growth.

The pathological appearances of IUGR are a small infarcted placenta with evidence of fibrin deposition around the villi. The fetus will be relatively long and thin with little subcutaneous fat, an increased head to abdominal circumference ratio and an absence of vernix. Its weight will be below the 3rd, 5th or 10th centile for gestational age depending on the definition used.

The invasion of trophoblast cells during early pregnancy and again at about 20 weeks of gestation into the media of spiral arterioles, making them soft and dilated, seems to be important in allowing an adequate flow of maternal blood at low pressure into the intervillous space. Platelet aggregation and subsequent fibrin deposition and reduced blood flow through the fetal placental circulation are well documented in cases of IUGR. The possibility that there is a deficiency of locally produced prostaglandins has been suggested, but the evidence is not conclusive. Recent evidence linking severe IUGR, leading to midtrimester fetal death and abortion, with the presence in the circulation of anticardiolipin antibodies is of considerable interest. These antibodies are thought to act by preventing the liberation of arachidonic acid from cell membranes and so, by reducing substrate availability, altering the quantity, and possibly range, of arachidonic acid metabolites produced. These antibodies are found in patients with a variety of connective tissue disorders, particularly those with thrombotic complications. They are present in women with recurrent abortions of the type described, but without evidence of connective tissue disorders, although some of these women may go on to develop these later in life.

Diagnosis

Clinical awareness of the problem and regular palpation of the uterus, preferably by the same individual, are of vital importance. Failure of maternal weight gain or increase in abdominal girth are not of significant prognostic value. A less than expected pubic symphysis to uterine fundal height may be of value. Ultrasound carried out at about 18 weeks to confirm gestation and to exclude fetal abnormalities is important. The subsequent diagnosis of fetal growth retardation is best made by ultrasound scan and an accurate assessment of duration of pregnancy is vital in making the diagnosis. Important measurements are the biparietal diameter, head circumference, abdominal circumference, femur length and an assessment of liquor volume (Fig. 9.4). In the symmetrically growth retarded fetus that has no congenital abnormalities, the pathology will have started early in pregnancy and be severe. All the measurements will have a similar relationship to each other. In the asymmetrically growth retarded fetus, the limb length will be appropriate for gestational age, while the circumference of the head will be reduced less than that of the circumference of the abdomen, thereby

increasing the ratio between them. In both instances, there will usually be reduction in liquor volume. Blood flow in the arcuate arteries, in the umbilical vessels and in the fetal aorta can be demonstrated using Doppler ultrasound. An alteration in these measurements precede fetal hypoxia and may be an indication for delivery.

Treatment

At present there is no treatment apart from bed rest, which seems to increase the uterine blood flow and improve fetal growth in mild cases. In more severe cases, with or without severe PIH, bed rest alone does not usually improve fetal growth. On the grounds that there is an enhancement of coagulation mechanism and fibrin deposition in the placental circulation, various combinations of dipyrimadole and heparin have been tried with

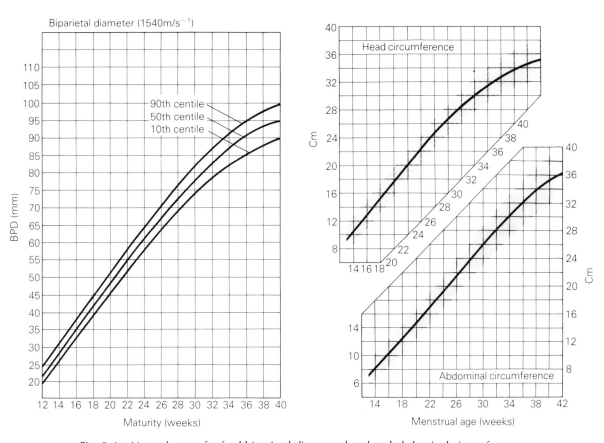

Fig. 9.4 *Normal range for fetal biparietal diameter, head and abdominal circumferences.*

some evidence of success. Low dose aspirin therapy (75 mg or less per day) which inhibits platelet thromboxane A2 synthesis and so diminishes platelet aggregation has also yielded some success, but both possible therapies need testing in large scale trials. However, the problems of setting up these trials in an appropriate manner are formidable. If there are anticardiolipin antibodies present in a significant titre immunosuppression using prednisolone in doses of up to 40–50 mg per day may be beneficial either with or without azothioprine and some form of antithrombotic therapy. Daily fetal cardiotocography is necessary to warn of the early onset of fetal hypoxia, any signs of which indicate delivery without delay by the most appropriate method if growth retardation is mild. When growth retardation is moderate or severe, delivery should be considered at an appropriate gestation, even in the presence of normal fetal heart traces so as to avoid the neonatal problems of a compromised low birth weight fetus. If the fetal weight, estimated by ultrasound, is less than 1.5 kg, delivery should probably be by lower segment caesarean section. Otherwise, if there is no fetal distress, a vaginal delivery can be considered.

The growth retarded baby is particularly vulnerable to hypoglycaemia and hypothermia. Blood sugar and calcium estimations should be carried out at birth and repeated during the first 24–48 h. Temperature control and adequate oxygenation either by head box administration or mechanical ventilation is important. Intravenous glucose may be necessary.

ANTEPARTUM HAEMORRHAGE

Placenta Praevia

This is defined as a placenta situated wholly or partially in the lower uterine segment. Its significance is that when the lower uterine segment is taken up and the cervix is effacing either before or during labour, placental separation, and thus inevitable haemorrhage, will occur. The aetiology of placenta praevia is not known, but it can be recurrent and is said to be more common in multiple pregnancies because of a larger placenta. Its presence is determined by the site of implantation by defective decidual reaction allowing the

placental site to extend. Traditionally, placenta praevia has been graded 1–4 as follows (Fig. 9.5):

Grade 1: placental edge in lower uterine segment;
Grade 2: placental edge reaches internal cervical os;
Grade 3: placental edge covers internal cervical os;
Grade 4: complete placenta central over the internal cervical os.

In practice, it is difficult to be so specific and, indeed, cases of grade 1 placenta praevia may never be diagnosed. A division into major and minor degrees of placenta praevia is a practical one, the major degrees being grades 3 and 4, where delivery by caesarean section is mandatory, while a minor degree of placenta praevia would encompass grades 1 and 2 in which vaginal delivery may or may not be possible, depending on the circumstances.

Presentation

Placenta praevia presents during the antenatal

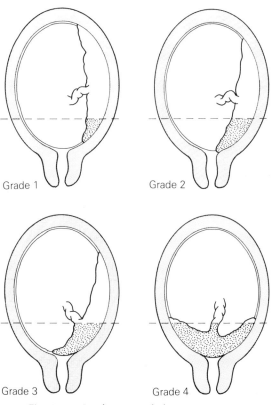

Fig. 9.5   *Grades 1–4 of placenta praevia.*

period with a relatively small, painless antepartum haemorrhage sometimes associated with intercourse, or with an unstable fetal lie. Occasionally, there are no warning signs until there is a brisk haemorrhage during labour. Bleeding from the lower genital tract should be excluded by a speculum examination using a Sims speculum to avoid stretching the vault and lower uterine segment.

Diagnosis

Diagnosis is nowadays by ultrasound, which is extremely accurate at localising the placenta and in determining its position relative to the internal cervical os. There is no place nowadays for other forms of imaging to localise the placenta.

Management

Admission to hospital during the last trimester of pregnancy is considered necessary because of the unpredictability and sometimes catastrophic nature of the haemorrhage. Crossmatched blood must be available at all times. As there is not a large area of placental separation, fetal growth is not usually impaired and pregnancy in the absence of severe haemorrhage may safely continue until 38 weeks. Delivery is usually considered at this time because of the increasing likelihood of the onset of labour with inevitable bleeding. A minor degree of placenta praevia, particularly if the placenta is on the anterior uterine wall, warrants assessment for possible vaginal delivery. An examination under anaesthesia in theatre prepared for immediate lower segment caesarean section will be carried out, followed by either rupture of the membranes and i.v. oxytocin to induce labour, or lower segment caesarean section, depending on the circumstances. For a major degree of placenta praevia, elective caesarean section is mandatory.

Accidental Haemorrhage (Abruptio Placentae)

This can be either revealed, concealed (retroplacental) or both together.

Revealed

This form of haemorrhage implies a variable degree of separation of the placenta with the blood tracking behind it to the vagina. Bleeding is usually painless

and the volume of blood lost probably reflects the extent of placental separation. Admission to hospital is necessary, and a diagnosis is made by exclusion of other causes of bleeding from the lower genital tract. A speculum examination should be carried out, but not a bimanual vaginal examination. Placenta praevia is excluded by ultrasound examination at which time a blood clot behind the placenta may be seen.

Management. If bleeding is not repeated and has been slight, the fetal prognosis is good. The mother can be discharged after a few days, if there has been no further bleeding and the pregnancy can be allowed to continue to 38 or 40 weeks, with a careful watch kept on fetal growth. If bleeding is persistent or repeated, however slight, then there will be increasing areas of placental separation and diminishing placental reserve. Fetal monitoring involving daily fetal cardiotocography and twice weekly ultrasound scans to determine fetal growth is essential. Biochemical monitoring is still favoured by some. The ability to diagnose fetal growth retardation by biochemical tests is limited and they are unable to predict acute fetal hypoxia. If used, they should not be instead of, but in conjunction with, biophysical monitoring. The volume, persistence, or recurrences of the haemorrhage, together with the state of the fetus, will determine the timing of delivery, usually at or before 38 weeks. If the fetus is uncompromised, or unless the bleeding is very heavy, delivery should be vaginally.

Concealed haemorrhage

Blood loss from a concealed antepartum haemorrhage is all retained retroplacentally or is extravasated into the myometrium. Revealed and concealed blood loss can occur from different parts of the placenta, these cases being called mixed antepartum haemorrhage. The aetiology is not clear, but concealed antepartum haemorrhage is more common in women with severe pregnancy induced hypertension when the increased pressure of the blood entering the intervillous space could be of importance. Other associations are with multiparity. Physical forces such as those of an external cephalic version, or after rapid reduction in size of a previously overdistended uterus, can lead to shearing between the placenta and its uterine attachment. Folate deficiency has been suggested as a factor in causing a possible inadequacy of vascular development. Occasionally, abruptio placentae can recur in successive pregnancies.

Diagnosis. The main symptom of concealed antepartum haemorrhage is uterine pain and tenderness, usually of sudden onset and sometimes getting progressively worse as the area of placental separation increases. In mixed cases, the above will occur together with overt vaginal bleeding. Retroplacental clot can be seen ultrasonically. In severe cases, there will be evidence of shock, namely peripheral vasoconstriction, hypertension and sometimes, paradoxically, a normal or slow pulse rate. Shock is due to the pain and to the blood loss. There can be up to 2 litres of blood lost quickly in retroplacental clot and extravasated into the myometrium. In these cases, the uterus is larger than expected, hard and tender. Fetal heart sounds may be absent or, if present, difficult to hear.

Management. In cases where only a very small abruption is diagnosed or where there is doubt about the diagnosis, expectant management in hospital is appropriate. Blood should be crossmatched as a larger haemorrhage may occur unexpectedly. Daily fetal monitoring should be carried out. If there are recurrent small concealed antepartum haemorrhages, delivery is the best option, as sooner or later there will be a large one, with potentially serious fetal and maternal consequences. In moderate or severe cases, delivery as soon as possible is appropriate, as further extension of the haemorrhage may be fatal to the fetus and dangerous to the mother. Shock must be treated promptly with i.v. blood, or plasma if blood is unavailable. Tranfusion should be as rapid as possible to retain normal jugular venous pressure measured by a central venous pressure catheter. Blood loss, particularly in cases of concealed antepartum haemorrhage, is usually underestimated and prolonged hypovolaemia and hypotension will increase fibrinolysis. Disseminated intravascular coagulation can occur due to release of placental thromboplastins into the circulation leading to hypofibrinogenaemia. The clotting time needs quick assessment while awaiting laboratory investigations which comprise measurement of fibrinogen, fibrin degradation products and platelet count. Treatment with i.v. fibrinogen and fresh platelets may be needed but, if blood transfusion is prompt and adequate, the coagulation abnormalities are rare. Urinary output may be impaired, so this must

be watched carefully, usually by means of an indwelling catheter. Prompt correction of hypotension and hypovolaemia will reduce the risks of renal problems. The mode of delivery depends on the circumstances, such as fetal viability, maternal blood pressure, extent of haemorrhage and cervical dilatation. Labour can be quick in such cases, as there are a lot of prostaglandins released from the damaged uterine and placental tissue initiating uterine contractions, but this is a risky approach as there are real dangers of intrauterine death. For most cases with a definite diagnosis, caesarean section is the best method of delivery.

Vasa Praevia

Rarely, antepartum haemorrhage may be slight and consist of fetal blood from rupture of a placental vessel overlying the internal os. This may happen at artificial rupture of the membranes. The umbilical cord may be inserted at the edge of the placenta. If the bleeding is recurrent or severe, the fetus may die from haemorrhage or suffer the effects of prolonged anaemia. Abnormal fetal heart traces, such as marked decelerations or fetal tachycardia, may suggest this type of haemorrhage. The diagnosis is confirmed by carrying out a Kleihauer test to differentiate maternal and fetal red blood cells within the blood lost.

HYDATIDIFORM MOLE

In this abnormal pregnancy, there is no fetus, but only an overgrowth of placental tissue with hydatidiform vesicular changes.

Hydatidiform degeneration of the chorionic villi can occur involving the stroma and blood vessels. The degenerate villi are swollen, due to stromal oedema. They become avascular and the epithelium is thickened over their surface. The chorionic epithelium of some vesicles proliferates. Very occasionally hydatidiform degeneration can occur in a normal placenta and is found more commonly in abortions. When the whole conceptus is involved, it becomes a hydatidiform mole. Depending on the state of the proliferative epithelium, moles can be benign or malignant (choriocarcinoma). There is an intermediate stage of invasive, but histologically non-malignant mole, which involves the myometrium, but does not metastasise. Hydatidiform mole is uncommon in Europe, the incidence being about 0.1%, but in South-East Asia the incidence can be as high as 1%.

Diagnosis

Hydatidiform mole is suspected if the uterus is large for dates, fetal movements are not felt, there is severe hyperemesis, pregnancy induced hypertension occurs before 20–24 weeks, or there is persistent slight bleeding during the first half of pregnancy. Diagnosis is by ultrasound scan when the appearances are very characteristic. Serum β HCG levels may be excessively raised by at least one order of magnitude.

Management

Expulsion of the mole can be induced medically using either oxytocin or prostaglandins. Suction curettage to complete the emptying of the uterus may be needed, but extra care must be taken to avoid perforation and haemorrhage due to uterine softening and atony. Histological assessment of the tissue is essential. Serum or urinary β HCG estimations are carried out for a period of 2 years to ensure complete removal of chorionic tissue and to check against a recurrence in the form of choriocarcinoma. Pregnancy should be avoided during this time. Choriocarcinoma can follow any form of pregnancy. It is a rapidly metastasising tumour, which can present with irregular vaginal bleeding (uterine tumour) or haemoptysis or other pulmonary symptoms (pulmonary secondaries). Diagnosis is by measuring elevated β HCG levels, histological confirmation from curettage or by characteristic cannonball appearances of the pulmonary metastases on chest x-ray. Late metastases can occur in any relatively vascular organ. Treatment is often successful if started early, with rapid elimination of the tumour using methotrexate and folinic acid, or other related cytotoxic agents. Long-term follow-up using urinary β HCG estimations is essential.

HYDRAMNIOS

This is defined as a significant excess of liquor amnii (greater than 1.5 l). The exact causes are unknown, but there may be an increased production of liquor from the membranes or there may be a reduction in its passage through the fetus or both. It can occur in either an acute or chronic form — the latter being the more common. Hydramnios is often found in association with congenital abnormalities in which the fetus cannot swallow, such as anencephaly, oesophageal atresia or severe muscular disorders. It is associated with diabetes and multiple pregnancy, often uniovular, in which case it may be acute. It can occur without any abnormality being detected.

Diagnosis

Diagnosis is made on clinical palpation when the uterus is tense and distended. Fetal parts are hard to feel, and a fluid thrill is present. Ultrasound examination will confirm this. The presence of fetal abnormalities should always be considered in cases of acute or chronic hydramnios. A thorough ultrasound examination of the fetus is very important.

Management

Premature labour due to uterine distension may occur and require treatment with drugs which inhibit myometrial contractions (tocolytic drugs). Amniocentesis to reduce pressure and relieve symptoms is not successful, as the fluid rapidly refills and the procedure may stimulate labour. Bed rest helps the discomfort, but this alone is rarely a cause for preterm delivery. Usually the patient will go into labour or is induced. If the latter, liquor volume should be reduced slowly to reduce the chances of shearing off the placenta and causing an abruptio placentae. After delivery, immediate examination of the baby for possible congenital abnormalities such as oesophageal atresia is very important.

MULTIPLE PREGNANCY

Multiple pregnancy may occur:

1. by the division of an ovum fertilised by one sperm, which then divides at the two-cell stage into two separate cell bodies. Chromatin is common, so twins will be identical.

2. by more than one egg being fertilised by more than one sperm. There is a familial tendency for this to happen. Although they may be of the same sex, these twins will not be identical.

Multiple pregnancies with more than two babies may be a combination of multiple fertilisation and division at the two-cell stage. The incidence of twins in Europe is 1 in 80, triplets 1 in 8000 and quadruplets 1 in 500 000. Multiple pregnancies are more common in some countries such as in Africa. Induction of ovulation using clomiphene or gonadotrophins leads to a higher incidence of multiple pregnancies. The same is true of in vitro fertilisation when often three or more embryos, fertilised in vitro, are replaced into the uterus to improve the chances of a successful pregnancy (*see* Chapter 23). Determination of whether twins are identical or not is difficult. Figure 9.6 depicts a logical scheme for such determination.

Diagnosis

The diagnosis of multiple pregnancy is suspected when the uterus is thought to be larger than

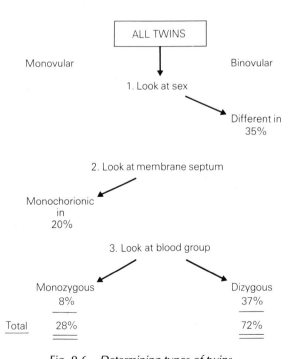

Fig. 9.6   *Determining types of twins.*

expected for the gestational period. Ultrasound scan is usually reliable at determining multiple pregnancies and the advent of routine scans at 16–18 weeks has detected most of these during early pregnancy. There is no role for x-rays in the diagnosis of multiple pregnancy.

Associated Problems

1. *Increased uterine size* and increased venous pressure lead to problems such as varicose veins of the legs and vulva, haemorrhoids and oedema of the legs.
2. *Anaemia* is more common due to the haemopoietic requirements of more than one baby. Iron and folic acid supplements are advisable.
3. *Congenital abnormalities* and *hydramnios* are more common and more often associated with uniovular twins.
4. *Pregnancy induced hypertension* is more common, but the reasons are not yet known. However, some fetal or placental factor may be involved.
5. *Intrauterine growth retardation* is another possible complication of multiple pregnancy. This may be equal in both babies due to inadequate uteroplacental circulation. On the other hand, there may be increased growth of one at the expense of the other twin, which is due to anastamosis of their placental circulations. The larger twin will be hypervolaemic and polycythaemic which may result in heart failure. The growth retarded twin will be correspondingly anaemic, also leading to heart failure in some cases. Regular ultrasound scans are needed to detect this problem and to deliver the babies before it becomes severe.
6. *Preterm labour* is the most important potential complication of multiple pregnancy. Most women with multiple pregnancy will go into spontaneous labour before 38 weeks and a number do so considerably earlier. Prophylactic bed rest or small doses of oral tocolytics do not seem reliable in preventing this. In threatened preterm labour, i.v. β sympathomimetic drugs, such as ritodrine, terbutaline or salbutamol are usually effective for some time. However, once the membranes have ruptured, delivery is usually imminent. For all these reasons more frequent antenatal care is necessary.

Mode of Delivery

Vaginal delivery is appropriate in most cases of twins, unless they present by the breech between 26 and 34 weeks' gestation, or unless there is a malpresentation with the first twin, when caesarean section may give a better fetal outcome. Three or more babies are usually delivered by caesarean section as the risks of malpresentation and obstruction to delivery increase, as do the risks of hypoxia from placental separation or cord compression during prolonged vaginal delivery. The conduct of labour until delivery of the first baby is the same as for a single fetus. After the delivery of the first baby, the lie of the second is checked and, if longitudinal, the membranes are ruptured. Intravenous oxytocin may be needed to expedite delivery of the second twin. If the lie is not longitudinal, an external cephalic version should be carried out before rupturing the membranes and using intravenous oxytocin. Postpartum haemorrhage due to uterine hypotonia is a potential problem, so continuation of intravenous oxytocin for some hours after delivery is advisable.

FETAL ABNORMALITIES

Congenital abnormalities are either genetic or environmental in origin. Major congenital abnormalities occur in about 1.5% of live births and account for a large part of neonatal mortality and morbidity. About one-half of perinatal mortality is currently due to congenital abnormalities: chromosomal disorders account for the majority of congenital abnormalities and disorders of chromosomal number in the autosomal structure account for the majority of these. They account for about three-quarters of chromosomal abnormalities and include trisomy 21, and those of the sex chromosome such as XYY; XXY; XXX; mosaics of these and XO. Disorders of autosomal structure account for about one-quarter of chromosomal abnormalities and include translocation (balanced or unbalanced) or deletion of chromosomes. Single gene disorders include the autosomal dominant conditions such as polycystic renal disease, achondroplasia, Huntingdon's chorea, polydactyly or the autosomal recessive conditions such as cystic fibrosis and β thalassaemia or other in-born errors of metabolism.

Examples of sex linked (X) recessive conditions are muscular dystrophy, mental retardation, haemophilia and Christmas disease and, of course, the most common, red/green colour blindness.

Environmental causes of congenital abnormalities include abnormal hormonal environment, infections, radiation, drugs or biochemical abnormalities induced by the diet. There are definitive examples of (1) hormones, such as testosterone or progestogens, causing virilisation of a female fetus; (2) of infections such as rubella and treponema, causing a variety of structural defects in the fetus; (3) radiation in high doses (50 rads) causing an increased incidence of a number of congenital abnormalities; (4) drugs such as warfarin causing a variety of fetal abnormalities (*see* Chapter 4).

There is no evidence that dietary deficiencies of certain vitamins or essential fatty acids cause congenital abnormalities, although it has been suggested that folic acid and vitamin supplements given from conception reduce the incidence of neural tube defects. Cause and effects are very difficult to prove and, unless there are large numbers of similar defects resulting from a common agent, the evidence will always be anecdotal.

The potential teratogen has to be involved at the critical time of organ development; for example active rubella infection at 6–10 weeks of pregnancy may result in eye or heart abnormalities, while at 16 weeks it is very unlikely to have any effect. Finally, the potential teratogen such as a drug may not act directly, but through an intermediate, metabolic step which could vary from person to person.

The subject is described in more detail in Chapter 4, and the diagnosis of these abnormalities is described in Chapter 7.

RHESUS ISOIMMUNISATION

Of the six main genes involved in the rhesus group, three are dominant and three recessive; these are C, D, E and c, d, e, respectively. A rhesus negative person must, therefore, be homozygus (c, d, e/c, d, e), while heterozygosity leads to being rhesus positive with D being present in any genetic combination. Fetal red cells can enter the maternal circulation at the time of abortion, during pregnancy or delivery, or during the third stage. These antigenic rhesus positive fetal cells may sensitise the mother so that, when there is a further similar stimulus in a subsequent pregnancy, anti-D antibodies will be produced. These cross the placenta causing fetal haemolysis and an increased fetal excretion of bilirubin into the liquor.

Diagnosis

All women have their rhesus and antibody status assessed at booking. A positive antibody titre indicates isoimmunisation, but it is not an accurate guide to the extent to which the fetus is affected. The reason for this is that the placental transfer of antibody from mother to fetus is variable. If the antibody titre is significant (1 in 16 or greater), then the severity of the condition is assessed by estimating the bilirubin content of the liquor collected by amniocentesis at 20 weeks. The higher the liquor content, the more severely the fetus is affected. The amniocentesis is repeated in 2 weeks and the two results plotted on charts prepared to determine the severity of timing of intervention (Fig. 9.7). In moderate or severe cases, the fetus will be anaemic and if severe and prolonged, cardiac failure will occur leading to peripheral oedema (hydrops fetalis). This can be seen on ultrasound or x-ray and is a late sign of severe disease indicating a bad prognosis for the fetus. Moderately affected cases warrant assessment twice weekly by amniocentesis, followed by delivery at the appropriate gestation while, in mildly affected cases, repeated amniocentesis may not be necessary and delivery could be as late as 38 weeks. Moderately affected cases will be delivered usually between 34 and 38 weeks, either by caesarean section or vaginally, depending on individual circumstances. Severely affected babies, if diagnosed before 28 weeks, will require intrauterine transfusion to prevent severe anaemia and its sequelae. O negative blood is injected under ultrasound control into the fetal peritoneal cavity by a needle passed through the maternal and fetal abdominal walls. Direct i.v. transfusion into the umbilical/placental vessels via the fetoscope or under ultrasound control is a better technique, if available. This is repeated twice weekly until the fetus is mature enough to be delivered and withstand the subsequent neonatal exchange transfusions, probably at 32 weeks, although delivery may need to be as early as 30 weeks if intrauterine transfusion is

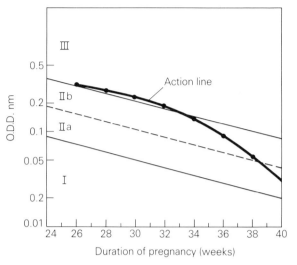

Fig. 9.7   *Optical density difference (O.D.D.) of liquor measured at 450 nm. Zone I = very mildly affected or unaffected fetus; Zone II (a & b) = moderately affected fetus; Zone III = severely affected fetus. When plot of O.D.D. reaches the action line, either intrauterine transfusion or delivery of fetus is required.*

proving difficult. Management in the neonatal period depends on the age of the baby. Phototherapy would commence if the bilirubin levels were 50–60 µmol/l within the first 24 h of life. After 48 h of age, treatment in the form of phototherapy or exchange transfusion is needed if the level reaches 150–350 µmol/l depending on the gestational age at delivery.

Prevention

The injection of anti-D gamma globulin (IgG) to all rhesus negative women after abortions and to those with rhesus positive babies within 48 h of delivery will destroy the fetal Rh positive cells in the maternal circulation and prevent sensitisation. The administration of anti-D gamma globulin during pregnancy has been shown to have some benefit in reducing the risk of immunisation.

FURTHER READING

Creasy R.K., Resnik R., eds. (1984). *Maternal-Fetal Medicine*. pp. 491–678. Philadelphia: Saunders.

Editorial (1986). Aspirin and pre-eclampsia. *Lancet*; **i**:18–20.

Kierse M.J.N.C. (1984). The small baby. In *Clinics in Obstetrics and Gynaecology*, Vol. II, No. 2. (Howie P., Patel N., eds.) pp. 415–36. London: Saunders.

10

Physiology, Mechanisms and Management of Normal Labour

PHYSIOLOGY OF THE UTERUS AND CERVIX

The human uterus is a muscular organ adapted to support the growth of the fetus during pregnancy and then to expel it when the fetus is mature. It is approximately pear-shaped and consists of two main parts, the body (or corpus) and the cervix (*see* Fig. 2.1. p. 9). The body is mostly composed of smooth muscle, comprising up to 90% of the upper segment. The lower segment contains a diminishing proportion of muscle, so that when it merges into the cervix, muscle fibres make up only 10% of the tissue. The remainder is made up of connective tissue with a large admixture of elastic fibres.

The uterus is covered with a layer of peritoneum (the serosa) and lined with a mucosa, the endometrium. The endometrium contains large numbers of glycogen secreting glands which serve to nourish the developing embryo before the development of the placenta.

The blood supply of the uterus is essentially from the uterine and ovarian arteries, derived from the internal iliac arteries and the aorta respectively. They feed a plexus in the myometrium from which a series of arcuate arteries pass up into the endometrium. These short, straight vessels pass through the basal endometrium and give rise to the spiral arteries which, in pregnancy, open into the maternal portion of the placenta (the intervillous space).

Like the smooth muscle of the bowel, uterine muscle is spontaneously contractile. A biopsy specimen, removed and suspended in a physiological solution, will contract every 2–5 min without being stimulated. This spontaneous activity can be suppressed by hormones, notably progesterone and β_2 agonists. It is thought that a major function of the secretion of progesterone in the luteal phase of the menstrual cycle is to suppress uterine activity and prevent the expulsion of a developing blastocyst. Once implantation has taken place, progesterone production is taken over by the placenta. Initially, chorionic villi cover the developing embryo, but by 6 weeks they begin to atrophy, except at the site of the developing placenta. As the conceptus and uterus enlarge, the area of the endometrium increases more rapidly than that of the placenta, and uterine muscle at a distance begins to escape from progesterone suppression. Thus, at between 20 and 24 weeks' gestation, spontaneous uterine contractility starts to reassert itself. At first, contractions are limited to single groups of fibres and produce only small rises in intrauterine pressure ('A' waves). However, as pregnancy progresses, oestrogen levels rise, resulting in the formation of 'gap junctions' between adjacent muscle fibres. These junctions provide low resistance pathways for the conduction of electrical activity from cell to cell and thus promote propagation and synchronisation of uterine activity. When large areas of muscle begin to contract in an organised fashion, they are able to raise intrauterine pressure to levels approaching those seen during menstruation and labour, ranging from 4 to 12 kPa (30–90 mmHg). These are termed 'B' waves which are commonly known as the 'uterine contractions' of labour. Because of the greater concentration of muscle fibres at the fundus, uterine contractions tend to start there and then sweep down the uterus towards the cervix. This is termed 'fundal dominance' and may be physiologically important in the stretching of the lower segment and the dilatation of the cervix during labour. There is some evidence that the insertion of the fallopian tube into the uterus is a common site for the origin of contractions and it is sometimes called the 'cornual pacemaker'.

The 'B' waves which occur during pregnancy are painless, because the cervix is not being dilated (see later discussion on the origin of pain in labour, p. 156). Nevertheless, they slowly stretch the lower segment of the uterus, which becomes elongated and thinned. In the third trimester, it balloons out during contractions, eventually allowing the descent of the presenting part into the pelvis. The contractions may also play a part in changing the consistency of the cervix prior to the onset of labour. Painless contractions occurring before the onset of labour are clinically termed 'Braxton-Hicks', after a 19th-century obstetrician.

The uterine cervix is predominantly composed of collagen and connective tissue with only a little muscle. In the non-pregnant state, the cervix has a firm consistency likened to that of the end of the nose. It usually acts effectively to retain the developing gestation sac within the uterus throughout pregnancy. However, during pregnancy there is a softening process which eventually allows the cervix to stretch up and permit delivery of the fetus, following which it reforms once again. How this remarkable feat is achieved is poorly understood, but it is thought to involve changes in the ground substance, particularly the breakdown of collagen by proteolytic enzymes and alterations in the relative amounts of the glycosaminoglycans, which normally bind the collagen fibrils together. There is also an increase in water content mediated by hyaluronic acid. It is thought that these changes are produced partly by alterations in oestrogen level and partly by other hormones such as prostaglandins. Prostaglandin E_2 is produced in increasing amounts by the amnion, chorion and decidua immediately prior to and during labour. It is known that disturbance of the membranes by vaginal examination in late pregnancy produces considerable transient local prostaglandin release. Relaxin, a hormone produced by the ovary, may also play a part in the cervical softening process (known clinically as 'ripening').

PHYSIOLOGY OF LABOUR

Onset of Labour

The mechanism of the onset of labour in the human is complex and, as yet, incompletely defined. Such evidence as we have points to fetal maturity being the main controlling factor, rather than, for example, parturition being triggered simply by the fetus reaching a particular size. The difficulty lies in discovering which particular fetal signal or signals acts upon the mother to start labour. In some species, such as the sheep, the fetal hypothalamic-pituitary-adrenal axis, in conjunction with the placenta, is clearly in control of the onset of parturition. A sharp increase in fetal cortisol acts on the placenta to reduce progesterone secretion, augment oestrogen production and, perhaps, to increase prostaglandin production. There is some evidence that a similar mechanism may operate in the human in that anencephalics, in whom the pituitary is missing, are more likely to be associated with prolonged gestation than those in whom the hypothalamus and pituitary are present. However, a sharp rise in fetal cortisol associated with the onset of labour has not been demonstrated in the human fetus, and attempts to induce labour with cortisol have met with very limited success. On the other hand, prostaglandins (notably PGE_2) are much more strongly associated with the onset of labour in the human than in many other animal species, and there is accumulating evidence that fetal production of oxytocin from the posterior pituitary is also involved by releasing prostaglandins from the fetal membranes and uterus.

Labour is divided into the first, second and third stages. The first stage begins with the onset of labour and ends when the cervix is fully dilated. The onset of labour is not an acute event, but a steadily accelerating process, whose origins can be traced back to the beginning of Braxton-Hicks contractions. Under their influence, the cervix 'ripens', becoming steadily softer and shorter (the latter is termed 'effacement'). Ripening normally becomes clinically apparent at about 36 weeks' gestation in the primigravida and even earlier in the multigravida, although the length of gestation is not affected by parity. Over the same period, uterine contractions become more frequent and regular, and may also become stronger. Eventually, the cervix begins to dilate progressively. This is the central event defining the onset of labour. The complete regularisation of contractions into the normal labour pattern frequently accompanies the onset of progressive dilatation, but may also precede it by a few hours or, less commonly, even days. Occasionally, the cervix may start to dilate before regular contractions are properly established. It is clear from this that it is often impossible to define a precise time for the onset of labour. The clinical

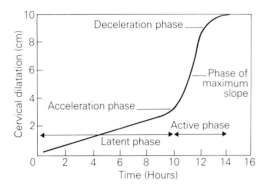

Fig. 10.1   *Latent and active phases of labour.*

aspects of the diagnosis of labour will be dealt with in more detail later in this chapter (p. 145).

First Stage

The first stage is divided into two main phases, the latent phase and the active phase (Fig. 10.1). The latent phase is that period when the cervix is exposed to regular uterine contractions, but is still softening and effacing. Cervical dilatation proceeds slowly, and does not normally reach more than 2–3 cm in this phase, which may last up to 12 h. Once the cervix reaches 3 cm dilatation, full effacement and softening have usually occurred. At this point the rate of cervical dilatation begins to increase (acceleration phase). From 4 to 9 cm the cervix goes through the most rapid rate of dilatation, after which there is often a deceleration phase. The mean rate of cervical dilatation over the whole of the active phase depends on the parity, with primigravidae dilating at a mean rate of about 1 cm per hour and multigravidae at about 1.5 cm per hour. This reflects differences in the cervix and pelvic soft tissues. The maximum rate of dilatation may be considerably more than 1–1.5 cm/h.

Effect of Contractions on Fetal and Placental Blood Flow, and on Oxygenation of the Fetus

The rise in intrauterine pressure during a contraction has no direct effect on the fetal circulation. This is because the whole of the fetal compartment is within the uterus, and thus changes in pressure occur equally at all points. The difference between arterial and venous pressures is, therefore, unchanged and flow is unaltered. The best analogy here is with a diver in a compression chamber whose circulation continues happily despite being exposed to three atmospheric pressures. The only exception to this is when there is direct pressure on a structure; for example cerebral blood flow may be reduced by direct head compression, or umbilical flow may be reduced by direct pressure on the cord if it is prolapsed alongside the head, or wrapped tightly round the neck. In general, the fetus is protected from these effects by the surrounding liquor which, like all fluids, is virtually incompressible. Direct pressure effects are, therefore, most likely during late first stage, as the fetus moves down through the pelvis, and following rupture of the membranes. It must be realised that rupture of the membranes usually releases only a small proportion of the amniotic fluid volume, as the head normally blocks the lower segment like a plug, preventing the escape of the majority of the liquor.

In contrast, the rise in intrauterine pressure during a contraction has a major effect on the circulation through the maternal side of the placenta. This is because the arterial pressure supplying the intervillous space is derived from the maternal circulation outside the uterus, and is therefore not increased by the same amount as the intrauterine pressure during a contraction. Between contractions, intrauterine pressure normally exceeds intra-abdominal pressure by about 1–2 kPa (7.5–15 mmHg). This is known as the 'baseline' or 'resting' tone. Arterial inflow pressure in the spiral arteries is usually about 4–6 kPa, being reduced and evened out by the unique structure of these arteries. Thus a pressure of about 3 kPa provides a steady blood flow through the intervillous space. Too high a pressure or flow rate would tend to dislodge the placenta.

The first event to occur during a contraction is that the rising intramyometrial pressure cuts off the low pressure venous drainage of the intervillous space. The arterial inflow continues, and the maternal pool of blood increases by up to 500 ml, as demonstrated using ultrasound, trapping a large reservoir of oxygenated blood in the placenta. When the intrauterine pressure rises to 4 kPa or more, the arterial inflow is arrested, and the maternal part of the placenta now becomes a closed system. The fetal circulation continues, and oxygen is extracted from the reservoir of maternal blood. Even so, the oxygen supply to the fetus declines

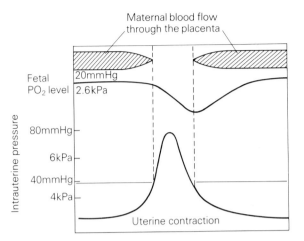

Fig. 10.2 *Effect of uterine contraction on fetal Po₂ level.*

steadily with time as the maternal blood becomes exhausted (Fig. 10.2). This decline continues until the intrauterine pressure once again falls below 4 kPa and fresh maternal blood can enter the placenta. It then takes some time for the oxygen depleted blood to be washed out of the intervillous space, and thus the oxygen supply to the fetus is not restored until about a minute or so after the contraction has worn off. The reduction in fetal oxygen supply resulting from contractions can be demonstrated using transcutaneous oxygen monitoring, and the resulting increase in anaerobic metabolism produces a small, but measurable, decline in fetal pH during labour. These regular episodes of relative hypoxia explain why labour is a stress for all fetuses, and are a particular problem for fetuses without much metabolic reserve (e.g. growth retarded) or with poor placental function

(e.g. after placental abruption). They also explain why an adequate interval between contractions is vital to the well-being of the fetus in labour, being literally a 'breathing space' and why excessively frequent contractions defined as more than one every 2–3 min are very dangerous (Fig. 10.3).

MECHANISMS OF LABOUR

First Stage

Engagement is defined as the descent of the presenting part of the fetus (the head in over 95% of cases) into the cavity of the pelvis. The head is said to be engaged when its widest diameter has passed through the brim. Two important points should be noted. Firstly, the brim is at an angle of 30° to the horizontal in the supine woman (Fig. 10.4). Thus the direction of engagement is backwards towards the mother's sacrum rather than down towards her feet. Secondly, the pelvic brim is normally heart shaped, as shown in Fig. 10.5, with its widest diameter in the transverse. The shape of the fetal head is such that the best fit is obtained in the oblique occipito-anterior (OA) position, and the majority of fetuses present in this way. The left

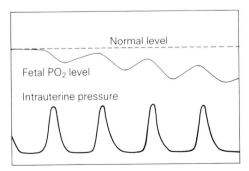

Fig. 10.3 *The effect of excessive frequency of contractions upon fetal oxygenation.*

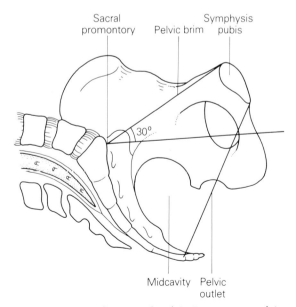

Fig. 10.4 *Lateral view of pelvis in a woman lying supine.*

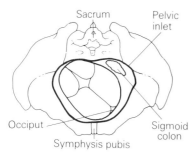

Fig. 10.5   *Relationship between the shape of the fetal head and the shape of the pelvic inlet.*

occipito-anterior position is the most common, possibly because the presence of the sigmoid colon on the left side of the sacrum takes up some of the available space in the other diagonal. It is thought that the fetus selects its position simply by moving about until it settles in the position of 'best fit', rather as a blind person fits together a jig-saw puzzle. This hypothesis is supported by the high rate of malpresentation in disorders which limit fetal movement (fetal abnormality, oligohydramnios) or reduce the pressure pushing the fetus down into the pelvis (polyhydramnios). Engagement can occur as early as 36 weeks in the primigravida, although, in most multigravidae and many primigravidae, it only occurs during the process of labour. In the African pelvis, where the brim is often almost horizontal in the supine woman, engagement may not occur until the second stage.

Once the fetal head has entered the midcavity of the pelvis, it is free to rotate in any direction. At this point, the shoulders encounter the brim. The baby will then move around until the shoulders find the position in which they will best fit into the brim, which is when they are transverse. Because the shoulders have their widest diameter at right angles to the widest diameter of the fetal head, the head is forced to take up a position in the anteroposterior plane (Fig. 10.6). This rotation of the head from the transverse to the OA plane is known as internal rotation. It is most likely to be occipito-anterior, because the shortest distance between the occiput and the neck is down the back of the baby's head, which fits neatly behind the pubic bone, the shortest side of the pelvis. Similarly, the long sloping part of the fetal head from the occiput down over the face fits best into the curve of the sacrum (Fig. 10.7). As the fetus continues to be pushed down by regular uterine contractions, it becomes 'compacted' by flexion of the trunk and neck, so that the vertex now becomes the presenting part, rather than the top of the head. The presenting diameter accordingly becomes the suboccipito-bregmatic rather than the occipito-frontal.

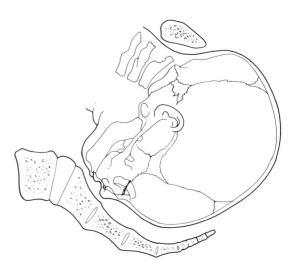

Fig. 10.7   *The fetal face adapts its position to fit into the sacral curve.*

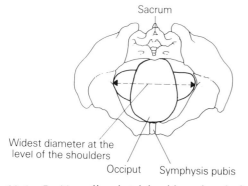

Fig. 10.6   *Position of head and shoulders when the head is in the midcavity and the shoulders are in the brim.*

As the fetus is pushed even further down, its head passes round the curve of the birth canal, extending its neck as it goes. Because of the process of internal rotation, it is in the correct position to pass through the outlet of the pelvis, whose widest diameter is in the OA plane. As the head emerges from the outlet, the shoulders enter the midcavity. They now have to rotate into the OA plane in order to negotiate the outlet. As they move round, the head naturally has to follow. This is known as external rotation. The anterior shoulder is normally the first to deliver, slipping under the symphysis pubis. The posterior shoulder is then born, followed easily by the rest of the body.

The corkscrew motion of the human fetus during delivery is often difficult for students to understand, but the most important point to remember is that the widest diameter of the fetal head is from front to back, while the widest diameter of the shoulders is from side to side. For the pelvis to allow delivery without being unduly wide, with consequential locomotional instability of the pelvis, it is necessary for the inlet and outlet to be separated by the length of the head, from vertex to shoulders, to be oval in shape, and to have their widest diameters at right angles to one another. This means that the head can be negotiating the outlet at the same time that the shoulders are passing through the brim, without twisting the fetus's neck into an impossible position. It is also appropriate for the widest transverse diameter to be at the brim, above the hip joints, rather than at the outlet, where the available transverse diameter is limited by the presence of the legs.

Second Stage

The second stage begins with full dilatation of the cervix, which is traditionally taken to be at 10 cm although, of course, the true dimension will vary with the size of the mother and fetus. It ends with the delivery of the baby. The median (most common) duration of the second stage is 50 min in primigravidae and 20 min in multigravidae.

Third Stage

The third stage of labour is from delivery of the baby to delivery of the placenta. The duration of the spontaneous third stage is about 20–30 min; the widely practised active management reduces this to about 5 min.

Once the fetus has been born, the uterus continues not only to contract, but also to retract. Retraction is a process whereby, following a contraction, the muscle fibres do not return to their previous length, but become progressively shorter. As a result, the internal surface of the uterus is greatly reduced, shearing off the attachment of the

placenta. Bleeding is controlled by the fact that the uterine muscle fibres are arranged in a criss-cross fashion around the perforating vessels supplying the placental bed. The retraction of the muscle fibres compresses the lumina of these vessels, the fibres thus acting as 'living ligatures'. Once the placenta is completely separated, it is squeezed out of the uterus by the continuing retraction of the upper segment. This process is often aided by maternal bearing down.

DIAGNOSIS AND MANAGEMENT OF FIRST STAGE LABOUR

Diagnosis of Onset of Labour

The primary signal that labour is occurring is progressive dilatation of the cervix in response to uterine contractions. There are three clinical signs, which are all related in some degree to this phenomenon.

A show

This is the passage of the plug of mucus which normally helps to seal the cervix during pregnancy against the ingress of infection. It falls out as the cervix begins to dilate, and may sometimes be mixed with a few streaks of blood (more blood than this should always be considered potentially abnormal). However, because cervical ripening occurs from about 36 weeks onwards in primigravidae (and even earlier in multigravidae), the passage of a 'show' often precedes active labour by many hours, and sometimes days. The diagnosis of labour should, therefore, never be made on the basis of a show alone.

Regular painful contractions

As previously mentioned, coordinated uterine activity can be demonstrated from about 24 weeks' gestation onwards. Normally, however, contractions only become painful once the cervix starts to dilate. The onset of regular, painful contractions is, therefore, an important indirect indicator that cervical dilatation is taking place. However, because women's pain thresholds vary, and the onset of labour is often not abrupt but can take place over several days, irrevocable clinical actions such as artificial rupture of the membranes should not be undertaken without evidence of appropriate cervical dilatation obtained by vaginal examination.

Spontaneous rupture of the membranes (SRM)

In about 10% of pregnancies, SRM is the first sign that labour is starting. Contractions and progressive cervical dilatation will follow within 24 h in 80% of cases. In the remaining 20%, there is a small risk of amniotic fluid infection occurring, usually with organisms derived from the vaginal flora. This can affect the fetus, causing intrauterine pneumonia and even septicaemia. For this reason, most obstetric units have a policy that labour should be augmented with oxytocics, if contractions do not commence within a specified time.

An urgent vaginal examination is sometimes recommended to exclude cord prolapse with SRM. However, in the absence of malpresentation, this is extremely rare and can effectively be excluded by a normal cardiotocograph (CTG) tracing.

In most cases, if membranes are intact at the onset of labour, they will rupture spontaneously as labour progresses. Some obstetric units have a policy of routine artificial rupture of membranes (ARM) at 4 cm dilatation. This has the advantage that meconium staining of the liquor can be detected, and a direct electrode can be applied to the fetus for CTG monitoring. It also promotes contractions in labours, where these are not yet fully established. Against this, many women feel ARM to be an unwarranted intrusion upon the normal progress of labour. Each case must, therefore, be dealt with on its merits.

Management

As explained above, the only irrefutable evidence that labour is established is progressive cervical dilatation. In all other cases, the diagnosis must be considered carefully before irrevocable action, such as ARM, is undertaken to avoid inappropriate induction of labour. The following procedures should help to clarify the situation where there is doubt.

Spontaneous rupture of membranes

A speculum examination, usually with a Cuscoe's speculum, is important to confirm that SRM has

actually occurred. Often the diagnosis is clear, and copious liquor containing white specks of vernix can be seen flowing through the cervix. Sometimes, however, the history is equivocal and, on examination, only a little or even no fluid is seen in the vagina. Asking the woman to cough may produce a spurt of liquor from the cervix. Sometimes, nitrazine sticks are used to test the pH of the vagina. At the normal vaginal pH of <5, the indicator is yellow, but it turns blue-green when the pH rises above 6.5. Because the pH of liquor is above 7, if the sticks turn black, it suggests the presence of liquor in the vagina. However, local infections due to organisms such as *Gardnerella* are also associated with a raised pH, and contamination with maternal urine can also produce this colour change. In doubtful cases, where there are no epidemiological risk factors for infection, and the cervix is unfavourable, it may be better to take a high vaginal swab (HVS) to check for the presence of potentially pathogenic organisms, such as beta haemolytic streptococci, and do nothing further if these are not found, rather than intervene with oxytocics and risk a failed induction of labour.

Contractions with an unfavourable cervix

The favourability of the cervix is normally described using the Bishop score (Fig. 10.8), published by E.H. Bishop in 1964 and devised by him to predict the outcome of induced labour. If the score is less than 4, 40% of induced labours in primigravidae will end in caesarean section for prolonged labour. In general, if the membranes are intact, it is unwise to intervene in labour (e.g. by ARM or the administration of oxytocics) if the Bishop score is

BISHOP SCORE				
CERVIX	0	1	2	3
Dilatation	0	1–2	3–4	5–6
Consistency	Firm	Medium	Soft	–
Canal lengths cm	>2	1–2	0.5–1	<0.5
Position	Posterior	Mid	Anterior	–
Station	–3	–2	–1, 0	+1 +2

Fig. 10.8   *Bishop score.*

less than 7. This applies even if the woman appears distressed with her contractions, since subsequent measurement of intrauterine pressure often shows that these women have weak contractions with a low pain threshold. It is better to assess the condition of the fetus carefully with CTG and to provide emotional support, and sometimes analgesia, to the mother. The active phase of labour normally starts at a Bishop score of 11, with the cervix 4 cm or more dilated and, if associated with contractions, it is then safe to diagnose labour.

Monitoring of labour progress

In current practice, a partogram is almost invariably used to monitor the progress of labour. This is a chart on which all the observations made in labour are recorded, its focal point being a graphical representation of the rate of cervical dilatation. Prior to 1970, it was common for labours to continue for many hours before recognition that adequate progress of cervical dilatation was not being made. Labours sometimes lasted several days with all the attendant risks of infection, progressive fetal asphyxia and maternal exhaustion. The pioneering work of Philpott in Zimbabwe, Studd in England, and O'Driscoll in Eire led to the concept of the 'active management of labour'. This philosophy involves regular monitoring of labour progress, allowing early intervention by oxytocin infusion or caesarean section, as appropriate, to prevent unduly prolonged labour. Current evidence suggests that failure of the Bishop score to improve by at least one point per hour in the latent phase, or of the cervix to dilate by at least 1 cm every hour in multigravidae or every two hours in primigravidae should be considered abnormal, and augmentation of labour by oxytocin infusion should be considered.

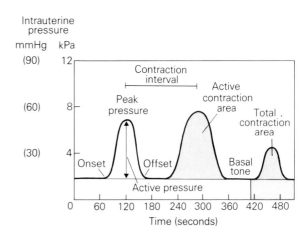

Fig. 10.9 *Terminology used when describing uterine contractions. Active pressure = peak pressure minus basal tone; active contraction area = area under contraction curve, but above basal tone; uterine activity integral (UAI) = active contraction area measured over a period of 15 min; kPa (kilo Pascal) = S.I. unit of pressure (13.3 kPa = 100 mmHg); kPas (kilo Pascal seconds) = S.I. unit of UAI (i.e. units of pressure × time).*

Augmentation of labour

The basic terminology of the description of uterine contractions is shown in Fig. 10.9. Mean values for the various parameters are shown in Table 10.1, as are the values below which it is generally agreed that slow progress is likely and oxytocin augmentation is warranted. Oxytocin is a potentially dangerous drug in that an overdose can cause prolonged and excessively frequent contractions, which will asphyxiate the fetus. In the multigravid patient, excessive contractions may cause the uterus to rupture. Oxytocin is structurally related to ADH, and having an antidiuretic action, it can

Table 10.1

Normal Values for Uterine Contractions

Measurement	Mean values (SD)	Lower limit below which augmentation with oxytocin is indicated
Frequency	3 per 10 min (1)	1.5 per 10 min
Active pressure	5 kPa (1.3)	3 kPa
	40 mmHg (10)	25 mmHg
Montevideo units	140 (65)	90
kPas/15 min	1100 (333)	700

cause water retention. In association with excessive i.v. fluid administration, fits can occur due to water intoxication. An increase in neonatal jaundice due to oxytocin has also been reported by many workers when large amounts have been used. Ideally, therefore, the need for and the response to oxytocin stimulation should be monitored using an intra-uterine catheter, in the same way that a hypotensive drug is monitored by measuring the blood pressure. However, due to lack of equipment and staff trained in its use, most obstetric units cannot do this. They must, therefore, rely on careful clinical monitoring of contractions and on observation of fetal con-dition, preferably by CTG. Clinical monitoring of contractions can be difficult; for example if the woman is obese, and studies show that observers' impressions of the intensity of contractions are often related more to the parturient's reaction to labour than to the true intrauterine pressure. Clinical monitoring, therefore, depends heavily on measur-ing contraction frequency and, unfortunately, this is poorly related to overall uterine activity. The major factor in determining the rate of cervical dilatation is the active pressure of contractions. Nevertheless, prevention of excessively frequent contractions, defined as more than 4 in 10 min, is an important safeguard for fetal oxygenation.

Intravenous oxytocin infusion is normally com-menced at a rate of 1–2 mU/min, and increased every 15–30 min until adequate uterine activity is achieved. It is unusual for more than 8 mU/min to be required, and once normal contractions are established, the infusion rate can often be consider-ably reduced or even discontinued. Oral and vaginal prostaglandin administration for the aug-mentation of labour have been investigated but appear to be more unpredictable in their efficacy. They do have the advantage of allowing the patient to be ambulant.

Maternal condition should be monitored carefully during labour, with measurement of pulse rate, blood pressure and temperature every hour (more often if abnormal). Urine output and fluid intake should also be charted.

MANAGEMENT OF SECOND STAGE LABOUR

Recent years have seen a major change in the approach to the management of the second stage.

Longitudinal studies of fetal acid-base status are all agreed that there is a slow decline in fetal pH in the first stage of labour, due to the mild hypoxia produced by contractions. This continues unchanged once full dilatation has occurred, but accelerates once maternal bearing down com-mences. Because of fears for fetal well-being, the practice grew up that, if the second stage, diagnosed from full dilatation, lasted longer than 30 min in a multigravida or 60 min in a primigravida, delivery should be expedited artificially. However, this practice has recently been widely modified to take into account two new factors: firstly, use of epidural anaesthesia and regular vaginal examination have resulted in the diagnosis of the second stage well before it would be reasonable to expect the mother to bear down; secondly, the use of CTG has enabled the accoucheur to be more objective about the diagnosis of 'fetal distress', and the second stage can be allowed to continue so long as there is no sign of fetal asphyxia and descent of the head continues. If it becomes evident that progress has stopped, or the mother becomes exhausted, a thorough search for the cause should be made. One or more of the following causes should be sought:

1. An overfull bladder or, rarely, rectum.
2. Malposition of fetus — commonly occipito-posterior or transverse or even, rarely, a malpresentation.
3. Too small a pelvis or a contracted outlet with a narrow subpubic angle and prominent ischial spines.
4. Inability of mother to push effectively.

The use of epidural anaesthesia has trebled the forceps rate in many units where it is used.

In most cases of halted labour, or prolonged labour, forceps or vacuum extraction offer a suit-able solution: caesarean section may be necessary if there is significant disproportion or fetal asphyxia. Operative delivery is covered in detail in Chapter 11.

MANAGEMENT OF THIRD STAGE LABOUR

If allowed to occur spontaneously, the placenta takes about 30 min to deliver. During this process, there is blood loss from the uterus, before the 'living ligatures' are fully effective. In about 10% of cases, this will exceed 500 ml and be by definition a 'primary postpartum haemorrhage' which is loss of >500 ml within 24 h of delivery. To prevent this blood loss, ergometrine, 0.25 or 0.5 mg, or more commonly 'syntometrine' (0.5 mg ergometrine and 5 iu oxytocin) used to be given i.m. or i.v. However, this produced a rapid and prolonged tonic contraction of the uterus, and unless averting action was taken, such a contraction could trap the placenta in the uterus, where it could be retained and would require 'manual removal'. The practice of 'active management' has, therefore, been developed whereby the placenta is withdrawn by careful traction on the cord as soon as separation is evident, care being taken to prevent invertion of the uterus by suprapubic pressure. Active management is the usual practice in most developed countries.

Complications of the Third Stage

Retained placenta

This may occur if the placenta is morbidly adherent to the uterus, or if the cord is pulled off due to excessive traction. The management plan that should be followed is:

1. Set up an i.v. infusion if one is not already in place.
2. Take blood and arrange for 2 units to be crossmatched.
3. Call an anaesthetist.

Do *not* attempt to remove the placenta until the anaesthetist has arrived and the blood is ready, as such an attempt may precipitate a severe haemorrhage. If bleeding is more than slight, it can usually be controlled by an i.v. infusion of oxytocin (10 units per litre at 30 drops per minute). When everything has been prepared, the operator should 'scrub up' and clean the perineum. The bladder should be catheterised and a gentle vaginal examination performed, as in many cases the placenta will have separated spontaneously and be lying in the vagina, in which case it can be delivered without further ado. If not, the woman is then given an anaesthetic. If an epidural is already in place, it may be appropriate to top this up, but some anaesthetists prefer general anaesthesia in this situation, because it is quicker, and more suitable should some further serious complication occur, requiring hysterectomy. The cervix is then dilated manually with the hand in a funnel shape and the placenta sheared off with the fingers, grasped and withdrawn.

Postpartum haemorrhage

This is usually due to uterine atony, which nearly always responds to oxytocin or $PGF_{2\alpha}$. If it does not, hysterectomy may very rarely be necessary. If haemorrhage continues despite a well contracted uterus, an assiduous search for lacerations in the genital tract must be made. Lithotomy position, good anaesthesia and a good light are all prerequisites for this manoeuvre.

LABOUR AND THE FETUS

The fetus is adapted in many ways to the relative hypoxia of the intrauterine environment. For example, the dissociation curve of fetal haemoglobin is shifted to the left compared with adult haemoglobin, which allows the effective delivery of oxygen at partial pressures much lower than in the adult. This is necessary because the fetus obtains its oxygen via its mother, rather than directly from the atmosphere, and operates at an arterial Po_2 of 3–4 kPa rather than the normal adult value of 12–14 kPa. This shift results in the preferential transfer of oxygen from the maternal blood to fetal blood across the placental interface and also means that significant amounts of oxygen are held in reserve in fetal haemoglobin even when the Po_2 falls as low as 1–1.5 kPa.

The low Po_2 at which the fetus lives has many important secondary effects. For example, it maintains the patency of the ductus arteriosus, which acts like a shunt allowing blood to bypass the lungs, which are not yet functional. It is also thought to maintain a high level of cerebral endorphins ('endogenous morphines'), a phenomenon also seen in severely hypoxic adults. A powerful action of endorphins is the suppression of breathing reflexes, an action also seen with 'synthetic endorphins' such as pethidine. The fetus does make some breathing movements *in utero* which are important in the proper development of the lungs, but these are sporadic and interspersed with long periods of apnoea. In labour, the further reduction of Po_2 produced by uterine contractions effectively abolishes regular fetal respiratory movement, replacing it with intermittent gasping. This gasping is important at delivery, since the rapid rise in Po_2 produced by gasping and expansion of the lungs switches off the production of endorphins and allows the establishment of regular respiration.

Endorphins may also play a part in regulating the cerebral state of the fetus. Ultrasound study of fetal heart rate and activity patterns, coupled with EEG recordings during labour, suggest that the fetus spends less than 5% of its time in a state which in the adult we would term 'awake'. Most of its time is, therefore, spent in various forms of 'sleep'. In view of the very limited environmental stimulation available to the fetus, this would seem to be an appropriate adaptation. Initially, there is no differentiation within the sleep state, but from about 30–32 weeks' gestation upwards, periods of 'active' sleep become distinguishable from periods of 'quiet sleep'. In quiet sleep, fetal activity is at a minimum. In active sleep, there is considerable fetal movement, usually associated with increased heart rate variability and accelerations in fetal heart rate. 'Rapid eyeball movements', which are associated with dreaming in the adult, can also be demonstrated. Fetal breathing movements are also more in evidence. Active and quiet sleep alternate at intervals of between 20 and 40 min and the transition between them is often abrupt. These alternating periods continue during labour and appreciating them is vital to the clinical interpretation of CTG traces.

Fetal Monitoring in Labour

In order to understand the analysis of fetal heart rate (FHR) patterns, it is necessary to appreciate how they are produced, using a cardiotocograph machine.

In such a machine, signals representing cardiac action, either electrical (the 'R' wave of cardiac depolarisation) or ultrasound (Doppler signals representing cardiac movement) are used to measure the duration of the cardiac cycle. This measurement is correctly expressed in milliseconds. However, clinical measurement of heart rate has traditionally been by counting the number of beats in a given interval, usually one minute. In order to convert the measurement of cardiac cycle length into a figure readily understood by clinical personnel, it has become customary to programme the CTG machine to divide the measurement in milliseconds into 60 000 (one minute), thus obtaining the rate which would be counted if that interval

continued unchanged for the next minute. For example, a beat-to-beat interval (one cardiac cycle) of 500 ms is equivalent to a heart rate of 120 beats per minute (bpm); one of 333.3 ms is approximately equivalent to 180 bpm, etc. In practice, of course, the fetal heart rate does not beat with such regularity, there normally being a variation of 0.4–1.2 bpm between beats, this being defined as the beat-to-beat variation. The significance of this has been studied for many years, but at present its clinical implication is obscure. Because of this, the normal CTG machine uses a chart recording system, which is not designed to demonstrate beat-to-beat variation, but rather the more gross fluctuations in rate known as baseline variability, accelerations and decelerations. The chart recorder is by convention operated at a paper speed of 1 (UK) or 3 (USA) cm per minute. The terminology used in normal CTG analysis is shown in Fig. 10.10.

Baseline rate

This is the lowest rate to which the fetal heart rate consistently returns. It is normally between 120 and 160 bpm. A rate slower than this is called bradycardia and a faster rate is called tachycardia.

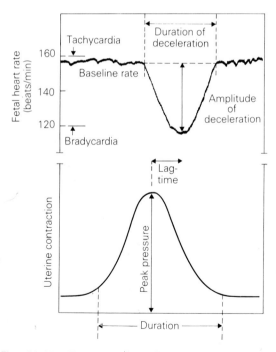

Fig. 10.10   *Terms used in the study of continuous records of FHR.*

Baseline variability

This consists of oscillations in rate which normally range between 5 and 15 bpm (Fig. 10.11). There are usually about 2–5 oscillations per minute. They reflect the fine adjustments of heart rate produced by the autonomic nervous system in response to fluctuations in the fetal environment.

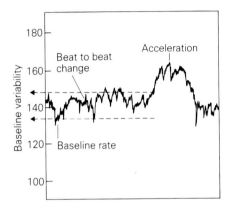

Fig. 10.11 *Beat-to-beat variation and baseline variability.*

Accelerations

Accelerations are increases in rate of more than 15 bpm which last for more than 15 s. They are usually associated with fetal movement, as both occur mostly in active sleep.

Decelerations

Decelerations are decreases in rate of more than 15 bpm for more than 15 s. There are two main types of deceleration.

Reflex decelerations are neurologically mediated via the vagus nerve. They are most often produced by head or cord compression. Head compression raises intracranial pressure. This activates the baroceptor mechanisms, which normally control intracranial pressure by regulating the pressure of the blood supply; blood pressure is, therefore, reduced via a vagally mediated bradycardia. Cord compression cuts off 25% of the fetal peripheral circulation producing a dramatic rise in peripheral resistance. Blood pressure rises as a consequence, and stretch receptors in the aorta act via the vagus nerve to produce bradycardia, limiting the rise in pressure. Both head and cord compression normally occur only during contractions. The resulting decelerations, therefore, occur synchronously with the contraction, with the nadir of the deceleration being at the peak of the contraction.

Hypoxic decelerations usually occur only if the Po_2 in fetal arterial blood falls below 1–1.8 kPa. At these levels, lactate produced in the myocardium has a direct effect to reduce FHR. The pattern of reduction in rate follows the Po_2 level, usually reaching a nadir at, or after, the end of a contraction (*see* Fig. 10.3). These decelerations are therefore delayed, or late, with respect to the contraction.

Techniques of monitoring the fetal heart

External FHR monitoring uses ultrasound (approximately 2.5 MHz) which is beamed from a piezo-electric transmitter towards the fetal heart. The movement of the heart alters the frequency of the reflected sound (Doppler effect), which is detected via a piezoelectric receiver. The transmitter and one or more receivers are usually combined in a single transducer. Air, which transmits ultrasound poorly, is excluded from the transducer-skin interface by a coupling medium, usually arachis oil or a proprietary gel. The Doppler signal, which reflects fetal heart activity, is used to trigger a rate meter and the rate is recorded continuously on a chart recorder. The signal is rather diffuse and, therefore, difficult to time, and so most CTG machines use various technical 'tricks', such as 'three beat averaging', to produce an interpretable trace. However, it should be noted that this produces a recording which is different in detail from a simultaneous trace produced using the R wave of the fetal ECG as a trigger for the rate meter. The fetal ECG can be detected from two electrodes placed on the mother's abdomen, but the signal strength is often poor and heavily contaminated with the maternal ECG and EMG noise. In labour, therefore, it is usually derived from an electrode placed directly onto the presenting part of the fetus, whose voltage is compared with an electrode in the maternal vagina. This technique usually produces a very clear and easily interpreted tracing, and, unlike ultrasound, recording is relatively insensitive to disturbance by maternal or fetal movement. The major disadvantage of using a direct electrode for electronic fetal heart rate monitoring (EFHRM) is that it requires the membranes to be ruptured. However, there are no proven deleterious effects of membrane rupture on the fetus other than an apparently innocuous increase in the incidence of synchronous decelerations due to head compression. In addition, ARM may speed desultory labour by encouraging contractions, and it also allows inspection of the liquor for the presence of meconium.

Techniques of monitoring contractions

The easiest method of recording contractions is to use an external 'tocodynamometer' or strain gauge. However, this instrument can only record accurately the frequency of contractions; relative intensity is also registered, but the true intrauterine pressure (IUP) cannot be measured reliably per abdomen. Thus the technique is satisfactory if the contractions only need to be recorded as an aid to interpretation of the FHR trace. If the true IUP needs to be measured to investigate slow labour or to allow accurate control of an oxytocin infusion, then an intrauterine catheter must be used, which usually requires that the membranes be ruptured. Two types are available: an open-ended fluid-filled catheter connected to an external pressure transducer, and a closed catheter with a pressure transducer mounted on its tip, so that the transducer is inserted into the uterine cavity. The latter system is easier to use and less subject to artefact, but can be expensive if the sensitive transducers are damaged frequently by careless use.

It can be seen from the above that for most routine monitoring, the external system of ultrasound FHR and tocodynamometer contraction recording is satisfactory but, in high risk cases, the more precise and reliable internal electrodes and transducers are preferable.

Normal traces. Fig. 10.12 shows normal baseline rate, variability and reactivity and the absence of decelerations.

If these criteria are fulfilled, the likelihood of a baby being born in poor condition (5 min Apgar score <7) is less than 2%. A baseline rate between 100 and 120 with no other abnormality can be considered normal (uncomplicated baseline bradycardia). Early decelerations (synchronous decelerations less than 40 bpm) with no other abnormality can also be considered normal in advanced labour, but should be considered as suspicious in early

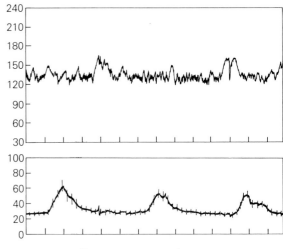

Fig. 10.12   *Normal trace.*

labour as they may indicate cord compression. Larger decelerations with no late component, and normal baseline rate and variability, can also be considered normal in the second stage of labour, as they are often due to head compression during descent through the pelvis.

Suspicious traces. These are defined as such when one or two of the descriptive components of the CTG are abnormal.

There are many permutations of the suspicious trace, and their implications are often different. However, some of the more commonly observed abnormalities are:

1. *Uncomplicated baseline tachycardia*, greater than 160 beats per minute with normal baseline variability and no decelerations, may be normal in some very preterm fetuses. This pattern is often associated with maternal pyrexia, which may be relatively harmless due to a hot room or interference with maternal sweating from epidural anaesthesia, but more seriously may be due to intrauterine infection. An uncomplicated baseline tachycardia may also represent the earliest sign of asphyxial stress and should, therefore, be investigated carefully.
2. *Uncomplicated loss of variability* may be physiological or due to drugs such as pethidine, diazepam or nitrous oxide (Fig. 10.13). However, it may be due to asphyxia and should, therefore, always be investigated if it persists for longer than 40 min.

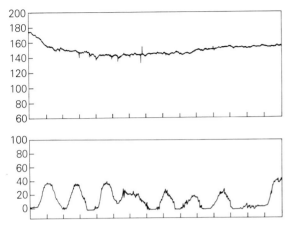

Fig. 10.13 *Uncomplicated loss of variability.*

3. *Uncomplicated variable decelerations* of >40 bpm with variable shape and timing most commonly reflect cord compression, usually due to cord entanglement around limb, body or neck, but occasionally indicate prolapse of the cord. They can also be produced by severe head compression. Acute problems with cord occlusion during delivery may occur. This pattern does not initially indicate asphyxia, but asphyxia may develop if the cord compression interferes significantly with fetal circulation.

4. *Late decelerations* always indicate fetal hypoxia, but this may be relatively mild and temporary, and many normal fetuses can tolerate mild asphyxia for several hours without coming to

serious harm. Nevertheless, when late decelerations are seen, attempts should always be made to identify the cause of the hypoxia and correct it. Common causes of reversible hypoxia are the supine position, uterine hyperstimulation with oxytocin and epidural hypotension. If late decelerations persist, further investigation is necessary (Fig. 10.14).

Abnormal traces. At least three, and sometimes all, of the descriptive components of the CTG are abnormal. This is very serious and carries with it up to a 50% risk of fetal acidosis and a 20% risk of a 5 min Apgar score <7. Such traces should be uncommon in modern practice, since they usually progress from normal traces through one of the milder abnormalities described above. Corrective action to relieve the cause of the abnormality or to deliver the fetus should, therefore, usually prevent the appearance of a severely abnormal trace.

The most common severely abnormal trace is a non-reactive tachycardia accompanied by decelerations (late or variable) (Fig. 10.15). If there is also loss of variability, then the trace is likely to be preterminal (the fetus is dying) and, even with prompt delivery, the risk of long-term neurological handicap is significant. It is followed by a fixed baseline bradycardia as the fetus actually dies.

Factors modifying the interpretation of the CTG

The predictive value of the CTG tracing taken alone is relatively low. For example, even using a

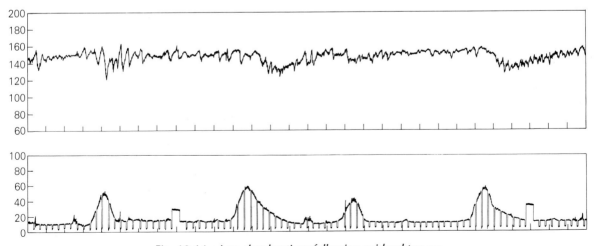

Fig. 10.14 *Late decelerations following epidural top-up.*

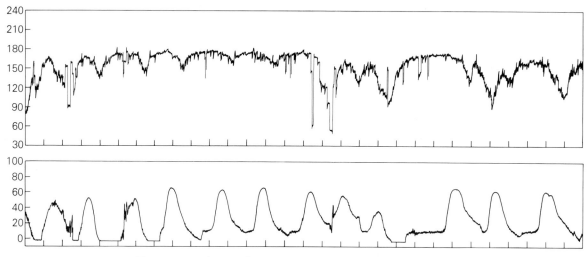

Fig. 10.15   *Abnormal trace showing non-reactive tachycardia.*

short-term measure of neonatal outcome, such as a 1 min Apgar score <7, only about 30% of fetuses with a suspicious trace will have an abnormal outcome, compared with about 10% if the trace is normal. Even if the CTG is severely abnormal, the predictive value only rises to about 50%. The predictive value of the CTG can, however, be improved if it is interpreted in conjunction with other indicators, such as meconium staining of the liquor, growth status of the baby, and pH of a fetal blood sample (FBS).

Meconium staining of the liquor. The passage of meconium by the fetus is a reflex response to stress which matures with age. Fetuses <34 weeks almost never pass meconium unless the bowel is directly irritated; for example, by infection with *Listeria monocytogenes*. On the other hand, one-third of fetuses of >42 weeks' gestational age will pass meconium in response to the normal stress of labour. It is, therefore, often a normal physiological event and, in the presence of a normal CTG, does not predict an abnormal neonatal outcome. How-ever, excessive stress does increase the likelihood of meconium passage, and the combination of an abnormal CTG and meconium staining of the liquor, therefore, has an enhanced predictive value of about 40%.

Intrauterine growth retardation (IUGR). Many studies have shown that babies weighing less than the fifth centile, corrected for sex, gestational age and birth order, are more susceptible to the effects of asphyxia than normally grown infants. The reasons for this are complex and not properly understood at the present time. Fortunately, a normal CTG in labour is just as predictive of normality in the growth retarded fetus as in the normally grown fetus. An abnormal trace, however, is almost twice as likely to be associated with an abnormal outcome in a growth retarded fetus com-pared with one that is normally grown. Moreover, the decline in pH in response to asphyxia is more rapid in the growth retarded infant. IUGR which is suspected on clinical, ultrasound or biochemical grounds before labour is, therefore, an important factor to be taken into account when interpreting the CTG trace.

Fetal blood sampling and pH measurement

CTG analysis is a screening technique, and cannot of itself quantify the effects of a stress on the fetus. If asphyxia is suspected, then the effects of this on the fetus should be quantified by taking a FBS for pH (and, if possible, blood gas) analysis. The scalp (or buttock in a breech presentation) is visualised via a metal tube called an amnioscope. This procedure cannot be performed if the cervix is less than 2 cm dilated. Ethyl chloride is sprayed on to cool the skin, following which a reactive hyperaemia occurs. This encourages the bleeding produced by piercing the skin with a 2 mm guarded blade mounted on a special holder. The blood is encouraged to form a discrete droplet by smearing the skin with silicone grease before the puncture is made. The blood is then drawn up into a preheparinised capillary tube, which is used to transfer the blood to a suitable blood gas/pH analyser.

The main objective of pH analysis of a FBS is to determine the degree of metabolic acidosis which has occurred as a result of asphyxial stress. Measurement of P_{CO_2} and base deficit helps to exclude the effects of transitory respiratory acidosis. If only pH measurement is available, then care should be taken not to take a FBS after an acute event when CO_2 is likely to be elevated.

The normal fetus has a pH between 7.30 and 7.45, a P_{O_2} between 3 and 4 kPa, a P_{CO_2} between 4 and 5 kPa and a base deficit less than 6 mmol/l. A pH between 7.25 and 7.30 suggests a stressed fetus, but is not dangerous in the short term. A pH between 7.20 and 7.25 is definitely abnormal, and operative delivery should be considered if spontaneous delivery is not imminent. A pH below 7.20 represents an emergency, and a pH below 7.15 in association with an abnormal CTG trace is likely to be associated with severe asphyxia in greater than 50% of cases and carries a concomitant risk of permanent neurological damage.

There is no doubt that use of CTG monitoring without a fetal blood sample results in an increase in the caesarean section rate, as operative delivery is undertaken in cases where the CTG is abnormal, but the outcome shows that the fetus was not, in fact, significantly asphyxiated. Even with the most abnormal CTG, a complicated baseline tachycardia, the likelihood of finding a significant metabolic acidosis on FBS is only about 50%. Unfortunately, FBS requires a level of equipment and staffing which is only available in about 20% of obstetric units

Risks Facing the Fetus in Labour

Asphyxia

At one time, asphyxia accounted for about 80% of all 'fetal distress' in labour. However, current studies have shown that, with careful management, this can be reduced to about 40%. Even so, asphyxia remains the most common single cause of distress. Asphyxia is biochemically defined as the combination of hypoxia, hypercarbia (raised CO_2 concentration) and acidosis. The earliest manifestation of reduced oxygen supply to the fetus is hypoxaemia which, if prolonged, will eventually lead to metabolic acidosis as lactate from anaerobic respiration accumulates. If the interference with oxygenation is acute and severe, it is usually accompanied by hypercarbia, which produces respiratory acidosis. The fall in pH due to hypercarbia can be reversed rapidly if gas exchange is restored, unlike the more persistent metabolic acidosis. Chronic asphyxia can be caused by inadequate placental function and may, therefore, be associated with intrauterine growth retardation. This combination is doubly dangerous, because the growth retarded fetus's ability to cope with asphyxia is often severely compromised. Acute asphyxia can be caused by events such as placental abruption or cord prolapse, or by iatrogenic insults such as maternal hypotension secondary to epidural anaesthesia or the supine position, and uterine hyperstimulation with oxytocics.

Trauma

The most obvious form of trauma is that which can be inflicted upon the fetus during delivery. For example, during injudicious vaginal breech delivery, the fetus is at risk of trauma to the limbs, visceral trauma, particularly rupture of the liver, traction injury to the brachial plexus, and intracranial injury, such as tentorial tears and intraventricular haemorrhage. Intracranical injury can also occur as a result of forceps delivery, particularly rotational forceps. The risk of intracranial damage is potentiated if there is cerebral oedema secondary to asphyxia, because the brain is 'stiff' and cannot cope normally with deforming forces. A less obvious form of trauma is due to severe and prolonged head compression; for example where there is cephalopelvic disproportion. This can be detected by assessing 'moulding' of the fetal head. If the sutures of the fetal skull are pressed closely together, there is said to be one '+' of moulding. If the sutures overlap, but can be reduced by finger pressure, the moulding is '++', and if it is irreducible, there is '+++' moulding. Prolonged severe head compression can lead to neonatal cerebral malfunction and should, therefore, be avoided. Moulding should not be confused with caput, which is simply oedema of the presenting part, and is much more common.

Meconium aspiration

The passage of meconium by the fetus in labour is not necessarily abnormal (*see* p. 154). However, when combined with gasping produced by asphyxia, it can lead to the inhalation of meconium with a resulting severe pneumonitis.

Infection

This is an uncommon, but potentially very serious, risk. It is associated with prolonged rupture of the membranes, and the presence of potentially pathogenic organisms in the vagina, such as beta haemolytic streptococci. The risk is increased if an excessive number of vaginal examinations are performed. The baby may be born with pneumonia or even septicaemia. The mother may also become ill from endometritis or septicaemia. A pyrexia or fetal tachycardia should always alert the accoucheur to the possibility of infection, which should be investigated with appropriate cultures, and if necessary treated with a suitable antibiotic.

Ventilation

Failure to establish proper ventilation after delivery is another risk. Delivery normally induces reflex expansion of the chest, filling the lungs with air and causing a rapid rise in arterial Po_2. This, in turn, produces closure of the ductus arteriosus and the establishment of the adult pattern of circulation. This reflex may be inadequately developed, for example in the preterm fetus, or suppressed, for example by drugs such as narcotics or general anaesthetics. In severe asphyxia, the fetus may already have passed the point at which it is capable of responding to delivery by taking a breath. In all these circumstances, which are mostly predictable, the presence of a skilled paediatrician capable of intubation is vital.

CONTROL OF PAIN IN LABOUR

Although some women are lucky and have relatively little pain in labour, for many women it is the most painful experience of their lives. A lot can be done to prepare women beforehand and to give them confidence. Understanding the birth process is in itself helpful in removing the fear of the unknown, and all women should be encouraged to attend appropriate antenatal classes. Some women may also benefit from techniques such as psychoprophylaxis, hypnosis and transcutaneous nerve stimulation (TNS). These all have the major advantage of being without significant side-effects. Their disadvantage is that they require considerable motivation and effort from all concerned over a fairly long period and are, therefore, seldom taken up by women in the poorer socioeconomic groups. They may also prove inadequate to deal with the pain, particularly if the labour is longer or more difficult than initially anticipated. There is, therefore, always likely to be a place for the pharmacological methods of pain relief.

The simplest and oldest agents used for analgesia in labour are the **narcotics**. Pethidine, 50–150 mg, is most widely used in the UK. Narcotics are generally estimated to relieve about 40–50% of the pain of contractions. In addition, they sometimes provide a feeling of euphoria, and often cause sleepiness which helps the woman to rest between contractions. On the debit side, they frequently cause nausea and are, therefore, often given with an antiemetic such as metoclopramide. Some women find the psychic effects unpleasant, and some find the pain relief simply inadequate. The other main disadvantage is that when given within 1–4 h of delivery, narcotics can suppress spontaneous neonatal respiration so that artificial ventilation is necessary, although this effect can be reversed rapidly with i.m. naloxone. Despite these drawbacks, many women find pethidine satisfactory and it is probably still the most widely used method of pain relief in labour.

The **inhalational anaesthetic agent**, nitrous oxide, can be used to supplement narcotics, or on its own. It is supplied as a 50/50 mixture with oxygen (Entonox) and is self administered via a hand held mask. It is not primarily an analgesic, but causes a feeling of detachment which many women find makes the pain more bearable. It is taken at the beginning of each contraction, and about four or five deep breaths are usually sufficient to provide the effect. It can be allowed to wear off between contractions as it takes effect very quickly. There are very few side-effects.

Pudendal nerve block coupled with local anaesthetic infiltration of the perineum can provide reasonable anaesthesia for a non-rotational forceps delivery. However, it is not helpful in the first stage of labour and almost never provides sufficient pain relief for rotational forceps delivery.

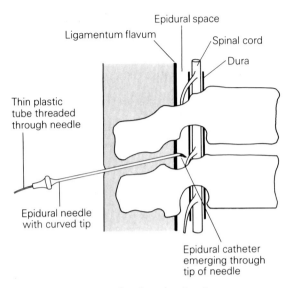

Ligamentum flavum

Epidural space

Spinal cord

Dura

Thin plastic tube threaded through needle

Epidural needle with curved tip

Epidural catheter emerging through tip of needle

Fig. 10.16   *Principle of epidural catheter insertion.*

Epidural Anaesthesia

A method of pain relief which has increased dramatically in popularity over the last 15 years is epidural anaesthesia. The basic anatomy of an epidural block is shown in Fig. 10.16. A plastic catheter is introduced into the epidural space and repeated injections of local anaesthetic can then be made. The aim is to stop transmission in the small pain fibres with, at the same time, minimal effect on the larger sensory and motor fibres. This is, however, somewhat unpredictable, and many women complain of numb immobile legs. Nevertheless, over 80% of women should experience complete relief of labour pain, and most of the remainder will obtain considerable effect. This is why it is so popular; in many hospitals about 35% of women choose to have an epidural, and in some hospitals the figure is as high as 60%. There are, however, some potentially serious side-effects from epidurals, and these should always be borne in mind when they are used.

1. *Dural tap*, which is inadvertent penetration of the spinal canal. This occurs in up to 2% of cases, depending on the experience of the anaesthetist. Because a large gauge needle has to be used to pass the catheter, a considerable leak of cerebrospinal fluid may occur with reduction of pressure and subsequent severe headache if the patient is not lying flat. More

seriously, if the puncture is not appreciated, direct injection of local anaesthetic into the subarachnoid space may occur, with resulting rapid anaesthesia of the whole spinal column, producing total paralysis and respiratory arrest. It can be treated with artificial ventilation until the anaesthetic wears off, but deaths have occurred before the nature of the problem was appreciated.

2. *Hypotension.* Paralysis of the lumbar sympathetic outflow causes loss of vascular tone in the lower limbs with consequent blood pooling, reduction of venous return, and severe maternal hypotension. If this is exacerbated by caval compression from the supine position, death can result. Minor degrees of hypotension can produce severe reductions in uterine blood flow with consequent fetal hypoxia. Many of these problems can be prevented by infusion of 500–1000 ml of colloid solutions, such as Hartmann's, before the local anaesthetic is given. This technique is called 'preloading'. All women having an epidural must, therefore, have an i.v. line *in situ*.

3. *Increased incidence of forceps delivery.* The epidural interferes with normal sensation, and so bearing down efforts are often impaired. About 50% of primigravidae will require forceps delivery for this reason if they opt for an epidural; this figure can be reduced by allowing longer second stages, with careful monitoring. However, 85% of multigravidae will achieve a spontaneous delivery despite having an epidural.

4. *Interference with bladder function.* Loss of sensation means that women frequently have to be catheterised in labour. Normal bladder function can take 24 h or even longer to return following delivery, and repeat catheterisations inevitably lead to an increased incidence of urinary tract infections.

5. *Long-term backache and paralysis.* Such complications can happen, but are extremely rare. Paralysis probably occurs in less than 1 in a million epidurals and is probably only due to the injection of the wrong material down the epidural catheter.

Absolute contraindications

1. Infection at or near the site of puncture.
2. Actual or anticipated serious maternal haemorrhage.

3. Coagulopathy, for example in fulminating pre-eclampsia or abruptio placentae; or anticoagulant therapy.
4. Fetal distress, which may be exacerbated disastrously if hypotension occurs.

Relative contraindications

1. Severe maternal hypertension.
2. Maternal neurological disease (e.g. multiple sclerosis).

It can be seen from the above that epidurals carry a significant medical risk; they should probably only be carried out when there is an anaesthetist and an obstetrician constantly available for the labour ward, and in a hospital with an intensive care unit.

Indications other than maternal request

Epidurals are undoubtedly of benefit in the management of twin labour, because the second twin may develop a malpresentation during the delivery of the first, which is uncorrectable except by internal podalic version (grasping the feet and delivering the baby as a breech). An epidural eliminates the delay required to institute general anaesthesia and,

if unsuccessful, the surgeon can proceed directly to caesarean section. A similar advantage accrues to the use of epidurals in prolonged labour, or breech presentation, where a vaginal delivery may have to be abandoned at short notice and resort made to caesarean section.

Epidurals also have many advantages for elective caesarean operations. They allow the mother and often also the father to enjoy the birth of their baby, there is less risk of anaesthetic complications such as aspiration pneumonia and chest infections and no depression of fetal respiration. The mother must be tilted laterally to about 30° to prevent fetal hypoxia due to inadequate placental perfusion during delivery.

FURTHER READING

Beazley J.M., Lobb M.O. (1983). *Aspects of Care in Labour*. Edinburgh: Churchill Livingstone.
Cohen W.R., Friedman E.A., eds. (1983). *Management of Labour*. Baltimore: University Press.
Crawford J.W., ed. (1985). *Risks of Labour*. Chichester: John Wiley.
Studd J., ed. (1985). *The Management of Labour*. Oxford: Blackwell Scientific Publications.

11

Abnormal Labour

Normal labour may be defined as the occurrence of regular uterine contractions with effacement and progressive dilatation of the cervix leading to spontaneous vaginal delivery of the baby between 37 and 42 completed weeks of gestation. Abnormal labour may be considered as all forms of labour which fall outside the limits of this definition thus providing a practical basis for discussing preterm labour, induction of labour, prolonged labour, operative delivery and malpresentations, each of which constitutes a form of abnormal labour.

Table 11.1

Percentage Survival by Birthweight

Birth weight %	Live birth	Neonatal death	% age surviving
0– 499	2	1	—
500– 999	20	5	75
1000–1499	57	4	93
1500–1999	50	1	98
2000–2499	102	1	99

PRETERM LABOUR

There is now general agreement that an infant weighing less than 2.5 kg be defined as low birth weight and that an infant delivered before 37 completed weeks (less than 259 days) from the first day of the last menstrual period should be classified as preterm. Less certain is what should constitute the lower limit for gestational age that reflects viability. With improved neonatal intensive care, the age and weight at which the fetus becomes viable is constantly dropping. Twenty-five years ago, it was unusual for an infant to survive if born before 28 weeks or if the birthweight was below 1000 g, and if the birthweight was less than 1500 g the chances of survival were only 50%. However, things are very different today and the figures in Table 11.1 depict the success achieved in a teaching hospital with a high rate of obstetric complications. Age of viability, however, remains ill-defined and a large survey is currently in progress. In practice, most units now accept 26 weeks' gestation as their lower limit, although a few consider it should be 24 completed weeks.

The diagnosis of preterm labour is problematical. Uterine contractions may occur which do not result in cervical dilatation and this false preterm labour may stop spontaneously or after treatment. Several publications testify to the effectiveness of placebo treatment, such as an infusion of 5% glucose. A survey at the John Radcliffe Hospital, Oxford, found that 3% of patients were admitted preterm with regular uterine contractions with or without ruptured membranes, a single live fetus and no vaginal bleeding, but only 50% delivered preterm infants. In those patients where the membranes remained intact, the cervix uneffaced and less than 2 cm dilated, only 25% delivered preterm. Unfortunately, there is no sure way to distinguish those who require therapy from those who do not.

In the United Kingdom, 6.9% of all babies weigh less than 2500 g at birth. It is estimated that approximately one-third of these births result from preterm labour, the remainder being due to elective preterm deliveries and small-for-dates term infants. Preterm delivery accounts for three-quarters of neonatal deaths not associated with congenital abnormalities.

Causes of Preterm Labour

Endocrine factors

The precise cause of labour at term remains unknown. Studies in sheep have demonstrated that an important step in the initiation of labour is an increased production of cortisol by the fetal adrenals. Results from human studies are not conclusive. Higher levels of cortisol found in umbilical cord plasma after delivery following spontaneous labour rather than delivery by elective caesarean section may be a response to the stress of labour.

The fetal brain may have an important role in the timing of normal parturition. When the fetus is anencephalic, and in the absence of hydramnios, the range of gestation at delivery is extended.

In some cases of preterm delivery of unknown aetiology, fetal adrenal hyperplasia has been described, which is consistent with the increased urinary levels of dehydroepiandrosterone sulphate (DHEAS) often found in preterm neonates.

It has been suggested that the immature fetal brain secretes fragments of ACTH, viz. α-melanotrophin (α-MSH) and corticotrophin-like intermediate lobe peptide (CLIP). As the fetal brain matures, the anterior pituitary produces 'real ACTH'. Preterm delivery may be associated with premature maturation of the fetal brain and result from an increased trophic stimulus to the fetal adrenal. Although this might explain the occurrence of adrenal hyperplasia in these infants, it is inconsistent with the high urinary levels of DHEAS which reflect adrenal immaturity.

There is no consistent abnormal change in the plasma concentrations of oestrogen or progesterone preceding preterm labour. However, it is interesting to note that during late gestation, a progesterone binding protein has been shown to appear in fetal membranes and a local withdrawal of progesterone may occur near term, which is undetected by plasma concentration measurements.

Oxytocin production from the posterior pituitary is thought not to be involved in the initiation of labour. It is certainly released during the second stage of normal labour. Increased levels in preterm labour have not been found. However, an increased myometrial sensitivity to oxytocin mediated via an increased receptor population cannot be excluded. There may be increased interaction between oxytocin and prostaglandins prior to the onset of labour.

In the sheep, oxytocin is known not only to act on the myometrium to enhance uterine activity, but also to increase prostaglandin F (PGF) secretion from both the myometrium and the maternal placenta. In normal human pregnancy the amniotic fluid contains PGE and PGF in amounts that increase markedly towards term. PGF is a powerful myometrial stimulant and its concentration in amniotic fluid rises steeply once labour is established. The levels of PGFM, (the metabolite of PGF), are not raised during early preterm labour, although levels do rise shortly before delivery.

The amnion is a major site of prostaglandin production, while the chorion and decidua produce much less, but are major sites for their metabolism. At term the amnion will metabolise arachidonic acid, mainly to PGE_2 and to lipoxygenase products. There is a strong association between preterm labour and genital tract infection. Bacteria can increase the production of PGE_2 by the amnion, thereby triggering labour. Changes in vaginal bacterial flora, or overt pathogenic infection are probably a more important cause of preterm labour than has been appreciated.

Epidemiological factors

Preterm birth has been associated with small stature (maternal height less than 155 cm), social classes IV and V, high parity and maternal age of less than 20 years. Obviously, these variables overlap considerably and, if short stature and low social class are combined, the preterm delivery rate is higher than for any other single variable. On the other hand, these variables must not be interpreted too rigidly as, for example, when height and weight are considered together, height is not of importance if the weight is appropriate. This reflects the importance of proper nutrition from birth to maturity in determining the stature and general health of the mother. The importance of adequate nutrition has been demonstrated by a study in New York, where nutritional supplementation in a poor black community resulted in an increased length of gestation and a reduction in the proportion of low birth weight infants in patients given a balanced diet. It may be that an inadequate intake of essential fatty acids is an important cause of some pathologies of pregnancy.

Smoking during pregnancy affects both birth weight (Fig. 11.1) and length of gestation. One study has suggested that the incidence of preterm delivery was doubled if the mother smoked. The influence of social class on spontaneous preterm birth applies whether or not mothers smoke in pregnancy. Not surprisingly, the incidence of preterm labour is higher in smokers than non-smokers for each social class.

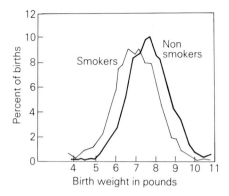

Fig. 11.1 *Distribution of birth weight by maternal smoking status. Smokers were those who consumed 20 or more cigarettes per day during pregnancy. (Adapted from E.J. Quilligan, 1981. Pathological causes of preterm labour. In* Preterm Labour. *M. Elder and C.H. Hendricks, eds., p. 65. London: Butterworth.)*

Previous reproductive history

The general reproductive capability of an individual is reflected by past events. The incidence of preterm labour in subsequent pregnancies is not increased by previous first trimester spontaneous abortions. However, a previous midtrimester abortion or preterm labour increases the risk of a subsequent preterm labour. Not surprisingly, those at greatest risk are mothers who have had two or more previous preterm deliveries (Table 11.2). The risks of preterm delivery after induced abortion are low provided the cervix is not dilated beyond 10 mm. The use of vaginal prostaglandin pessaries preoperatively to soften the cervix could virtually eliminate cervical trauma.

Previous cervical conisation

There is some evidence that an increased incidence of preterm labour occurs following cone biopsy of the cervix and that the risks may increase with parity. Cone biopsy is now less commonly performed than it used to be because of the success of more local forms of treatment for cervical disorders.

Cervical incompetence

The causes of cervical incompetence are trauma, as with forceful dilatation, lacerations in childbirth or previous cervical surgery, and congenital, probably due to a connective tissue defect. There is little doubt this condition causes midtrimester abortion and, to a lesser extent, preterm delivery. The history is classically one of painless, rapid labour and the diagnosis is often retrospective. Cervical cerclage is effective in those cases where the diagnosis is correct, but the condition is overdiagnosed and the true value of cervical cerclage is difficult to assess. The presence of a foreign body in the form of the suture material can increase the likelihood of infection which, in turn, may cause the membranes to rupture and cause abortion/preterm delivery.

Uterine abnormality

Congenital anomalies of the uterus are well known causes of preterm labour and abortion. Their incidence is small, but when such anomalies as septate uterus and uterus didelphys occur, the incidence of preterm delivery may be as high as 30%. Ultrasound scanning is proving of value in diagnosing these conditions and it is claimed that surgical correction gives excellent results.

Table 11.2

The Risk of Preterm Birth in Subsequent Births

First birth	Second birth	Number of mothers	Numbers	%	Relative risk
Not preterm		25 817	1128	4.4	1.0
Preterm		1 860	320	17.2	3.9
Not preterm	Not preterm	24 689	637	2.6	0.6
Preterm	Not preterm	1 540	88	5.7	1.3
Not perterm	Preterm	1 128	125	11.1	2.5
Preterm	Preterm	320	91	28.4	6.5

Based on 27 677 mothers with their first three singleton births, Norway 1967–1976. (From L. S Bakketeig and H. J. Hoffman, 1981. In *Preterm Labour* M. Elder and C. H. Hendricks, eds. London: Butterworth.)

Asherman's syndrome, in which synechiae form within the uterine cavity, has been reported as causing a high incidence (50%) of abortion and preterm delivery.

Medical problems

Elective preterm delivery is often carried out in cases of pregnancy induced hypertension, antepartum haemorrhage, intrauterine growth retardation, rhesus isoimmunisation and, occasionally, in severe diabetes. Other medical conditions thought to precipitate preterm labour include severe urinary tract infection, hyperthyroidism, alcoholism, drug habituation, heart disease and glomerulonephritis. These conditions are also likely to result in the delivery of a small-for-dates infant.

Multiple pregnancy

The length of gestation of multiple pregnancy is known to be shorter than singleton pregnancies. On average, twins are delivered 3 weeks before their singleton counterparts. It is thought the overdistension of uterine muscle fibres enhances contractility.

Polyhydramnios

As in multiple pregnancy, polyhydramnios causes excessive uterine distension. Its incidence has been reported to lie between 0.4 and 1.6%, and may occur in diabetes and rhesus isoimmunisation. The high fetal mortality of up to 70% is caused by congenital anomaly, low birth weight and prematurity.

Fetal malformations

Various congenital malformations of the fetus are associated with preterm labour. Their diagnosis is important when deciding the management of preterm labour. These abnormalities include those associated with hydramnios such as tracheo-oesophageal fistula, anencephaly, neural tube defects, gastrointestinal abnormalities such as omphalocele, renal agenesis, etc. Good ultrasound scanning during the second trimester as well as serum AFP estimations will detect many of these cases, but there should always be a high level of suspicion for congenital abnormalities in all cases of preterm labour, particularly if there is evidence of symmetrical fetal growth retardation.

Premature rupture of the membranes

It is generally held that a high percentage of preterm labour and delivery follows premature rupture of the membranes. This may be caused by genital tract infection, but in many cases the cause is unknown. However, abnormally thin membranes with reduced elasticity has been suggested as another possible cause. Prolonged ruptured membranes commencing at from 16 to 24 weeks of pregnancy is likely to cause pulmonary hypoplasia, as liquor in the lungs is necessary for the development of tertiary bronchioles and alveoli.

Bleeding in pregnancy

Bleeding in both early and late pregnancy predisposes to preterm delivery. Studies which have reviewed cases of threatened abortion have shown that although the pregnancy may continue after the initial bleed, the rate of preterm delivery is increased by up to three times that for the normal obstetric population. Antepartum haemorrhage (i.e. bleeding after 28 weeks' gestation) due to abruptio placentae and non-specific causes are associated with preterm delivery. The latter is surprising and underlines the need for continuously cautious management even when placenta praevia and abruptio placenta have been discounted as causes for antepartum haemorrhage.

Placental factors

The morphology of the placenta delivered after preterm labour is normal in the vast majority of cases. However, it is interesting to note that up to 10% may show accelerated maturation of the villi, reflecting the features of a term placenta.

Management of Preterm Labour

Until the complexity of the aetiology of preterm labour is unravelled, its effective prevention will remain elusive.

General measures such as using scoring systems to predict the risk of preterm delivery and to identify patients at high risk, nutritional supplementation, antismoking advice and extra bedrest for mothers with multiple pregnancy may be of marginal, if non-specific, value.

It is not surprising, therefore, that great interest

has been shown in the inhibition of uterine contractions, especially since the pharmacological agents to do so are readily available and, in high enough dosage, are effective.

β-*sympathomimetics drugs*

In 1948 it was shown that the uterus contained stimulatory α-receptors and inhibitory β-receptors. Subsequently, it was suggested that two types of β-receptor were present in the body; β_1 receptors which, when activated, caused stimulation of the cardiovascular system; and β_2 receptors which inhibited smooth muscle. Pharmacological agents followed which were capable of specifically stimulating β_2 receptors, provoking a lesser response on β_1 receptors and thus reducing their effect on the cardiovascular system.

The drugs most commonly used in current obstetric practice are isoxsuprine, ritodrine, salbutamol, terbutaline and feneterol. All produce unwanted cardiovascular side-effects which restrict the dose used to inhibit uterine contractions, but on the whole they are quite efficacious.

In addition to decreasing myometrial activity, β-sympathomimetics may have other useful effects. It has been shown that uterine blood flow may be increased with the use of ritodrine. Whether this actually promotes improvement in placental perfusion awaits proof. There is also some evidence to suggest these drugs may promote acceleration of fetal lung maturity. It is postulated that the drugs act on cyclic AMP in the type II pneumocyte within the fetal lung promoting the production of surfactant.

Tachycardia, palpitations, tremor and anxiety may prove intolerable to the patient. The heart rate should not be allowed to exceed 130–140 beats/min. The drugs are hazardous in patients with known cardiac and hypertensive disease and fatalities have been reported when used in patients with cardiomyopathy. When used in combination with steroids and excessive i.v. fluids, serious pulmonary oedema has occurred in a few cases. The drugs also have a hyperglycaemic effect by inducing gluconeogenesis in the liver. Hyperinsulinaemia follows as a result of the increased plasma glucose and a direct effect of the drugs on pancreatic islet cells. Care, therefore, is required with use in diabetics. Hypokalaemia may also be produced, due to a shift of potassium from the extracellular to the intracellular compartment. Antepartum haemorrhage is considered a contraindication to the use of these drugs. The effect of peripheral vasodilation caused by β-sympathomimetics incapacitates the usual compensatory mechanisms for controlling haemorrhage. One possible exception may exist in the case of haemorrhage from placenta praevia in the presence of preterm labour where short-term tocolytic therapy may help to arrest labour and the consequent worsening haemorrhage. This remains controversial, as β-sympathomimetics are known to increase uterine blood flow.

Although these drugs are far from perfect, they are the agents most often used in the treatment of preterm labour.

Prostaglandin synthetase inhibitors

These compounds are effective in reducing uterine activity (tocolytic drugs). Prostaglandins are known to be strong uterine stimulants and, if their production is inhibited, the major stimulus for uterine activity is removed. Indomethacin and naproxen have been infrequently used in practice. This is because of concern that, by inhibiting fetal prostaglandin production, these drugs promote closure of the ductus arteriosus *in utero* with resultant neonatal pulmonary hypertension.

Calcium antagonists

Compounds such as nifedipine should theoretically be effective by blocking intracellular calcium transfer and so myometrial contractions. In practice, they have not yet been used to any extent.

The use of steroids in preterm labour

Betamethasone administration, 24 mg over 48 h to the mother, has been shown to reduce the incidence of respiratory distress syndrome (RDS) in the preterm infant by one-third. The advantages are greatest between 28 and 32 weeks' gestation and commence 24 h after administration of the drug, lasting for approximately 7 days. Repeated courses may be necessary.

The routine use of betamethasone in this situation is not accepted by all. There is concern about the possible effects of large doses of corticosteroids on fetal brain development and a possible increased risk of infection in the mother due to immunosuppression. Neither of these has been proven and it is unlikely that such short-term dosage could have significant effects on what are long-term processes.

Mode of Delivery of the Preterm Infant

Once the cervix achieves a dilatation of more than 4 cm, especially in the presence of ruptured membranes, treatment for preterm labour is likely to fail. The mode of delivery becomes an issue in this situation and the best course remains contentious. Almost all studies are retrospective and contain such varying elements that their comparison is virtually impossible. All appreciate the importance of avoiding asphyxia and trauma during delivery and this applies particularly to the preterm infant. Thus arose a vogue for delivering all preterm infants by caesarean section. The figures available, however, have failed to show a dramatic difference in outcome. Some of the most recently published reports suggest that when the fetal weight is between 1000 and 1499 g caesarean section offers a better outlook for the fetus presenting by the breech in terms of reduced mortality and morbidity as measured by incidence of neonatal intraventricular haemorrhage. Caesarean section may offer no advantage to fetuses with a cephalic presentation weighing less than 1500 g, except a lowered incidence of ultrasonically diagnosed intraventricular haemorrhage. The long-term clinical significance, if any, of these usually small haemorrhages is not yet known.

Should Preterm Labour be Treated?

When the means to treat preterm labour became available, a new day was thought to be dawning in obstetric practice. It was hoped that such a development would further improve perinatal mortality and morbidity. In effect, the case has not been proven and the question now posed is whether preterm labour should be treated at all. The obstetrician is unable to predict which case of preterm labour will stop spontaneously and which case will benefit, in terms of improved fetal outcome, from treating preterm labour. The drugs used are potentially hazardous to the mother and prolongation of the pregnancy may prove more hazardous to the baby than preterm delivery. Neonatal intensive care has improved dramatically in the last decade, with the result that more small and less mature

infants are surviving and subsequently developing normally.

One aspect which has been generally accepted relates to the place of delivery of the preterm infant. Good neonatal intensive care facilities must be available to ensure the best possible outcome for the fetus. Transfer of the fetus *in utero* to centres which can provide such facilities is increasingly frequent and the use of tocolytic therapy is of value in postponing delivery until transfer of the mother can be accomplished. Truly effective treatment of preterm labour must await the identification of its cause. In the meantime, the improvements in neonatal care and the delivery of the baby in the best possible condition avoiding hypoxia and infection in particular offer the most realistic hope for the pregnancy complicated by preterm labour.

INDUCTION OF LABOUR

Induction of labour is the initiation of uterine activity by an independent stimulus to achieve vaginal delivery of the fetus prior to the onset of spontaneous labour.

Since 1948, when the administration of oxytocin by i.v. infusion to induce uterine contractions became feasible, induction of labour has become a practical reality and a part of usual practice in every obstetric unit. At first, the availability of induction of labour was accepted enthusiastically by obstetricians with the genuine aim of reducing both maternal and perinatal mortality and morbidity. However, the last three decades have seen enormous swings in the frequency with which induction is used and this perhaps reflects that its use has not produced the dramatic improvement in perinatal mortality that was expected. Currently, there is a downward trend in the frequency of induction of labour, but there remains a marked variation from one obstetric unit to another.

Indications

Indications for induction of labour may be obstetric or non-obstetric. A list of indications can never be complete, as obstetricians vary considerably in their views on acceptable reasons for induction of labour. Also, individual patients present differing circumstances which might make induction of labour appropriate or inappropriate.

Obstetric and medical conditions

Well defined complications such as pre-eclampsia, hypertension in pregnancy, intrauterine growth retardation, antepartum haemorrhage, multiple pregnancy, prolonged pregnancy, diabetes mellitus, rhesus immunisation, gross congenital fetal abnormality and fetal death *in utero* are generally accepted to warrant planned elective delivery. Table 11.3 lists the recent indications for induction

Table 11.3

Indications for Induction of Labour

Indication for induction	Number (%)
Postmaturity	344 (41.8)
Pre-eclampsia/Hypertension	232 (28.2)
Static maternal weight/weight loss at term	72 (8.8)
Previous Caesarean section/hysterotomy	46 (5.6)
Breech presentation	34 (4.0)
Antepartum haemorrhage	33 (4.0)
Placental insufficiency	25
Poor obstetric history	20
Diabetes/abnormal GTT	15
Spurious labour	23
Intrauterine death	10
Haemolytic disease	4
Congenital malformations	1
Multiple pregnancy	7
Others	34

of labour and their frequency in one obstetric unit. It is worth noting that not all of these indications would receive universal approval throughout the United Kingdom.

Relative indications

Individual patients will present differing features which are peculiar to themselves but which will influence a decision to deliver electively. Maternal age, poor obstetric history, previous infertility and a child suffering from the effects of traumatic childbirth or postmaturity are examples. Often a patient will have a combination of these factors and, although each factor on its own may constitute

insufficient reason for induction of labour, their cumulative effect cannot be ignored.

Social indications

On the whole, social convenience for both patient and obstetrician has not been generally accepted in Britain as an indication for the induction of labour. This was not the prevailing attitude in America and, since 1978, the Food and Drug Administration has required the pharmaceutical companies to include the following information with oxytocin supplied to hospitals:

> *Important Notice:* Pitocin is not indicated for the elective induction of labour because available data and information are inadequate to define the benefits-to-risks considerations in the use of the drug's product. Elective induction of labour is defined as the initiation of labour in an individual with a term pregnancy who is free of medical indications for the initiation of labour.

More recently, the American College of Obstetricians and Gynaecologists (1982) have recommended that induction of labour with oxytocin should be initiated only if required for the benefit of the mother or fetus.

There are occasional situations in which planned delivery may be necessary to provide the best level of care for the baby and/or mother. Such planned delivery allows for the availability of anaesthetic, paediatric and nursing personnel and also intensive care facilities with laboratory back-up for investigations. These are usually more easily achieved if delivery occurs during the normal working day.

Suitability for Induction of Labour

The approach to deciding if labour should be induced should be as logical and rational as possible. The first question to be answered is: 'should the pregnancy be interrupted before the onset of spontaneous labour?' If so, then the next questions are: 'what is the most appropriate method of induction and mode of delivery?' Although simplistic, such an approach at least lends itself to clarity of thought.

When the indication to induce labour is maternal, it must be certain that the process of labour will not place her at unnecessary risk. When fetal indications predominate, the ability of the fetus to cope with the physiological and mechanical stresses of labour and vaginal delivery must be assessed. Antenatal assessment of the fetus will include cardiotocography, fetal movement counts, estimation of fetal weight by head and abdominal circumference measurements by ultrasound scan, Doppler assessment of blood flow patterns in fetal and utero placental circulations, etc. Intrapartum continuous fetal heart rate monitoring will be employed to monitor fetal well-being after labour has been induced.

Once the decision is made that labour should be induced and that vaginal delivery is reasonable, an assessment of the likelihood of induction of labour being successful is of value. Bishop devised a scoring system based on the findings at vaginal examination in relation to the state of the cervix and the level of the presenting part, and a modified version is shown in Fig. 10.8, p. 146. Normal labour, as discussed in Chapter 10, is conveniently considered in two phases, namely prelabour, which is slow and time-consuming, and active labour, which is efficient and progressive. The Bishop score provides the clinician with information about the time required to complete the prelabour phase (Fig. 11.2) and the likelihood of success of the procedure to induce labour. The higher the score, the less time required for prelabour and the greater the likelihood of successful induction of labour. It is worthy of note, however, that this system describes a trend and even with a Bishop score as low as 2, 80% of patients will still have a successful induction of

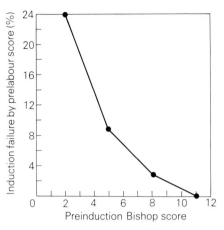

Fig. 11.3   *High preinduction Bishop score is a good predictor of successful induction. (From data of Friedman et al., 1966. C. H. Hendricks, 1983. Second thoughts on induction of labour. In* Progress in Obstetrics and Gynaecology, *Vol. 3. John Studd, ed., p. 105. London: Churchill Livingstone.)*

labour (Fig. 11.3). Nevertheless, when the cervix is found to be totally unfavourable and/or the presenting part is high, and the indication for delivery is fetal, the obstetrician may feel that delivery by elective caesarean section is more appropriate.

Methods of Induction of Labour

Methods of induction of labour may be conveniently divided into surgical and medical categories. In practice, a combination of methods is often employed, but each will be considered separately for ease of reference.

Surgical

Traditionally, high and low amniotomy were the accepted methods of surgical induction of labour. The former has virtually disappeared from modern obstetric practice, but in the presence of a ripe cervix, both methods successfully induce labour in 80–90% of patients. In order to achieve artificial rupture of the membranes (ARM), the cervix must be 1–2 cm dilated and this, of course, improves the Bishop score for predictability of successful induction. Also, the membranes are routinely swept digitally from the lower uterine segment at the time of ARM and this will cause the local release of prostaglandins, thus enhancing the onset of uterine contractility. The

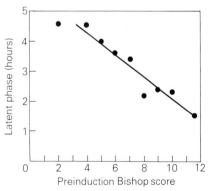

Fig. 11.2   *The longer 'latent phase' associated with a low preinduction Bishop score is an accurate indicator of the amount of prelabour which needs to be completed before active labour can proceed. (From data of Friedman et al., 1966. C. H. Hendricks, 1983. Second thoughts on induction of labour. In* Progress in Obstetrics and Gynaecology, *Vol. 3. John Studd, ed., p. 104. London: Churchill Livingstone.)*

membranes are ruptured by grasping them with a toothed forceps or using an amniotomy hook to tear a small hole. Care must be taken not to traumatise the fetal presenting part. Liquor should be allowed to drain slowly. The fetal heart must be checked immediately following the procedure.

The true value of amniotomy is twofold. It sensitises the uterus to the action of syntocinon and allows more direct intrapartum surveillance of the fetus.

Medical

Syntocinon. Syntocinon is the commercially synthesised compound which is chemically similar to naturally occurring oxytocin.

When syntocinon became available, the methods of induction commonly employed were ARM alone or syntocinon alone with the membranes intact. While there was no doubt that uterine contractions occurred following syntocinon administration, the success rate of inducing labour was not as high as when the membranes had ruptured. Also with amniotomy alone, the rate of 90% successful induction of labour only occurred with up to a 48 h delay and considerable risk of intrauterine infection. When amniotomy and syntocinon infusion were combined, 80–90% of patients were delivered within 12 h. As a result, the modern practice of induction of labour combines these procedures, although there is variation among obstetricians in regard to the timing of syntocinon infusion relative to amniotomy and to the dose schedule used. Most dose regimens would commence syntocinon at the time of ARM or within 6 h of the procedure.

The sensitivity of individual patients to syntocinon varies widely and the importance of titrating the dose administered against uterine response must be appreciated. Most regimens commence with a dose of 1 milliunit/ml which is doubled every 15–30 min until effective uterine contractions occur. Once active labour and cervical dilatation have begun, the dose rate may be held constant or, more likely, reduced as the endogenous production of prostaglandins effectively maintains the labour. The majority of patients whose labour is induced by this method can be expected to deliver within 12 h of induction.

Side-effects of syntocinon infusion are rare. Water intoxication may occur with high dosage, due to the antidiuretic effect of syntocinon or when large volumes of fluid are used to administer a suitable dose of the drug. With awareness of this problem it should not occur. Syntocinon may cause haemolysis in the fetus and an increased incidence of neonatal jaundice after its use has been reported, but this is rarely serious.

Although the results of this method of induction of labour are satisfactory, there are certain drawbacks. The method remains unpopular with patients. Some find the amniotomy painful, and dislike the restriction of movement imposed by the i.v. infusion. A minority of patients show a poor response to this method of induction of labour. In particular, primigravidae with an unripe cervix at induction tend to have long painful labours, with fetal distress developing more often. (Table 11.4).

Prostaglandins. Although prostaglandin preparations have been available for use in clinical

Table 11.4

Details of Labour and Delivery of 125 Primigravidae Analysed by the State of the Cervix at the Time of Amniotomy

Cervical score	Number	Induction delivery intervals (hours) mean ± s.d.	Mode of delivery		
			Caesarean section	Forceps	Spontaneous
0–3 (unripe)	31	14.9 ± 5.5	10 (32%)	16 (52%)	5 (16%)
4–7 (intermediate)	69	8.9 ± 3.0	3 (4%)	38 (55%)	28 (41%)
8–11 (ripe)	25	6.4 ± 2.2	0 (0%)	11 (44%)	14 (56%)

practice for at least a decade, their widespread use for induction of labour has been slow to develop. This has been due mainly to their side-effects after systemic administration. A single prostaglandin may have several actions throughout the body. Prostaglandin $F_{2\alpha}$ ($PGF_{2\alpha}$) will stimulate the smooth muscle of the lungs, intestine and uterus. On absorption into the bloodstream, 90% of the drug is rapidly metabolised in the lungs and thus large doses are required to gain an effect on the uterus with a consequent increase of unwanted effects.

The production of an oral tablet PGE_2 0.5 mg aroused interest and when used in conjunction with amniotomy in those with favourable Bishop scores (>4), it has proved reasonably effective using doses of 0.5–1.5 mg hourly. The absence of an i.v. infusion is attractive, but the side-effects of nausea, vomiting and diarrhoea experienced with doses of 1.5 mg hourly are unpleasant.

Local administration of prostaglandin within the genital tract avoids these side-effects and PGE_2 vaginal tablets and gels are now commercially available. It is known that natural prostaglandins are involved in the process of cervical ripening and, when induction of labour is indicated and the cervix is unfavourable, administration of PGE_2 vaginally is of benefit. Not only will such treatment ripen the cervix, but labour will satisfactorily follow in up to 60% of patients. Even when the cervix is favourable, vaginal administration of prostaglandin may be preferred, thus deferring the need for an i.v. infusion and perhaps amniotomy. In multigravidae with a Bishop score of more than 4, a single vaginal tablet of 3 mg PGE_2 and amniotomy 6 h later achieves delivery in up to 90% of cases.

Individual obstetricians vary widely in their choice of methods for induction of labour (Table 11.5). As with syntocinon, patients vary in their

sensitivity to prostaglandin and the finer control of dose that i.v. infusion of syntocinon allows may be preferred. Prostaglandin and syntocinon should not be used concurrently as prostaglandins are known to sensitise the uterus to oxytocin. Excessive uterine activity may occur with hypertonus severe enough to endanger the fetus from asphyxia or the mother from uterine rupture.

Complications of Induction of Labour

The complications following induction of labour will be considered briefly.

Mode of delivery

It is generally accepted that there is a greater incidence of operative delivery following induced labour than spontaneous labour (Table 11.6) which will to some extent reflect the reasons for induction of labour.

Method of induction

Amniotomy. Prolapse of the cord is thought to occur in 0.5% of cases, which is very similar to the incidence following spontaneous rupture of the membranes. Rupture of the membranes above the presenting part, or hindwater amniotomy can sometimes cause damage to a posteriorly situated placenta.

Syntocinon. Uterine hypertonus causing fetal asphyxia and water intoxication has already been discussed (p. 167).

Prostaglandins. When given i.v. or orally, diarrhoea, nausea and vomiting may occur. Uterine

---

Table 11.5

*Method of Induction of Labour at
Northwick Park Hospital*

ARM only	151 (18.4%)
ARM and syntocinon	27 (3.3%)
ARM and oral prostaglandins (PGE_2)	213 (25.9%)
ARM and oral prostaglandins and syntocinon	17 (2.1%)
Prostaglandin pessaries	220 (26.7%)
Prostaglandin pessaries and ARM	194 (23.6%)

Table 11.6
*Complications of Spontaneous and Induced Labour.
Peninsula Maternity Services, Cape Town*

Nature of complication	Spontaneous labour %	Induced labour %
Caesarean section	10.7	19.8
Forceps delivery	7.6	10.7
Failed induction or failure to progress in labour	0.9	4.6
Fetal distress	3.9	11.9
Prolapsed cord	0.3	0.6
Rupture of uterus	0.03	0.0
Total number of patients	9014	1022

(From V. K. Krutzen, H. Tanneberger and D. A. Davey, Sept. 1977. *S. Afr. Med. J.*, **52**, 12: 482–5.)

hypertonus may occur in occasional patients who are very sensitive to prostaglandins.

Failure of induction

Following amniotomy, there is a significant risk of intra-uterine infection if delivery is delayed for more than 24 h. Caesarean section must be considered then if vaginal delivery is not imminent.

Prematurity

Preterm infants may be delivered intentionally for obstetric reasons or in error due to incorrect assessment of gestational age. Such errors are avoided if confirmation of gestational age in early pregnancy by ultrasound scanning is available.

Neonatal complications

Neonatal asphyxia may follow delivery of the at-risk fetus unable to cope with the stress provoked by a normal uterine contraction. Hypertonus provoked by uterine overstimulation will very rapidly produce fetal asphyxia.

Neonatal jaundice may be caused by the use of syntocinon in labour as a result of haemolysis. It is thought the antidiuretic effect of syntocinon influences the water content of the red cell in the neonate, altering its shape and promoting its destruction.

PROLONGED LABOUR

One of the most notable changes in obstetric practice over the last 15 years has been the reduced incidence of prolonged labour. The length of labour is now normally hours rather than days. The definition of prolonged labour varies from >12 to >24 h. One large teaching hospital in Dublin has defined labour as being abnormal when its duration exceeds 12 h. The dangers of prolonged labour are well appreciated and threaten both mother and baby. In brief they are intrauterine infection, fetal asphyxia, metabolic changes in the mother from dehydration and ketosis, and loss of morale which may have devastating effects on the mother's approach to future pregnancies. Dangers also occur as a result of a cause of prolonged labour, namely obstructed labour, and to cephalopelvic disproportion causing uterine rupture.

Causes of Prolonged Labour

The causes of prolonged labour are traditionally classified as:

Faults in the powers
Faults in the passages
Faults in the passenger.

The Powers: Inefficient Uterine Action

The function of uterine contractions is twofold: to dilate the cervix during the first stage of labour and to cause the presenting part of the fetus to descend to the pelvic floor during the second stage of labour. Uterine efficiency can be assessed by the time taken to achieve delivery of the baby. The normal expectations may be depicted in graphic form by plotting the rate of dilatation of the cervix. Partograms which depict the progress of labour by cervical dilatation and descent of the presenting part are now generally accepted and are discussed in Chapter 10, p. 147.

Once labour is established, the cervix should dilate by at least 1 cm per hour. Inefficiency of uterine action occurs more often in primigravidae than multiparae and other causes of slow labour must be carefully considered in the latter.

During the first stage of labour, inefficient uterine action may present in one of two ways. Most commonly, the cervix dilates slowly right from the onset of labour. This, of course, assumes the initial diagnosis of labour has been correct. Less frequently, inefficient uterine action occurs late in the first stage of labour, when the rate of cervical dilatation slows down after a normal start. This may reflect cephalopelvic disproportion and careful assessment is required.

During the second stage of labour, inefficient uterine action may occur when the presenting part fails to descend through the birth canal to the pelvic floor, following full dilatation. Again, careful assessment is required as the lack of progress may reflect cephalopelvic disproportion.

Treatment of inefficient uterine action

Amniotomy. When the membranes have remained intact, amniotomy alone will often improve uterine contractions. This improvement is probably mediated via the local release of prostaglandins.

Syntocinon. Syntocinon may be given by i.v. infusion in gradually increasing dosage until contractions are occurring regularly. In general the diagnosis of cephalopelvic disproportion can only be justified in the presence of efficient uterine action. Care and regular assessment of the patient is required. The primigravid uterus virtually never ruptures, whereas the parous organ is more prone to rupture and so the use of syntocinon in multigravid women requires caution.

The Passages: Cephalopelvic Disproportion

True contraction of the pelvis nowadays is very uncommon and reflects better nutrition in child-

hood years. Only very occasionally are congenital anomalies of spine or pelvis encountered and acquired defects, due to fractures, for example, only rarely affect pelvic capacity. The size of the baby is usually related to parental characteristics and small women tend to produce babies which are in proportion. Generalised fetal enlargement may be hereditary or acquired, such as in diabetes and rhesus isoimmunisation. Localised fetal deformity, such as hydrocephalus, usually proves an obstruction to vaginal delivery.

It is difficult to diagnose with certainty most cases of cephalopelvic disproportion in advance of labour. The labour is abnormal if there is poor dilatation of the cervix during the first stage or failure of the head to descend during the second stage. Inefficient uterine action in the primigravid patient must be excluded or treated, otherwise a diagnosis of cephalopelvic disproportion is likely to be wrong. Efficiency of uterine action will often safely overcome minor degrees of cephalopelvic disproportion due to the ability of the fetal head to mould and the ability of the pelvic ligaments to stretch a little. When the cervical dilatation ceases and/or the head remains high in the presence of efficient uterine action, recourse to delivery by caesarean section is necessary. In the multigravid patient, abnormally slow labour is much more likely to reflect cephalopelvic disproportion and very careful assessment is required.

The Passenger: Occipitoposterior Position

It is well known that when the fetal head adopts the occipitoposterior position, labour is likely to be prolonged. It is easily diagnosed by abdominal and vaginal examination. Labour may be abnormal in that cervical dilatation is slow or the head fails to descend and rotate. If rotation is incomplete, deep transverse arrest of the head may occur in the second stage of labour. Inefficient uterine action as the cause of the poor labour may be excluded by the use of syntocinon during both first and second stages of labour. If labour remains abnormal, then recourse to operative delivery is indicated.

Augmentation or acceleration of labour is often confused with induction of labour. The former is used to expedite a labour already commenced, whereas the latter is used to interrupt the pregnancy. Augmentation reduces the incidence of operative delivery, which is more prevalent for various reasons following induction of labour.

OPERATIVE DELIVERY

The procedures involved in operative delivery are necessarily of a practical nature and, therefore, best learnt by seeing them performed. The student is encouraged to spend as much time as possible in the delivery suite to witness all forms of delivery. An understanding of the mechanisms of normal spontaneous, vaginal delivery is essential to comprehend the mechanics and rationale of forceps delivery.

Forceps Delivery

The idea of using instruments to expedite the delivery of the baby is approximately 400 years old. Modern forceps include a pelvic curve to the blades to allow easier introduction to the curved birth canal, a locking mechanism to join the blades together and a traction handle to allow the direction of pull to be applied in an efficacious manner. Slight differences of design and attendant gadgetry have led to the availability of a large number of different forceps, estimated by one source as being in excess of 600. However, we shall simply consider the essentials which allow a classification of three types:

1. Long-shanked forceps, e.g. Simpson, Neville-Barnes;
2. Short-shanked forceps, e.g. Wrigley;
3. Kielland forceps.

The constituent parts of the obstetric forceps and their types are illustrated in Fig. 11.4. The instrument consists of two blades, usually fenestrated to avoid excess weight and held together when assembled by a simple locking mechanism akin to that of scissors. The blades are curved on the edge to fit the curve of the pelvis and on the flat to accommodate the baby's head.

Long-shanked forceps (Fig. 11.4a). These were originally designed for application when the baby's head was still at the pelvic brim and unengaged and had a traction device attached to ensure that the direction of pull was applied in the axis of the birth canal. In modern obstetrics, 'high forceps' is not

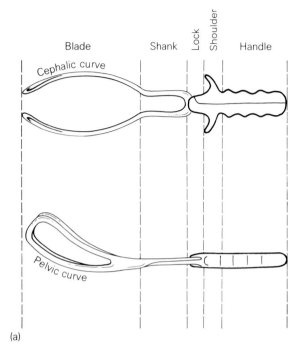

(a)

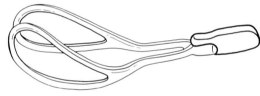

(b)

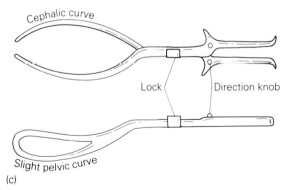

(c)

Fig. 11.4 *Types of forceps. (a) Simpson's; (b) Wrigley's; (c) Kielland's. (Adapted from Derek Llewellyn-Jones, 1969. Fundamentals of Obstetrics and Gynaecology, vol. 1, 'Obstetrics'. London: Faber and Faber.)*

practised due to the unacceptably high risk of damage to both baby and mother. The forceps are now used for delivery when the head has descended at least to the midcavity of the pelvis and the fetal sagittal suture lies in the anteroposterior diameter of the pelvis. The instrument is also of great value in controlling the delivery of the after-coming-head in a breech delivery and, because of the length of the forceps, the operator's hands are well removed from the maternal perineum allowing the assistant ready access to clear the baby's mouth, nose and nasopharynx of liquor and mucus.

Short-shanked forceps (Fig. 11.4b). These forceps are very light and used to deliver the baby's head when it has descended to the maternal perineum and vulval outlet. They can be applied relatively painlessly.

Kielland's forceps (Fig. 11.4c). The use of these forceps remains controversial. Some would claim their only place in obstetrics is in the museum. All would agree their use should be treated with respect. Originally introduced to deliver the unengaged head, these forceps are now exclusively used when the head has descended at least to the midpelvis (the level of the ischial spines) and has remained in the transverse or posterior diameter of the mid or lower pelvis. The blades have minimal pelvic curve and, after application, the forceps are used to rotate the head so that the sagittal suture lies in the anteroposterior diameter of the pelvis in the occipitoanterior position. The locking mechanism allows the shanks of each blade to slip on each other, permitting the correction of asynclitism of the fetal head which arises due to lateral tilting.

Indications for forceps delivery

The indications for forceps delivery are:

Delay in the second stage of labour. It is traditional teaching that the second stage for a primigravid patient should last no more than 1 h and for a multigravida, 30 min. This timing has required reconsideration with the extensive use of epidural anaesthesia. Providing the fetal heart rate remains normal, it is reasonable to allow the second stage to continue for longer if epidural anaesthesia is being used and provided the labour continues to progress in the absence of maternal complications.

In general, however, the causes of delay in the second stage of labour are transverse arrest of the head in the midcavity, persistence of an occipitoposterior position of the head in the midcavity, inadequacy of the uterine powers and minor degrees of cephalopelvic disproportion.

Maternal distress. Delivery of the baby may be indicated in the situation where the mother has become extremely distressed and is failing to cope with the second stage of labour. This is now an infrequent occurrence with better management during the first stage of labour and effective means of pain relief.

Associated maternal conditions. When the mother has associated conditions, such as pre-eclampsia, hypertension and cardiac disease, which may deteriorate if 'pushing' is prolonged during the second stage, forceps delivery may be performed as an elective procedure.

Fetal distress. If the baby is showing signs of distress during the second stage, delivery may be expedited by the use of forceps. The head should have descended to a level below the ischial spines.

Breech delivery. As the aftercoming head of the breech traverses the pelvic outlet and perineum, forceps may be used to control its delivery so that a sudden change in pressure is avoided as this may cause cerebral damage.

The indications for forceps delivery in a major UK hospital are shown in Table 11.7.

Table 11.7

Incidence and Indications for Forceps Delivery

	Number (%)
Number of cases	169
Incidence per cent	13.0
Indications:*	
Delayed second stage	92 (54%)
Fetal distress	90 (53%)
Eclampsia/hypertension	0
O-P position/Deep transverse arrest	22 (13%)
Prematurity	1

* In some cases more than one indication were recorded.

Conditions necessary for forceps delivery

The following list of conditions are generally accepted as absolutely necessary to allow a forceps delivery:

Full dilatation of the cervix. Delivering the head through a non fully-dilated cervix with forceps may lead to extensive trauma of the cervix, vagina and lower uterine segment. Severe haemorrhage can result from such damage. A small, thin rim of remaining cervix may cause little trouble in the application of forceps by an experienced operator, but if the other factors permitting an easy delivery are absent, tissue damage is highly likely. The base of the broad ligament and uterine vessels may be involved and laparotomy may be required to control the resulting haemorrhage. The risks are, therefore, great and, if delivery prior to full dilatation of the cervix is judged appropriate, use of the vacuum extractor (p. 174) is required.

Engagement of the fetal head. Engagement is considered to have occurred when the widest diameter of the presenting part has passed through the pelvic brim. The application of forceps when the head is still high in the pelvis has no part in modern obstetric practice. Correct application of the forceps is extremely difficult to achieve in such circumstances and the non-dilatation of the soft tissues of the birth canal affect considerable resistance to delivery. Damage to the baby and mother is extremely likely. Rarely, a high forceps delivery is justified in the multiparous patient when the cord prolapses or a second twin needs expeditious delivery in the absence of facilities for immediate caesarean section.

Cephalic presentation. Forceps can only be reliably applied to the fetal head and, in general, with vertex and face presentations.

Position of the fetal head. When the vertex presents, forceps may be applied with the occiput in an anterior, lateral or posterior position. The most common position by far in spontaneous vaginal delivery is occipitoanterior reflecting the optimum position of the head for delivery. Forceps delivery should mimic this as far as possible and occipitoposterior positions should generally be rotated to the anterior position. However, when the head is deep in the pelvis and in the occipitoposterior position, proceeding to delivery in this position may be more advantageous than exposure to the risks attendant with upward displacement and rotation of the fetal head. The vertex presentation in an occipitolateral position requires rotation to occipitoanterior. The rotation may be performed manually or with Kielland's forceps, both of which require skill and experience.

Rupture of the membranes. The membranes should be ruptured before application of the forceps blades.

Empty bladder. Ensuring that the bladder is empty is important for two reasons. Firstly, all the space within the pelvis is available for the fetal head when the bladder is empty and, secondly, it minimises the chances of bruising the bladder neck either by the forceps or the fetal head.

No cephalopelvic disproportion. The pelvis below the level of the fetal head must be adequate to allow vaginal delivery. The head should *never* be pulled past an obstruction. In these circumstances, delivery by caesarean section is required.

Complications following forceps delivery

The complications following delivery with forceps are as follows:

Fetal damage. Serious fetal damage caused by forceps can be avoided if the conditions required for forceps delivery outlined above are observed.

Immediately after delivery, the baby may have erythematous marks where the forceps blades have been applied. Occasionally, there may be slight bruising in these areas or to the lobe of an ear, but this is seldom serious.

A facial palsy may result from compression by the blades of the forceps on the facial nerve just as it runs in front of the baby's ear. While the paralysis may last a few days, it always recovers spontaneously and completely.

Intracranial haemorrhage in the baby may occur if the forceps blades are applied incorrectly or excessive traction is used.

Maternal damage. Despite the use of episiotomy, further perineal and vaginal tears may occur, or the episiotomy extend. Occasionally, these tears may extend up to and through the anal sphincter.

Occasionally, the cervix may be torn, especially when it is not fully dilated at the time of application of the forceps. The cervix should be carefully checked after all rotational forceps deliveries.

After forceps delivery, there may be oedema in the proximal urethra/bladder neck region. This can cause acute retention of urine, but invariably settles with catheter drainage of the bladder.

Episiotomy

Episiotomy is virtually always performed before operative deliveries to prevent tearing of the perineum and vagina. It is also performed in other vaginal deliveries and is currently performed in about 25–35% of cases. It involves incision by scissors of the perineal muscles and lower vagina at the end of the second stage of labour. It is usually made in a posterolateral direction following infiltration with plain local anaesthetic. Some operators favour a midline incision, although the risks of this incision extending posteriorly into the anal sphincters and rectum are greater.

The indications for episiotomy are:

1. to expedite delivery of the fetal head if there is fetal distress during the late second stage of labour;
2. to reduce trauma to the fetal head in cases of prematurity (<34 weeks) and breech presentation;
3. to minimise risks of large perineal and vaginal tears if forceps are used, if the fetal head is very large or if the perineum is fibrotic and likely to tear during delivery.

The operation should never be performed without a clear indication that it is really necessary.

Repair of an episiotomy is not always easy. The vaginal incision should be repaired by a continuous plain catgut suture. Interrupted chromic catgut sutures should be used to bring the perineal muscles together. The perineal skin should be closed with a subcutaneous continuous suture of fine catgut.

Postoperative pain is common because of the sensitivity of the perineum, the presence of oedema and chafing of sutures while walking. Good surgical technique and a subcutaneous skin incision should minimise discomfort, but perineal ice-packs and analgesics or occasionally ultrasound may be necessary for a few days.

It has been claimed that a number of suture materials other than catgut cause less tissue reaction and so are better. They dissolve more slowly and may cause long-term infection and expulsion of suture material many weeks after delivery. In the author's opinion a good surgical technique using plain and chromic catgut is the best.

Vacuum Extraction

Delivery of the baby by vacuum extraction is an old idea that only became a reality in obstetric practice in the early 1960s. The vacuum extractor is shown in Fig. 11.5. A metal or plastic cup is applied to the fetal scalp. When a vacuum is applied, the soft tissues of the scalp are sucked into the cavity of the cup forming a dome (chignon). Traction is then applied to the cup and, if excessive, causes detachment of the cup (Fig. 11.6), a feature considered to protect the baby from the effects of excessive traction.

Indications for vacuum extraction

1. **During the first stage of labour**
   Slow progress in cervical dilatation. It has been claimed that vacuum extraction may be safely undertaken if the cervix is 5 cm or more dilated and the presenting part has descended to the midcavity of the pelvis. This is particularly true for the multiparous patient. There must be no cephalopelvic disproportion. Traction is applied intermittently, bringing the head into contact with the undilated part of the cervix. Delivery can be effected safely within 20 min in the majority of cases.

   When the level of the fetal head lies above the ischial spines, there is a danger of trauma to the mother and fetus and a high incidence of failure to deliver. As with forceps delivery, a high vacuum extraction is to be avoided. An exception to this rule may be the delivery of the second twin. Where the tissues of the birth canal have already been dilated by the delivery of the first twin, application of the vacuum extractor to the head of the second twin, even if still high, may result in safe delivery.

   Fetal distress in the first stage of labour. Much controversy surrounds the use of vacuum extraction in this situation. Once cervical dilatation has reached 7 cm, delivery can be effected quickly

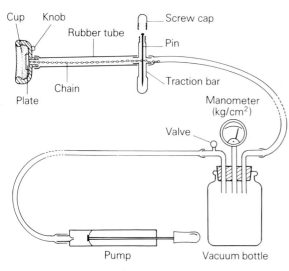

Fig. 11.5 *The vaccum extractor.*

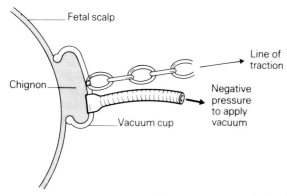

Fig. 11.6 *The application of the vaccum cup to the fetal scalp to permit traction. (Adapted from G. Chamberlain, 1980. Forceps and vaccum extraction. In Clinics in Obstetrics and Gynaecology. I. MacGillivray, ed. London: Saunders.)*

and safely. More often than not, delivery is achieved long before the time taken to organise and commence a caesarean section. Here, more than ever, the experience of the operator is vital.

2. **During the second stage of labour.** The vacuum extractor may be used as an alternative to forceps for delivery when the cervix is fully dilated and operative delivery indicated. Its use in such situations is popular in many European countries. There is probably little to choose between the

methods, given skilled operators. The vacuum extractor may be safer than rotational forceps when the head is occipitoposterior or transverse. Also its use may produce less discomfort for the mother, avoiding the additional distension of the soft tissues and perineum incurred with forceps delivery.

Complications of vacuum extraction

The complications of vacuum extraction are described below.

Fetal. The chignon which remains after removal of the cup from the fetal scalp looks formidable, but invariably settles quickly. There may be a circular area of bruising which dissipates within 3–4 days. When traction has been ill-directed or excessive, superficial scalp abrasions may occur. These heal rapidly and without treatment.

In approximately 1% of cases, cephalhaematoma occurs which is not very different from the figure for all deliveries. As the haematoma resolves, neonatal jaundice may occur.

Maternal. Damage may occur to the cervix and walls of the vagina if they are inadvertently included during application of the cup to the fetal scalp. Proper technique avoids this.

Very rarely the cervix has been lacerated when the instrument is used during the first stage of labour. Such lacerations require suturing, but heal well.

Dilatation of the cervix using the vacuum extractor does not cause cervical incompetence.

Contraindications of vacuum extractor

The major contraindication to the use of the vacuum extractor is cephalopelvic disproportion. In this respect, the instrument offers greater safety than forceps in that, when excessive traction is applied, the cup detaches, thus protecting the baby's head.

In malpresentations, the vacuum extractor is used with caution. It may be of benefit in brow presentation, but has no place in the management of face presentation. In such a presentation, the vacuum would be applied over the eyes, causing severe damage.

Caesarean Section

Elective caesarean section is performed prior to the onset of labour and implies that vaginal delivery is contraindicated. Emergency caesarean section is performed after the onset of labour and implies that safe vaginal delivery has become impossible.

Lower segment caesarean section describes the placement of the incision of the uterus in its lower segment, usually in a transverse direction and is by far the most common procedure performed (Fig. 11.7). Classical caesarean section describes the placement of the incision of the uterus in the upper segment, invariably in a longitudinal direction.

Indications for elective caesarean section

It is virtually impossible to draw up a list of specific indications for caesarean section that would gain universal approval.

The indications may be categorised in a general sense. Often these categories combine fetal and maternal interests.

Cephalopelvic disproportion. Where there is an obvious discrepancy between the size of the baby and the birth canal, the risk of birth trauma may warrant delivery prior to the onset of labour.

Complications of pregnancy. This group includes conditions which cause placental insufficiency and render the infant incapable of withstanding the physiological stress of labour. Severe intrauterine growth retardation may warrant elective section solely in the interests of the fetus. Elective section in the presence of fulminating preeclampsia or severe abruptio placentae may combine both fetal and maternal interests.

Presentation of the fetus. A body of opinion firmly believes elective caesarean section is warranted in all breech presentations for fear of birth trauma. A greater proportion of obstetricians accept that a breech presentation combined with any other complication, such as hypertension, intrauterine growth retardation, prematurity (estimated fetal weight <1.5 kg) or maternal diabetes, should not be allowed to deliver vaginally.

Obstruction to the descent of the presenting part. This group of indications includes cephalopelvic disproportion. The presence of placenta prae-

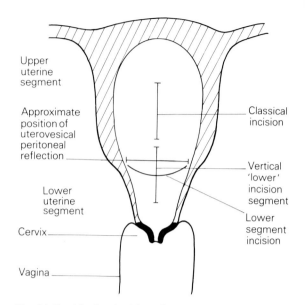

Fig. 11.7   *Uterine incisions for caesarean sections.*

via, cervical fibroid or ovarian cyst may prevent the presenting part from entering the pelvis. The occurrence of an unstable lie at term is accepted by many as an absolute indication for elective caesarean section.

Previous surgical incision of the uterus. In the past, previous hysterotomy or myomectomy were considered to be indications for elective caesarean section. However, views are now favouring a more conservative approach and these patients are usually allowed to deliver vaginally. Multiple myomectomy would be an indication for abdominal delivery.

Previous lower segment caesarean section for a non-recurring cause has generally been accepted as a poor reason for repeat elective section. However, if two or more caesarean sections have been performed previously, the risks of the conservative approach must be carefully considered as the incidence of uterine rupture will be increased.

Labour following a previous classical caesarean section is also cause for concern as the risk of uterine rupture is six times as high as with the lower segment counterpart (Table 11.8).

Poor obstetric history. Most obstetricians accept that there are circumstances in which previous reproductive/obstetric performance warrants elective caesarean section in a subsequent pregnancy. The would-be mother, particularly over 35 years of age, who has had several previous pregnancies ending in early or late spontaneous abortion, or the mother who has a handicapped child as a result of intrapartum asphyxia provide examples.

Delivery of the preterm infant. With the improvement in neonatal care, there has been marked improvement in the outlook for the small, preterm infant. What risk these babies face, especially if presenting by the breech, in vaginal delivery poses a real dilemma for the obstetrician. There has been a marked increase in the use of elective caesarean section in these cases specifically to avoid fetal asphyxia and trauma (intracranial haemorrhage) during labour and delivery. Published figures are both confusing and contradictory, but it has been suggested on retrospective evidence that caesarean section is of value when the infant weighs between 1000 and 1499 g and presents by the breech. Caesarean section *per se* does not seem to benefit the preterm infant weighing 1000–1499 g whose presentation is cephalic.

Multiple pregnancy. Triplets and quadruplets are rare events in obstetrics. However, most obstetricians accept that such multiple pregnancies are best delivered by elective caesarean section. With the increasing use of in vitro fertilisation for infertility, there is likely to be a small rise in the incidence of such multiple pregnancies.

Indications for emergency caesarean section

Fetal or maternal distress. Fetal distress in the first stage of labour may be severe enough to warrant prompt delivery. As outlined previously, delivery may be effected by use of the vacuum extractor if the cervix is nearly fully dilated, but the majority would advocate delivery by lower segment caesarean section.

Maternal distress during the first stage of labour is rarely, if ever, an indication for caesarean section due to the availability of adequate methods of providing analgesia.

Prolonged labour. As has been previously discussed, failure of labour to progress despite efficient uterine action may warrant delivery by caesarean section to reduce fetal and maternal risks.

Cephalopelvic disproportion/obstructed labour. This is an important diagnosis and may not be apparent until after labour has commenced. Caesarean section is indicated to avoid fetal injury and uterine rupture.

Type of caesarean section

The vast majority of caesarean sections performed in modern obstetric practice are of the lower segment variety. An incision so placed heals better, provides less risk to the integrity of the uterus in subsequent labour (Table 11.8), is associated with less haemorrhage at the time of surgery and is less likely to cause intraperitoneal adhesions.

However, the use of the classical procedure will never disappear entirely. Major degrees of placenta praevia may render the lower segment so vascular that an incision in the upper segment provides a safer option. An anterior wall fibroid in the lower segment may render access impossible. Compound presentation of the fetus, especially if the arm has prolapsed through the cervix into the vagina, or a transverse lie with the uterus contracted, may require an incision in the upper uterine segment to provide sufficient access to permit manipulation of

Table 11.8

The Incidence Rate of Rupture of the Uterus in Patients Previously Delivered by Caesarean Section

	All cases %	Cases in labour %	Cases delivered vaginally %
Lower segment incision	0.5	0.8	1.2
Classical incision	2.2	4.7	8.9

Table 11.9

Estimated Fatality Rate per 1000 Caesarean Sections in England and Wales

Year	Rate per 1000 Caesarean Sections
1966	1.9
1967	1.4
1968	1.4
1969	1.0
1970	1.1
1971	1.1
1972	1.0
1973	1.0
1974	0.7
1975	0.7

(From *Report on Confidential Enquires into Maternal Deaths in England and Wales, 1973–1975*. London: HMSO.)

the baby to enable delivery. These are rare occurrences, but deny any option in the type of procedure performed.

Complications of caesarean section

Maternal mortality. The risk of fatality following caesarean section is now less than 1 in 1000 (Table 11.9). The operation can, therefore, be considered as relatively safe. When the causes of death are scrutinised (Table 11.10), it can be appreciated that the administration of an emergency anaesthetic together with other causes of death, such as hypertensive diseases of pregnancy, increase these risks for an individual.

Haemorrhage. Haemorrhage is the most common complication of the operation. The average blood loss is between 300 and 600 ml, mainly due to the large venous sinuses within uterine muscle, which become even larger in the presence of placenta praevia. After delivery of the baby, the uterus naturally retracts and contracts, providing a very effective, mechanical means of controlling haemorrhage. Intravenous syntocinon (10 u) is given as a bolus routinely after the delivery of the baby to aid this process and to overcome any relaxing effect the anaesthetic may have on uterine retraction.

Excessive haemorrhage is most often associated with extension of the uterine incision laterally causing damage to the uterine vessels. It can be avoided by using a curved incision, properly placed in the lower segment, and unhurried delivery of the head and shoulders. Suturing of this region is hazardous and requires extreme care to avoid damaging surrounding structures such as the ureter and sigmoid colon.

Very rarely, haemorrhage is excessive and uncontrollable, but occasionally occurs with multiple fibroids, placenta praevia and uterine rupture. In these circumstances, hysterectomy may offer the only hope of vascular control.

Bladder damage. Given proper surgical technique, this should occur only very rarely. In repeat caesarean section, the bladder is often very adherent to the lower uterine segment and requires careful, sharp dissection. When the bladder is damaged, recognition is essential as repair is usually straightforward, with good results.

Table 11.10

Proportion of Maternal Deaths Connected with Caesarean Section, Classified According to Immediate Cause of Death

Cause of death	1967–69 %	1970–72 %	1973–75 %	1976–78 %
Haemorrhage	11.3	7.2	9.9	11.1
Pulmonary embolism	14.5	15.3	7.4	10.0
Sepsis and paralytic ileus	8.9	14.4	9.9	8.9
Hypertensive diseases of pregnancy	4.8	13.5	14.8	13.3
Anaesthesia	25.8	17.0	21.0	22.2
Other conditions (including associated diseases)	30.6	32.4	37.0	34.4

(From *Report on Confidential Enquiries into Maternal Deaths in England and Wales, 1976–1978*. London: HMSO.)

Deep venous thrombosis/pulmonary embolism. Pregnancy causes increased coagulation potential, with increases in factors I, VII, VIII and X from approximately 14 weeks' gestation. This, associated with any circumstances which reduce venous blood flow or damage the intima of the vessel wall, increases the potential for developing deep venous thrombosis and/or pulmonary embolism.

Many of the hazards are avoidable, such as prolonged labour, failure to correct dehydration and blood loss, misuse of lithotomy poles, failure to relieve calf pressure by ankle support at caesarean section and delay in mobilisation postoperatively. Early treatment of pelvic infection minimises the risk of pelvic vein thrombosis.

Postoperative ileus. Postoperative abdominal distension is common after caesarean section. The majority recover within 24–48 h with simple measures such as intravenous fluids and aspiration of gastrointestinal contents.

Infection. As with operative procedure, infection may occur within the pelvis or abdominal wound, but should occur in less than 4% of patients.

MALPRESENTATIONS

These include breech presentations, face and brow presentations, transverse lie with possibly the arm or shoulder presenting and finally cord presentation.

Breech Presentation

The incidence is about 30% at 28–30 weeks' gestation and reduces to about 3% at term. The incidence of breech delivery varies between 2 and 3% depending on various factors such as the incidence of prematurity. The more common type of breech presentation is shown in Fig. 11.8. The hips are flexed, the buttocks and sacrum fill the lower uterine segment and so cord prolapse is not very likely. The knees may be fully extended, splinting the body. The other form of breech presentation is when one or both hips are extended with the knees in varying degrees of flexion, consequently a knee or foot may present. The risk of cord prolapse in these cases is increased considerably.

External cephalic version

It is debatable as to how much a policy of external cephalic version actually reduces the incidence of breech delivery. If it is carried out, it should be between 34 and 36 weeks, because prior to 34 weeks the breech may turn spontaneously, while after 36 weeks it gets progressively more difficult to perform the version. The breech should be out of the pelvis, the uterus relaxed (tocolytics can be used) and no undue force should be exerted. The direction of rotation should be such as to encourage flexion of the fetus. The version may only be temporarily successful, it may cause placental separation, rupture of the membranes or, particularly if performed more than once, cord entanglement. It should only be attempted in singleton pregnancies and must not be carried out if there is (1) a scar on the uterus; (2) hypertension; and (3) a history of antepartum haemorrhage.

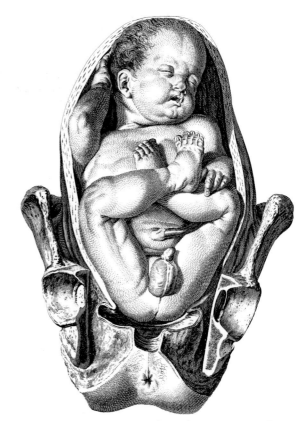

Fig. 11.8 *Common types of breech presentation. (From William Smellie's Anatomical Tables. Facsimile of 1754 edition published by University of Auckland, 1971.)*

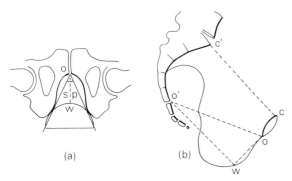

Fig. 11.9   *Radiograph of (a) outlet of pelvis, sp = subpubic angle; ow = waste space; (b) erect lateral view. cc' = shortest conjugate; ow = waste space between fetal head and subpubic arch; o'w = available antero-posterior diameter of pelvic outlet.*

Assessment of mode of delivery

Labour should only be allowed to proceed with a breech presentation if there is adequate room within the pelvis for easy passage of the after-coming fetal head. There will be no time for moulding and while minor degrees of cephalopelvic disproportion can be dealt with naturally by mould-ing when the head presents, this can lead to disastrous fetal damage in breech presentations.

The pelvis is assessed radiologically and clini-cally. An erect lateral film gives most information with one x-ray. Details are given in Fig. 11.9. Clinical pelvimetry is necessary to assess the outlet and, in particular, the width of the pelvis, the prominence of the ischial spines, and the angle of the subpubic arch. If the pelvis is normal with prominent ischial spines and a narrow subpubic angle, it suggests an android type of funnel-shaped pelvis. Breech delivery in those circumstances should only be considered if the fetus is preterm. Assessment of fetal size, including biparietal dia-meter and head and abdominal circumferences, should be made with ultrasound. A vaginal breech delivery in a primigravid patient should only be considered if the baby is not excessively large (<3.5 kg) and the diameters of the pelvis are good. The anteroposterior diameter of the pelvic brim should be at least 11.5 cm and that of the pelvic outlet equally good.

Attitudes to breech delivery have changed consi-derably throughout the developed world during the last 10 years, with an increasing trend towards caesarean section, because of the increased fetal mortality and morbidity with breech delivery and a more litigious general public and legal profession.

The current practice in many developed coun-tries is to allow vaginal breech delivery if the pelvis is obviously adequate and if there are no other abnormalities of pregnancy. Otherwise, lower seg-ment caesarean section is the mode of delivery.

Management of labour in breech presentation

The membranes should be left intact for as long as possible, particularly if it is a footling breech pres-entation, as cord prolapse is more likely than when the presenting part fits snugly into the pelvis. Progress in labour in terms of descent of the presenting part and cervical dilatation should be steady and if this is not the case in the presence of a frank breech, then serious consideration should be given to delivery by caesarean section before the second stage is reached. In breech presentation, the duration of the first stage of labour is usually longer than normal. The technical details of breech deli-very are outside the scope of this book. However, some important principles for delivery of the frank breech should be known. These are:

1. Adequate relaxation and analgesia are nec-essary in order to carry out the necessary manoeuvres — epidural anaesthesia is ideal.
2. The breech should be allowed to descend to the perineum before any intervention takes place.
3. An episiotomy should be performed.
4. The breech and legs should deliver sponta-neously as far as possible before there is any assistance.
5. Once the legs are delivered, the umbilical cord is revealed and a loop pulled down to ensure that it is not too short to allow completion of the delivery.
6. The trunk is delivered either spontaneously or by gentle traction on the fetal pelvis. The shoulders are then rotated into the anterior-posterior plane, the anterior arm is delivered by flexion and traction at the elbow followed by the posterior arm. Should there be difficulty, this is likely to be due to extended arms. They are brought down by first getting the shoulders into the anteroposterior plane and then rotat-ing the fetus with its back uppermost through 180°. This brings the previously posterior arm to behind the pubic symphysis and it is then delivered. Rotation back through 180° again

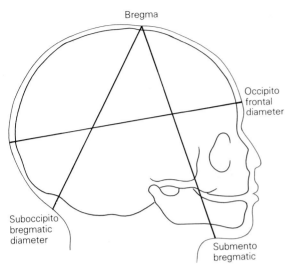

Fig. 11.10 *Fetal diameters presenting in face and brow presentations.*

Shoulder Presentation

This presentation may often lead to cord prolapse. It can occur if there is hydramnios, uterine abnormalities, minor degrees of placenta praevia or, spontaneously, in grand multiparae with uterine hypotonus.

If there is a tranverse lie, an arm may decend through the cervix. Vaginal delivery is, therefore, impossible as can be seen from Fig. 11.11. Delivery by caesarean section is necessary, otherwise the uterus may rupture.

Cord Presentation and Prolapse

Occasionally, loops of cord will present behind intact membranes. Caesarean section is necessary to prevent cord prolapse when the membranes rupture. More often the cord will prolapse as a result of some other malpresentation, such as a footling breech or transverse lie. Management of this obstetric emergency requires keeping the cord warm and moist by replacing it into the vagina, keeping pressure off it to prevent mechanical

with the back uppermost, allows delivery of the other arm (Lovset's manoeuvre).

7. Once the trunk, shoulder and arms are delivered, the body should be allowed to hang for a few seconds to encourage descent and flexion of the head.
8. Delivery of the head is by low cavity forceps or with manual control of flexion of the head (using Mauriceau-Smellie-Viet manoeuvre).

Face and Brow Presentations

These represent varying degrees of extension of the normally well flexed fetal head. Partial extension results in a brow presentation with the presenting diameter being the largest, namely the occipito-frontal. Obstruction during labour is very likely and so delivery should be by caesarean section.

Full extension of the fetal head leads to the submento-bregmatic diameter being the presenting one and this approximates to the normal subocci-pito-bregmatic diameter which presents when the head is well flexed (Fig. 11.10). Vaginal delivery is therefore possible, particularly if the chin is anterior (mentoanterior). If the presentation is mentoposterior, rotation to mentoanterior followed by a vaginal delivery may occur. If rotation fails, then the chin gets obstructed within the hollow of the sacrum and delivery by caesarean section is necessary.

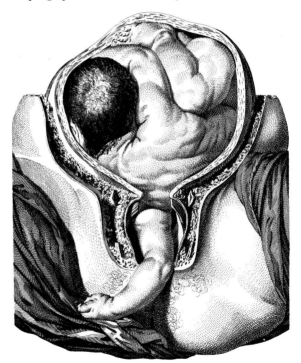

Fig. 11.11 *Transverse lie with arm descending through the cervix. (From* William Smellie's Anatomical Tables. *Facsimile of 1754 edition published by University of Auckland, 1971.)*

obstruction to the blood flow and to minimise its handling. Caesarean section should be carried out as soon as possible. Alterations in temperature and Po_2 cause chemical constriction of the cord vessels. Occasionally, if cord prolapse occurs when the cervix is fully dilated, immediate operative vaginal delivery may be appropriate.

FURTHER READING

Anderson A., Beard R., Brudenell M., Dunn P., eds. (1977). *Proceedings of the Fifth Study Group of the Royal College of Obstetricians and Gynaecologists.* London.

Beard R., Brudenell M., Dunn P., Fairweather D., eds. (1975). *Proceedings of the Third Study Group of the Royal College of Obstetricians and Gynaecologists.* London.

Beazley J.M. ed. (1975). Active management of labour. In *Clinics in Obstetrics and Gynaecology*, Vol. 2, No. 1. London: W.B. Saunders.

Elder M., Hendricks C.H. eds. (1981). *Pre-term Labour.* London: Butterworth.

MacGillivray I., ed. (1980). Operative obstetrics. In *Clinics in Obstetrics and Gynaecology*, Vol. 7, No. 3. London: W.B. Saunders.

12

Puerperium and Lactation

Puerperium is derived from the Latin *puerperus* meaning childbirth. It refers to the period of time from the end of the third stage of labour until most of the changes of pregnancy have reverted to normal, usually six weeks. Some of these changes such as involution of the uterus are obvious and occur rapidly, while others, such as the reversion to normal of the urinary tract, are much more gradual and less obvious.

PSYCHOLOGICAL CHANGES AND REACTION

The postpartum depression or 'blues' is a relatively common event reflecting a mixture of emotions. Prolonged anticipation and excitement culminating in delivery has a rebound effect. Additionally, fatigue, anxiety about the baby and the effect on the brain of the big reductions in circulating oestrogen and progesterone levels following delivery, all contribute. The 'blues' may present as emotional instability or mild depression and should not last for more than 2 weeks. Support and reassurance that these events are normal is usually sufficient treatment. Pre-existing psychotic illness can present during the puerperium for the first time as a result of stress, but it is not caused primarily by childbirth. Persistent postnatal depression is a manifestation of pre-existing endogenous depression and needs appropriate investigation and management. Antidepressant drugs are not usually appropriate therapy. Attention to the woman's physical state, together with sympathetic support and counselling with formal psychotherapy, if necessary, are normally better forms of treatment.

ANATOMY OF BREAST AND LACTATION

The development and anatomy of the mammary gland is described in Chapter 16. During preg-

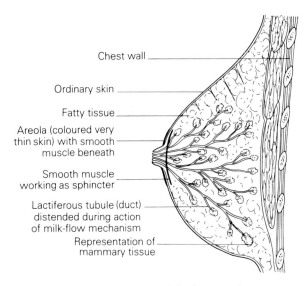

Chest wall

Ordinary skin

Fatty tissue

Areola (coloured very thin skin) with smooth muscle beneath

Smooth muscle working as sphincter

Lactiferous tubule (duct) distended during action of milk-flow mechanism

Representation of mammary tissue

Fig. 12.1 *The structure of the lactating breast.*

nancy, growth of lobules and alveoli proceeds. Mammary growth during pregnancy is stimulated by oestrogen, human placental lactogen, progesterone, growth hormone and cortisol. The structure of the lactating breast is shown in Fig. 12.1.

Antenatal Assessment of the Breast

During midpregnancy, the protractility of the nipple should be assessed by a finger and thumb on either side at the edge of the areola and squeezing gently to see whether the nipple and tissues under the areola pull forward. If the nipple and tissues remain flat, the baby may have difficulty in obtaining milk. Treatment should be started in the middle of pregnancy with breast shells (also called shields). These work by exerting gentle pressure on the breast while the nipple projects through the hole in the shell. Gradually, the nipple and areola become more protractile. The shells require support from a well-fitting brassiere and the hole should be large enough for the nipple and about one-third of the areola to be free. The mother should start off wearing the shells an hour a day and then for as many hours as convenient during daytime (Fig. 12.2).

Milk Production

Milk is produced by the alveolar cells taking up precursors from the blood and synthesising the milk constituents, which are then passed into the lumen of the alveolus. This process is independent of neurological control, but is under endocrine control.

Prolactin

Prolactin is a polypeptide hormone produced in the anterior pituitary. Its amino acid sequence has some similarities to growth hormone. Human placental lactogen (HPL) is secreted throughout pregnancy by the placenta, but the high levels of oestrogen and progesterone block the lactogenic effect. After birth, the levels of oestrogen and progesterone fall. This removes the block and allows a full secretory response. With the delivery of the placenta, HPL levels fall. If the mother does not breast feed, serum prolactin remains at around 10 ng/ml but, in mothers who breast feed, prolactin levels rise to 20–50 ng/ml. The sucking stimulus brings a rapid rise to about 1000 ng/ml.

The pathway for prolactin secretion is from two origins. One is from the frontal cerebral cortex and the other is the sensory innervation of the nipple.

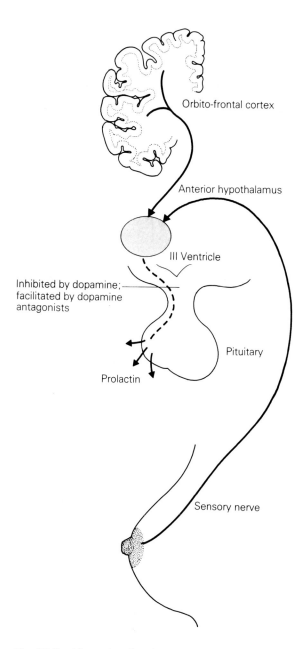

Orbito-frontal cortex

Anterior hypothalamus

III Ventricle

Inhibited by dopamine; facilitated by dopamine antagonists

Pituitary

Prolactin

Sensory nerve

Fig. 12.3 *Necessity of prolactin secretion for the initiation and maintenance of lactation.*

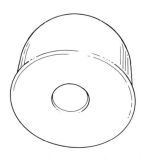

Fig. 12.2 *Woolwich breast shell.*

Both inputs go to the anterior hypothalamus close to the third ventricle. From there, neurotransmitters are conveyed to the anterior pituitary by the hypophyseal portal system (Fig. 12.3).

Prolactin secretion is inhibited by the neurotransmitter, *dopamine*. L-dopa inhibits lactation in this way. Bromocriptine, a dopamine agonist, is a more powerful inhibitor of lactation and can be used therapeutically in doses of 2.5–5.0 mg daily to mothers who do not wish to breast feed. Oestrogens can also be given to inhibit lactation as they block the effect of prolactin. Secretion of prolactin can be increased by the administration of hypothalamic thyrotrophin-releasing-hormone (TRH). Dopamine antagonist drugs such as the phenothiazines stimulate prolactin and this has been used to increase milk production in mothers who cannot supply all their baby's needs. Chlorpromazine, metoclopramide and sulpiride have all been used in this way.

Milk Removal

Milk, when produced, is stored in the alveoli, ducts and cisterns of the breast. The milk in the larger ducts and sinuses is available to the baby sucking. Milk is transported from the alveoli by the contraction of myoepithelial cells which envelop the alveoli. Contraction is stimulated by oxytocin from the posterior pituitary gland in response to the stimulus of the baby sucking on the breast. This sudden availability of milk is known as the 'milk ejection', 'draught' or 'let down' reflex. The reflex can also be stimulated by the sight and sound of the baby and

by gentle touch on the breast. This pathway is from the sensory nerve endings in the nipple to the spinothalamic tract, then the paraventricular nuclei from which neurosecretory axons run to the posterior pituitary. The reflex takes less than a minute from stimulation.

Oxytocin is released in repeated bursts and produces pressure waves of over 15 mmHg in the ducts of the breast. These changes occur in both breasts while the baby is sucking from only one. Thus some milk usually drips from the opposite breast even when no sucking is applied.

Continued breast feeding may result in amenorrhoea and thus provides some degree of contraception, particularly when suckling is frequent. Once night feeding is reduced or stops, ovarian follicular function commences, and ultimately so does ovulation. Contraception is advisable during lactation.

Composition of Breast Milk

Table 12.1 shows the composition of mature human milk compared to cow's milk. The protein content of cow's milk is higher and much of the protein is casein which tends to form large curds in the stomach. The sodium and phosphate content of cow's milk is much higher than human milk. The carbohydrate content of cow's milk is lower and the fat content varies according to the breed of cow (being very high in Channel Island cows, for example). The composition of mature human milk is ideal for human babies' growth. The high sodium content of cow's milk may result in a baby becoming dangerously hypernatraemic if fluid loss from diar-

Table 12.1

Composition of Milk

	Mature breast milk	Preterm breast milk	Cow's milk	
Protein	1.0	1.9	3.3	g/dl
Fat	3.8	3.5	3.7	g/dl
Carbohydrate	7.0	7.1	4.8	g/dl
Sodium	15	32	58	mg/dl
Calcium	33	30	125	mg/dl
Phosphorus	15	15	96	mg/dl
Energy	67	67	66	kcal/dl

(From T.E. Oppe, 1974. *Present Day Practice of Infant Feeding*. DHSS Report on Health and Social Subjects. London: HMSO.)

rhoea or fever occurs. The high phosphate content may give excessive plasma phosphate levels with reciprocal hypocalcaemia and convulsions.

Preterm babies, especially those born before 32 weeks, have different requirements from full-term babies and need larger amounts of sodium, calcium and phosphate. Breast milk from mothers who deliver preterm has a different composition from mature breast milk, having significantly higher protein and sodium levels, but no change in phosphate content.

Human milk has a number of important *protective substances* of which the most important is IgA globulin fraction. During the first few days, the initial milk, known as colostrum, is particularly rich in IgA. Lactoferrin is a protein which binds iron in the lumen of the intestine and makes it unavailable for bacterial growth, while intestinal absorption can continue. Lysozyme is a non-specific antibacterial protein. An antiviral substance has also been demonstrated in human milk. White blood cells are present in breast milk and may also have a protective effect in the body. Cow's milk and artificial formulae have no protective effect on human babies.

Cow's milk protein allergy

This is a cause of some cases of failure to thrive, infantile eczema and perhaps colic. While allergy to human milk is much less common, it is still possible for a baby to react to very small amounts of antigens (cow's milk, egg, etc.) from the mother's diet which have passed into the breast milk.

Nutritional Requirements

All the requirements of a full-term baby are supplied by breast milk if the volume of fced is approximately 150 ml/kg/day. Sufficient protein, calories, electrolytes, minerals, trace elements and essential fatty acids are provided.

No supplementation is needed until the baby is at least four months of age when solid foods such as rice cereal and puréed apple may be given for variety and to space out the meals, but are not nutritionally essential.

The only nutritional supplement which is advisable is *vitamin K*. This is essential for the synthesis of coagulation factors. If no vitamin K is given at birth, a small but definite number of breast fed infants become deficient and develop a clinical bleeding disorder towards the end of the first week of life.

If the mother's diet is grossly deficient, then the breast milk may be reduced in volume rather than protein and calorie content. Vitamin D and vitamin B_{12} may be deficient in breast milk if the mother's diet is severely reduced in these nutrients.

Technique of Breast Feeding

The mother should be in a comfortable position. She can be sitting upright or lying down (Fig. 12.4). If she is sitting up, it may help to lean forward slightly. The breast should be quite free of the brassiere. The baby can be held in one arm (left arm for left breast, right arm for right breast) with the arm supporting the neck and head and holding his mouth and nose level with the nipple.

If the mother is lying down, the baby can be laid on his side parallel to her trunk. The breast can then be moved so that the nipple is level with the baby's mouth.

The baby can be put to the breast within minutes of delivery. The release of oxytocin may be helpful in contracting the uterus. Subsequently, the baby can be put to the breast for a few minutes every three or four hours. There will be small volumes of colostrum released in the first two days, but by the 3rd or 4th day the volume of milk increases.

The baby obtains milk by:

1. the milking action of the baby's jaw and tongue;
2. suction with each swallow;
3. by the milk ejection reflex.

The nipple should go right to the back of the mouth so that the areola comes between the jaws and milk is obtained by compression of the ducts under the areola. This milking action of the jaws and tongue is the most important mechanism, because it obtains milk and also stimulates oxytocin secretion. With the milk ejection reflex, the rate of flow from the breast may be 30 ml or more per minute early in a feed. The position of the baby's head may have to be adjusted, close to the breast with the chin against the skin and the head slightly extended.

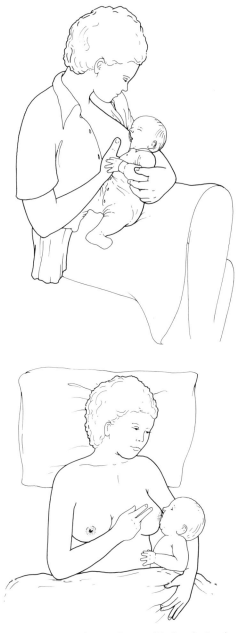

Fig. 12.4 *Positions for mother and baby during breast feeding.*

Problems of Lactation

Some common problems are:

1. **The nipple is not far enough into the mouth.** The milk ducts are not compressed and there is inadequate stimulation of the milk ejection reflex.

2. **The mother is afraid or anxious.** If the baby feeds for a short time and then stops, feel the breast. If the breast is empty, it is soft. If the milk ejection reflex has not been stimulated, the breast will feel full. If there is insufficient milk production, extra feeding may stimulate prolactin secretion. Helping the mother to relax mentally and physically, and maintenance of the fluid intake, will help with breast feeding. Dopamine antagonist phenothiazines, such as metoclopramide, have been shown to increase milk production, but emotional support, explanation and encouragement are probably more helpful.

3. **Fighting the breast** is the term used to describe the baby turning his head away from the nipple, crying, arching his back and pushing with his fists. This upsetting behaviour is usually due to difficulty with breathing, the upper lip riding up and covering the nostrils. This is more likely to happen if the nipple protracts poorly.

4. **Engorgement** is a painful accumulation of milk which may occur on the 3rd or 4th day. By the 3rd day, milk production may exceed the baby's capacity and the milk-ejection reflex may not be working satisfactorily. If the pressure within the breast rises, obstruction to the lymphatic drainage may occur, causing oedema. The lax tissues beneath the areola may swell and harden, thus making it more difficult for the baby to take the areola into his mouth. Engorgement should be prevented by the baby emptying the breast at each feed. The treatment for engorgement is to give analgesia and empty the breast using a pump. Manual expression is not easy for many mothers to learn and a hand or electric pump will empty the breast more efficiently.

5. **Acute intramammary mastitis.** This condition occurs when an excessively distended set of alveoli leak milk into the surrounding tissues. An inflammatory reaction occurs with local swelling, tenderness, redness and a fever. Early emptying of the breast by pump may resolve the problem. If the condition has established itself over two days, milk suppression, analgesia, local application of warmth and anti-staphylococcal antibiotic cover will be necessary.

If not controlled early, secondary invasion with staphylococci may lead to a *breast abscess*, with segmental redness and oedema.

Suppression of Lactation

Suppression of lactation after it has commenced is seldom necessary, but it may be required if the nipples become very cracked and sore, a breast abscess develops or there is bleeding from the nipple. A dopamine agonist inhibiting prolactin secretion such as bromocriptine is the most effective treatment and it is used in doses of 2.5 mg b.d. for up to two weeks. The use of large doses of oestrogens is no longer acceptable because of side-effects, including an increased risk of venous thromboembolism. Preventing lactation from starting may often be achieved by avoiding emptying the breast, using firm supports, analgesics if required, and fluid restriction for two to three days. If this conservative approach is unsuccessful, bromocriptine is again recommended.

Breast Feeding Small-for-Gestational-Age Babies

Babies below the 10th centile for birth weight may have low stores of carbohydrate and fat. There is a need for a substantial nutritional intake to prevent hypoglycaemia. Milk production may be much less than the 80–100 ml/kg/day that the baby requires, especially if the mother is primiparous. Hypoglycaemic convulsions at 24–48 h may permanently damage the baby. Thus extra effort is required to help mothers with such babies and blood glucose must be monitored every 4–6 h.

Breast Feeding and Preterm Babies

Babies born before 35 weeks' gestation are not usually able to breast feed for themselves. Tube feeding is required either by the use of an indwelling nasogastric tube, indwelling orogastric tube or intermittent orogastric tube (gavage). Mother's milk can still be given by using an electric or hand pump to express the milk which can either be given fresh or may be frozen to be thawed and given later. Boiling breast milk (to kill any bacteria) destroys all the protective substances and milk lipase. If decontamination, such as milk donated by other mothers, is considered necessary, pasteurisation at 62°C for 30 min should provide adequate sterilisation while preserving most of the protective substances.

Drugs and Breast Feeding

Many drugs may enter breast milk and so be ingested by the infant. However, the significance of this to the infant depends on the nature of the drug, degree of protein binding and the quantity in which it is transferred. Protein bound drug is not transferred. Transfer to breast milk usually takes place by diffusion. Drugs that ionise and have a basic pH diffuse more readily than acidic ions, as the pH of milk is weakly acid compared to that of maternal plasma, which is weakly alkaline. Some drugs are actively transported into breast milk. Drugs with large molecular size do not, as a rule, pass into breast milk. These include heparin and insulin. Some maternal drugs which may have harmful effects on the breastfed baby sufficient to contraindicate breast feeding are shown in Table 12.2.

Table 12.2

Maternal Drugs which Contraindicate Breast Feeding

Methotrexate
Cyclophosphamide
Iodine and radioiodine
Amiodarone
Lithium
Thiouracil
Phenindione
High dose benzodiazepines

A number of other drugs can cause side-effects in the baby, but may not be completely contraindicated. These are listed in Table 12.3 together with their possible effects on the infant.

High doses of progestogens, if given to the mother as injectable contraception, will transfer to the breast milk and be ingested. Daily amounts are tiny, but these drugs should not be used during the first six weeks of lactation.

Table 12.3

Maternal Drugs Causing Side-effects on Infant

Drug	Side-effect
Alcohol	Drowsiness
Various antibiotics	
Gentamicin	
Streptomycin	Ototoxicity
Kanamycin	
Tetracycline	Discoloured teeth
Septrin	Folic acid deficiency
Chloramphenicol	Feeding problems
Barbiturates	Sleepiness
Antithyroid drugs (carbimazole)	Nodular goitre
Tolbutamide	Hyperglycaemia
Laxatives	Diarrhoea

UTERINE INVOLUTION AND OTHER CHANGES

The uterus reduces in weight from about 1 kg at term to about 50–100 g in the non-pregnant state. Contractions occurring after delivery and throughout the puerperium are stimulated by oxytocin. These are particularly strong and sometimes painful during breast stimulation, i.e. suckling. Muscle fibres remain constant in number, but are reduced in size, losing intracellular constituents in the form of amino acids which are excreted. The puerperal woman is, therefore, initially in negative nitrogen balance. Fibrous tissue undergoes hyaline degeneration. Veins thrombose and undergo hyaline degeneration, while arteries have their lumen occluded by subendothelial swelling. Withdrawal of progesterone leads to autolysis and shedding of the decidua. The placental site is obliterated by the following processes: (a) vascular constriction and occlusion causing haemostasis; (b) ischaemic necrosis; (c) hyalination; (d) autolysis. The endometrium regenerates from the basal layers (decidua basalis) and by growing in from the margins of the placental site.

Lochia

These consist of the autolytic products of the degenerating decidua from the placental site. Until haemostasis is complete, blood is present in the lochia and so they are red for the first two or three days of the puerperium. Blood is replaced by a serous exudate, while leucocytes, mucus, vaginal epithelial cells and non-pathogenic sapprophytic bacteria appear in increasing amounts. The lochia are, therefore, brown from Days 3–6 approximately as the number of red cells decline and, thereafter, become cream coloured. Passage outwards of the lochia and their alkalinity protect against ascending uterine infection. Vaginal douches, therefore, should not be used.

Cardiovascular Changes

The increased blood volume and cardiac output that occur during pregnancy revert to normal during the first few days of the puerperium, a diuresis frequently being obvious. Coagulation factors VII, IX and X are all raised during pregnancy, and there is a further rise during the first few days of the puerperium before a gradual return to non-pregnant levels. There is an increase in venous tone and gradual reduction in varicose veins commonly found in pregnancy. However, they will persist for some time into the puerperium. Increased coagulation factors and increased platelet adhesiveness found postoperatively mean that the puerperal woman who has undergone an operative delivery is at risk for venous thromboembolism. Adequate hydration, prevention of anaemia, good surgical technique and, above all, early and active mobilisation reduce the risk of thromboembolism to one that is very small (1–2 per thousand deliveries). Superficial thrombophlebitis is more common, but less serious as subsequent embolism is very rare.

Treatment of anaemia in the puerperium is usually by oral iron. Folic acid will be needed if there is a macrocytic anaemia. If oral iron is poorly tolerated, then consideration should be given to using i.m. iron sorbitol, or citric acid complex, or rarely as a total dose i.v. infusion of irondextran in saline. Deep venous thrombosis must be treated promptly with anticoagulants, namely i.v. heparin for 48 h, while oral anticoagulation with warfarin is being established.

Alimentary Tract

Constipation is common during the puerperium because of reduced food intake, perineal pain due to episiotomy and/or haemorrhoids, lax abdominal muscles and intestinal atony persisting from pregnancy. Treatment is by increasing fluids, bulk in the diet and use of a bulk laxative (bran, agar) if necessary.

Urinary Tract

The increased glomerular filtration rate, ureteric hypertrophy and dilatation of renal calyces, pelvis, and upper ureter which occur during pregnancy, revert gradually to normal. An intravenous urogram (IVU) should not be performed within three months of childbirth, as residual effects of pregnancy such as ureteric dilatation will make interpretation difficult. Mild trauma to the bladder neck causing oedema may occur during delivery and this, together with bladder atony and perineal pain, may lead to urinary retention during the first few days of the puerperium. Intermittent catheterisation as necessary is the correct management. Indwelling catheters and use of parasympathomimetic drugs should be avoided, because of the increased risk of vesico-ureteric reflux and so infection. Urinary tract infection is more common during the puerperium for the reasons already stated. Awareness of the potential problem, prompt diagnosis and treatment with appropriate antibiotics will prevent the more serious complication of chronic pyelonephritis.

Puerperal Pyrexia

The common causes of puerperal pyrexia are uterine infection, urinary tract infection, breast engorgement — with or without infection — and pelvic or lower limb deep vein thrombosis.

Normally, the flow of lochia prevents ascending infection from the vagina to the uterus. However, the presence of pieces of placenta or blood clot within the uterus can encourage the growth of bacteria, leading to infection. A subinvoluted tender uterus with offensive lochia are diagnostic, and treatment is by emptying of the uterus and antibiotics.

Ascending urinary tract infections may occur in the puerperium as a result of diminished local resistance secondary to trauma and urinary stasis. Stasis allows bacteria a longer incubation time and interferes with the host's natural defence mechanism such as phagocytosis or destruction of bacterial cell walls by leucocytic lysozymes. Diagnosis is by the symptoms and from culture, and treatment is by the appropriate oral antibiotic.

Deep vein thrombosis can occur in the puerperium, particularly after an operative delivery, due to tissue damage and/or infection in the presence of increased coagulability of the blood which is a feature of pregnancy and the early puerperium. Deep vein thrombosis in the pelvic veins may only present by a mild fluctuating pyrexia and pelvic tenderness. Deep vein thrombosis in the lower limbs need not be associated with infection and presents with pain, swelling and localised tenderness in the calf and a positive Homan's sign. Diagnosis can be made using Doppler ultrasound or venogram. Treatment should be with anticoagulants and antibiotics if necessary.

IMMUNISATION

Rubella vaccine should be given to all non-immune mothers during the puerperium. The immunity induced may be impaired if a blood transfusion is given during the puerperium. It is important that efficient contraception is used during the subsequent three months.

Anti-D γ globulin should be given to all rhesus negative women delivering rhesus positive babies. Anti-D must be given within 72 h of delivery and preferably sooner if isoimmunisation is to be avoided. If the Kliehauer count indicates a greater than normal transfer of fetal cells into the maternal circulation, a double dose of immunoglobulin should be given.

POSTPARTUM CONTRACEPTION

Lactating women do not ovulate until the frequency of suckling starts to diminish, particularly when night feeds are cut out or spaced to 4–6 h intervals. Hormonal contraception such as progestogen only pills, progestogens given by injection, implant or vaginal ring are suitable as they do not affect milk production. The combined pill may reduce milk volume. All hormonal methods should be avoided during the first few weeks of lactation, as trace amounts of the steroid will reach the infant and theoretically may affect its future sexual behaviour. For the non-lactating woman, any form of hormonal contraceptive that is appropriate can be initiated soon after delivery. Insertion of intrauterine devices in the immediate postpartum period is best avoided as the incidence of expulsion or removal for bleeding is higher than when the device is inserted six weeks after delivery.

STERILISATION

Sterilisation is quite often performed during the puerperium for convenience. The failure rate is increased twofold due to a greater chance of recanalisation of the tubes. It should also be remembered that the first week of life is the most dangerous and an unexpected neonatal death following sterilisation may cause the decision to be bitterly regretted.

Diaphragms should not be fitted until involution of the genital tract is complete.

FURTHER READING

Bowes W.A. ed. (1980). The puerperium. In *Clinical Obstetrics and Gynaecology*, pp. 971–1142. Hagerstrom: Harper & Row.

Gunther M. (1973). *Infant Feeding*. Harmondsworth: Penguin.

Hartmann P.E. (1986). The breast and breast feeding. In *Scientific Foundations of Obstetrics and Gynaecology*, 3rd edn. (Phillip E., Barnes J., Newton M. eds.), pp. 286–96. London: Heinemann Medical.

Oppe T.E. (1974). *Present Day Practice of Infant Feeding*. DHSS Report on Health and Social Subjects. London: HMSO.

13

Adaptation to Extrauterine Life

Within a matter of minutes of delivery, the fetus has to change from gas exchange, continuous i.v. nutrition and removal of waste products, all being managed by the placenta, to pulmonary gas exchange and intermittent orogastric feeding with intestinal digestion. The baby's kidneys have to take over the elimination of waste products and the baby has to control its entire metabolism independently (Table 13.1).

In this chapter the normal processes of adaptation will be described. Failure to adapt to extrauterine life leads to many serious problems for the baby and death may result.

FETAL CIRCULATION

Oxygenated blood from the placenta returns to the fetus via the umbilical vein, bypasses the liver via the ductus venosus and enters the right atrium. The right atrial pressure is higher than the left atrial pressure in fetal life and this keeps the foramen ovale open, thus allowing oxygenated blood from the umbilical vein to cross into the left atrium. From there, the oxygenated blood crosses the mitral valve, enters the left ventricle and is pumped via the ascending aorta to the brain and other organs.

The deoxygenated blood from the brain flows along the jugular veins and superior vena cava to the right atrium. Some mixing with oxygenated blood occurs, but most flows through the tricuspid valve into the right ventricle from where it is pumped to the pulmonary artery. The fetal pulmonary circulation is vasoconstricted and has a high vascular resistance. Pulmonary artery pressure is slightly higher than aortic pressure during fetal life, in contrast to postnatal life when aortic pressure is normally considerably higher than the pulmonary artery pressure. As a result of the high vascular resistance, only 10% of the blood flowing along the pulmonary artery perfuses the lungs, 90% flowing through the ductus arteriosus into the descending aorta.

Fetal arterial P_{O_2} is approximately 4 kPa and P_{CO_2} 6 kPa. To help the fetus to transport oxygen around the body in the presence of relatively low P_{O_2}, the haemoglobin concentration is raised to 16–22 g/dl and consists of fetal haemoglobin (HbF). HbF has a higher affinity for oxygen than adult

---

Table 13.1

Adaptation of Vital Functions to Neonatal Life

	Fetal	Neonatal
Gas exchange	Placenta	Lungs: expansion circulation respiratory control
Nutrition	Placenta	Sucking, swallowing Gastric emptying Intestinal digestion
Elimination of waste products		
Urea	Placenta	Kidneys
Creatinine		
Bilirubin	Placenta	Liver

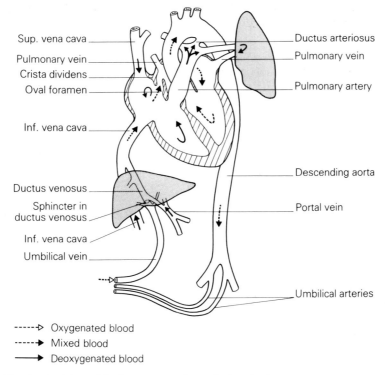

Fig. 13.1   *Plan of the human circulation before birth. Arrows indicate the direction of the blood flow.*

haemoglobin and can thus take up more oxygen in the placenta at a relatively low Po_2. The fetal circulation is shown in Fig. 13.1.

FETAL LUNG DEVELOPMENT

By 26 weeks' gestation, respiratory bronchioles with a rich capillary supply have developed. From this time, alveoli develop as clusters of thin walled sacs lined by flattened epithelium (type I pneumonocytes). Type II pneumonocytes are present at this gestation also (Fig. 13.2). Their cytoplasm contains layered inclusions which stain densely with osmium tetroxide and contain surfactant (Fig. 13.3). This phospholipid-lipoprotein complex lowers the surface tension in the fluid film which lines the alveoli once the lungs are expanding and being aerated.

Surfactant also has the property of further lowering surface tension within an air-filled space as the area is reduced. The pressure within a bubble required to prevent collapse due to surface tension is inversely proportional to its radius. The terminal

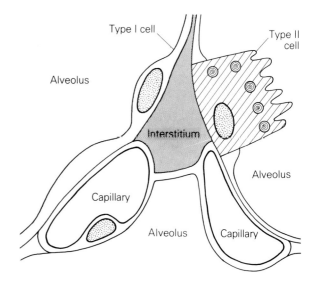

Fig. 13.2   *An alveolus with type I and type II pneumocytes.*

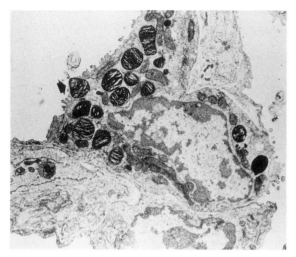

Fig. 13.3   *Electron micrograph of a type II pneumocyte showing the lamellated osmiophilic bodies which are thought to contain surfactant.*

bronchioles of babies born at 28 weeks are very small and would thus have a strong tendency to collapse in expiration. This collapse on expiration is inhibited by surfactant.

During fetal life, the lungs are filled by a fluid secreted by the lungs. Despite the relatively low arterial Po_2 and high Pco_2, the fetus makes only gentle shallow respiratory movements. Severe hypoxia and acidosis may stimulate the fetus to make gasping respirations.

Lung liquid contains surfactant and is 'breathed' out by the fetus into the amniotic fluid. Lecithin is an important constituent of surfactant and measurement of the ratio of lecithin to sphyngomyelin (which is not part of surfactant) gives a useful indication of adequate surfactant if the ratio is greater than 2.0. The presence of phosphotidyl glycerol is also powerful confirmation of surfactant. Experiments with pregnant ewes have shown that giving ACTH or glucocorticoids induces earlier production of surfactant. Further studies with fetal lambs have shown that, during labour, adrenaline is secreted by the fetal adrenal medulla. This inhibits the secretion of lung liquid and stimulates the absorption of lung liquid.

The First Breath

Why does a baby cry vigorously after delivery having breathed quietly and regularly for months in utero? Sudden loss of weightlessness and compression, exposure to cold and physical squeezing followed by release are the most likely stimuli to initiate breathing. After birth, the chemoreceptor control of respiration is changed, Pao_2 normally being maintained around 10 kPa and Pco_2 around 5.3 kPa. During vaginal delivery some lung fluid is squeezed out of the larynx by thoracic compression and the rest is absorbed over a period of hours by the pulmonary lymphatics. The first breath in a full-term baby is about 30 ml and requires a negative intrathoracic pressure of -40 to -100 cm H_2O. Very soon a tidal volume, which is the volume of each breath, is established and a negative pressure of only -5 cm H_2O is required.

CIRCULATORY CHANGES AFTER BIRTH

The umbilical vessels constrict in response to thromboxane released by natural stimuli such as animals chewing at the cord of their offspring or to cold, drying and increased oxygen tension. Filling the lungs with air produces a fall in pulmonary vascular resistance, a drop in pulmonary artery pressure and a large increase in pulmonary blood flow. Thus ventilation and perfusion of the lungs increase in parallel. *The pulmonary circulation converts from high resistance low flow to low resistance high flow.*

The tying of the umbilical cord removes a low resistance circuit from the circulation and the systemic arterial pressure rises above that of the pulmonary artery, thus reversing the flow through the ductus arteriosus.

As the pulmonary blood flow increases, blood returning to the left atrium increases and the left

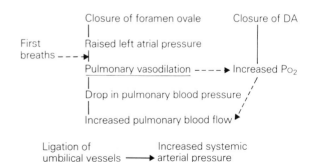

Fig. 13.4   *Key changes in transition from fetal to neonatal circulation.*

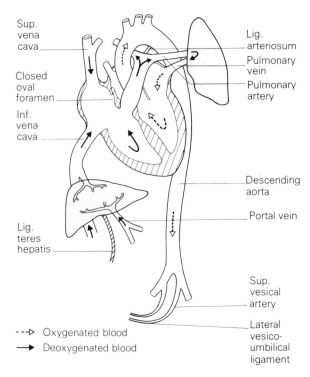

Sup. vena cava

Closed oval foramen

Inf. vena cava

Lig. teres hepatis

Lig. arteriosum

Pulmonary vein

Pulmonary artery

Descending aorta

Portal vein

Sup. vesical artery

Lateral vesico-umbilical ligament

- - -▷ Oxygenated blood
→ Deoxygenated blood

Fig. 13.5 *Plan of the human circulation after birth. Note the changes occurring as a result of the beginning of respiration and the interruption of the placental blood flow.*

atrial pressure rises above that of the right atrium. When this happens, there is no more right-to-left shunt between the atria, and the foramen ovale closes as a simple flap.

As the arterial P_{O_2} rises, the ductus arteriosus constricts. The ductus venosus constricts soon after umbilical flow ceases (Fig. 13.4). Neonatal circulation is shown in Fig. 13.5.

DISORDERS OF CARDIOPULMONARY ADAPTATION

Respiratory Distress Syndrome (RDS)

This is the condition affecting preterm infants deficient in surfactant. Lacking the surface-tension-lowering phospholipid, the terminal bronchioles and alveoli tend to collapse in expiration and remain collapsed. Worsening hypoxaemia occurs as more and more alveoli are non-ventilated and the

work of breathing increases as the lungs become stiffer. Clinically, the baby develops increasing tachypnoea, grunting, subcostal and sternal recession and cyanosis. As the baby fatigues, respiratory and metabolic acidosis increase.

Chest x-ray shows a granular pattern throughout both lungs (Fig. 13.6). Treatment within a neonatal intensive care unit consists of monitoring arterial blood gases and giving increased O_2 to maintain an adequate P_{AO_2} (7–10 kPa). Mechanical ventilation with positive-end-expiratory pressure is needed for persistent hypoxaemia, respiratory acidosis and prolonged apnoea (Fig. 13.7). Survival in RDS has improved over the last ten years, but many deaths still occur from complications such as pneumothorax and cerebral periventricular haemorrhage.

At autopsy, the lungs are very poorly expanded

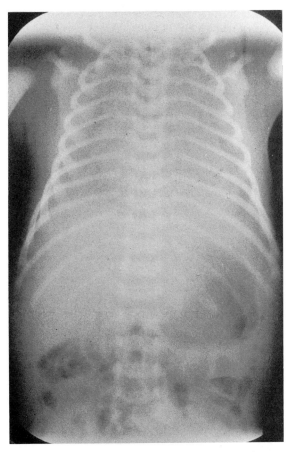

Fig. 13.6 *Chest x-ray of a preterm infant with RDS showing a generalised granular pattern throughout both lungs.*

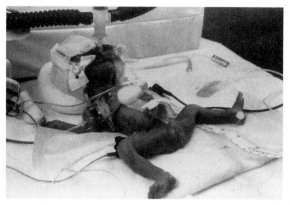

Fig. 13.7   *A 26-week gestation infant connected to a ventilator.*

and histologically there is a pink hyaline membrane lining the alveoli and terminal bronchioles (Fig. 13.8). Hyaline membrane disease is used as a synonym for respiratory distress syndrome, but strictly, it is a pathological diagnosis.

Advances in obstetrics have decreased the sever-

ity and frequency of RDS. Asphyxia damages the type II pneumocytes and increases the risk of RDS. Thus careful monitoring with operative delivery to avoid asphyxia reduces the chances of RDS in preterm infants. The risk increases as gestational age shortens and is greater in male than female infants. Prolonged rupture of the membranes or 48 h of maternal treatment with glucocorticoids such as dexamethazone 24 mg in 2 or 3 divided doses is thought to have a maturing effect on surfactant if the infant is delivered between 28 and 34 weeks' gestation.

Retained Fetal Lung Fluid

This condition affects babies at all gestational ages including term and is more common following elective caesarean section, when the fetus has not experienced any thoracic squeezing or adrenaline secretion to expel lung liquid. The breathing is rapid (over 60/min), but there is little or no grunting or recession. Hypoxaemia is frequent, but is easily relieved by a moderate increase in inspired oxygen

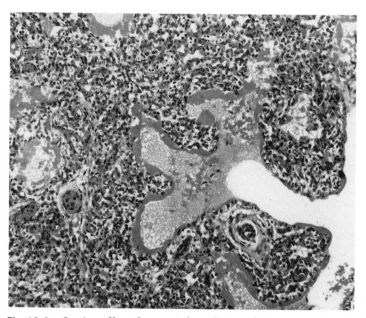

Fig. 13.8   *Section of lung from an infant of 29 weeks' gestation who died with respiratory distress syndrome at 30 hours of age. There is a dilated bronchiole with several branches containing red cells and proteinaceous material and lined with thick layers of amorphous hyaline membrane. The surrounding cellular tissue comprises the collapsed air spaces. Haematoxylin and Eosin stain. Magnification × 90.*

without the need for mechanical ventilation. The condition is also known as 'transient tachypnoea of the newborn' and may resolve within 24 h, occasionally taking 48–72 h.

Intrapartum Asphyxia

If the fetus is asphyxiated by significant hypoxia from obstetric complications, such as prolapsed cord or placental abruption, metabolic acidosis from accumulation of lactic acid occurs. Systemic vasoconstriction may result in blood being shifted from the baby's side of the fetal circulation to the placenta. After delivery, there may be systemic hypovolaemia as a result. The hypoxic fetus may pass meconium into the amniotic fluid and, if severely distressed, may gasp, thus inhaling meconium into the airways. Meconium aspiration is most common in postmature babies and the respiratory problem may be severe.

The particles of meconium exert a chemical irritant effect, but they also have a ball-valve effect so that inspiration may be obstructed much less than expiration. Air trapping with air leaks in the mediastinum and pleural space are common complications.

If intrapartum asphyxia persists before delivery, worsening acidosis, bradycardia and hypotension will subject all the baby's vital organs to hypoxia and ischaemia. This includes the brain, kidneys, intestines and heart. Treatment is, of course, emergency delivery and resuscitation to restore oxygenation, correct acidosis and to improve perfusion. For the baby who is limp, has bradycardia and is apnoeic, endotracheal intubation and manual ventilation at 40 breaths/min are the most effective means of oxygenation. If bradycardia persists, external cardiac massage should be started at 120/min. If the circulation remains poor, plasma, sodium bicarbonate and glucose should be given into the umbilical vein. The Apgar score is the universally acknowledged system of marking a baby's state at birth and response to resuscitation (Table 13.2).

An Apgar score of 4 or less necessitates active resuscitation. If the score is still 6 or less after 5 min, the response to treatment has not been good. If the baby takes more than 10 min to establish respiration, then it is likely that convulsions, transient renal failure, ileus and even myocardial ischaemia may follow.

If a full-term baby (without maternal sedative drugs) does not establish respiration after 30 min of vigorous resuscitation, that baby is so likely to have severe brain damage that further treatment may justifiably be stopped.

Persistent Pulmonary Hypertension (Persistent Fetal Circulation)

Following severe asphyxia and in severe respiratory distress syndrome, hypoxaemia and acidosis may stimulate pulmonary vasoconstriction. This results in pulmonary hypertension, reduced pulmonary blood flow and reduced pulmonary venous return to the left atrium. The reduced left atrial pressure results in right-to-left shunting through the foramen ovale. Thus deoxygenated blood shunts into the systemic circulation further worsening the hypoxaemia. The pulmonary hypertension may additionally cause pulmonary-to-systemic shunting through the ductus arteriosus which opens as a

Table 13.2

Agpar Score

Clinical feature	0	1	2
Heart rate	Absent	<100	>100
Respiration	Absent	Gasping or irregular	Regular or crying lustily
Muscle tone	Limp	Diminished or no movements	Normal with active movements
Response to pharyngeal suction	Nil	Grimace	Cough
Colour of trunk	White	Blue	Pink

response to hypoxaemia. Thus a vicious circle of hypoxaemia stimulating futher hypoxaemia characterises persistent pulmonary hypertension. Treatment involves giving high concentrations of oxygen, restoring the blood volume, correcting acidosis with buffer and using pulmonary vasodilator drugs such as tolazoline.

Patent Ductus Arteriosus (PDA)

Normally, the ductus arteriosus constricts within hours of birth. If the baby is very preterm (less than 32 weeks), this is often delayed for days or weeks. Usually the systemic arterial pressure is higher than the pulmonary arterial pressure after birth, and this causes blood to shunt left-to-right, i.e. aorta to pulmonary artery.

If the ductus arteriosus is patent, this can cause serious problems to very preterm infants because:

1. Pulmonary blood flow may be increased to the levels where the lungs are 'wetter' and stiffer. Thus more effort is required to breathe. Babies below 1500 g may become fatigued and apnoeic.
2. A large fraction of the left ventricular output is wasted in that it does not perfuse the systemic circulation. Thus the left ventricle has to increase its output substantially to keep up with the demand. Cardiac failure may result.

The frequency of PDA can be minimised in babies under 32 weeks by avoiding excessive fluid intake, hypoxaemia and anaemia. If PDA causes a clinically significant shunt with symptoms and signs, indomethacin, which inhibits the production of vasodilatory protaglandins is effective in closing most PDAs. If a troublesome shunt persists, then surgical ligation of PDA can be safely carried out even in tiny infants.

Pulmonary Hypoplasia

The lungs may fail to grow and develop if there is deficiency of amniotic fluid, a mass occupying space in the chest, or if severe neurological abnormalities inhibit respiratory movements (Fig. 13.9).

Normal lung growth and development requires fetal breathing movements with adequate space in the chest, amniotic fluid to breathe and muscle power. Clinically, pulmonary hypoplasia presents

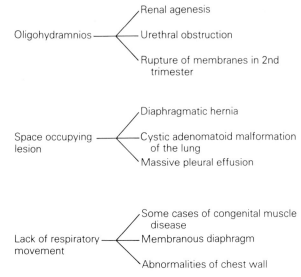

Fig. 13.9   *Causes of pulmonary hypoplasia.*

as severe respiratory difficulty which responds poorly to endotracheal intubation and ventilation. Even high pressures achieve poor ventilation and tension pneumothorax is a common terminal event.

NUTRITION

The fetus receives a continuous supply of glucose, amino acids, electrolytes, minerals and essential fatty acids via the umbilical vein. The fat intake is relatively small, most of the calories being supplied by glucose. Subcutaneous fat, which is white adipose tissue, is laid down in the fetus from 26 weeks' gestation, most of the triglyceride being synthesised from glucose.

After delivery, the baby changes from a continuous high carbohydrate diet to an intermittent high fat diet. Fetal blood glucose is normally slightly lower than maternal blood glucose. After birth, there is a fall in blood glucose during the first few hours, but this stabilises above 2 mmol/l when milk feeding starts.

The neonatal brain uses 50% of the total consumption of oxygen and calories. At birth, the carbohydrate store (glycogen) is only sufficient for about 12 h in a full-term infant. However, glycerol derived from the breakdown of fat in adipose tissue can be converted to glucose in the liver. By studying arteriovenous differences, it has been possible to show that the neonatal brain may take up not only glucose, but also acetoacetate and β hydroxybutyrate which are formed in the liver from fatty acids. Free fatty acids lactate, pyruvate and glycerol are not utilised directly by the brain. After birth, free fatty acid levels rise and double by 12 h. Vital organs, such as the heart, can utilise free fatty acids and within hours of birth the respiratory quotient falls from 1.0 to 0.7, indicating a switch from carbohydrate to fat utilisation.

Digestion

Fifty per cent of calories from breast milk are in the form of *lactose*. This is hydrolysed by lactase on the brush border of the intestinal mucosa to glucose and galactose. This enzyme is present even in very preterm infants. Lactase deficiency may occur as a result of injury or infection in the small intestine. Profuse watery diarrhoea results.

Protein digestion

Pancreatic peptidases such as trypsin, chymotrypsin and elastase are present even in very preterm infants. Further digestion occurs by proteases on the brush border. There is evidence that some animal species can absorb intact proteins in the neonatal period. It is not clear how important this process is in humans, but absorption of immunoglobulins from breast milk may give some protection, and absorption of antigens (in cow's milk, egg and wheat) may stimulate allergic responses. Over 80% of babies with *cystic fibrosis* have a deficiency of pancreatic enzymes because of obstruction of pancreatic ducts. Trypsin is normally detectable in neonatal stools Absence of trypsin from stools, or an excessive level of trypsin in blood, is suggestive of cystic fibrosis.

Fat digestion

Triglycerides are hydrolysed by pancreatic lipase into monoglycerides and fatty acids. Bile salts facilitate the absorption of monoglycerides and fatty acids. Breast milk contains a lipase which is activated by bile salts in the duodenum. Boiling breast milk to sterilise it, destroys the lipase and thereby reduces fat absorption.

Apart from congenital abnormalities of the gut,

such as atresias at various levels, the most serious gastrointestinal disorder in the neonatal period is *necrotising enterocolitis*. This condition occurs mainly in small, sick infants. The pathogenesis involves: (a) an injury to the integrity of the intestinal mucosa, usually hypoxic-ischaemic, from respiratory failure, cardiac failure, shock, catheters in the arteries or veins supplying the gut and (b) invasion of the wall of the gut by gas-forming anaerobic bacteria. The ileum and jejunum are most commonly affected.

Clinically, there is abdominal distention, bile-stained vomiting, and bloody diarrhoea. If infarction of the intestine or perforation with peritonitis occurs, there is considerable mortality. Most at risk are babies in neonatal intensive care units with severe respiratory distress syndrome, severe congenital heart disease, or those requiring exchange transfusion.

RENAL FUNCTION

The main function of the fetal kidney appears to be as a source of amniotic fluid. In renal agenesis, there is extreme oligohydramnios and severe pulmonary hypoplasia (Potter's syndrome). After birth, there is normally obligatory loss of water which gives a 5–10% weight loss in the first four days. This is partly due to continued excretion of water and sodium despite a small intake.

At birth, glomerular filtration rate and renal blood flow are both about one-third of that expected and gradually increase with age. Renal tubular function is also immature in that sodium excretion is limited and the maximum concentration is 700–800 mOsm/k, whereas an older child can excrete urine with osmolality of 1200–1400 mOsm/k. Apart from regulation of fluid and electrolyte balance, another important renal function is the elimination of drugs. Aminoglycoside antibiotics, such as gentamicin, are entirely cleared in the urine and elimination is significantly slower in the first week of postnatal life than later. To avoid potentially toxic accumulation of these drugs, the doses need to be less frequent than in older children.

In preterm babies, especially those below 32 weeks, all aspects of renal function are less mature than at term. Not only is sodium excretion limited, but sodium retention is also impaired. These babies may continue to excrete sodium-rich urine despite the low sodium content of human breast milk, a low plasma sodium and high plasma levels of aldosterone. Thus the care of sick and small infants involves very careful calculation of changes and requirements of fluid and electrolytes because of the limited ability of the newborn to maintain correct balance.

BILIRUBIN

Bilirubin is formed by the breakdown of haem from old red blood cells. In fetal life, this is removed by the placenta and accumulation only takes place in the fetus if there is extremely severe haemolysis as in rhesus incompatibility. After birth, the neonatal liver has to remove bilirubin. Bilirubin is initially released from the reticulo-endothelial cells as unconjugated bilirubin. This is more fat-soluble than water-soluble and cannot be excreted effectively by the kidneys. Plasma albumin has a considerable capacity to bind bilirubin and only a small fraction is actually unbound in plasma. Unconjugated bilirubin is taken up by specific receptors in the liver and by a series of steps is conjugated to bilirubin glucuronide. This is more water-soluble and is normally excreted in the bile. The process of conjugation frequently fails to keep up with need in the first week after birth and unconjugated bilirubin accumulates without there being any disease present (Table 13.3). This 'physiological jaundice' occurs in about one-third of all normal full-term babies and is usually fading by ten days of age.

High plasma levels of unconjugated bilirubin in plasma are potentially harmful because the binding capacity of albumin may become saturated by bilirubin. Thus free bilirubin may enter the brain and damage the basal ganglia and VIII nerve nuclei. This pattern of brain damage (kernicterus) gives choreo-athetoid cerebral palsy and sensorineural deafness.

Some breast fed infants remain mildly, but definitely, jaundiced for several weeks with unconjugated bilirubin. They thrive well and investigation reveals no other pathology. This is breast milk jaundice and is thought to be due to other substances inhibiting glucuronyl transferase. It is not necessary to stop breast feeding.

In full-term infants, plasma levels of bilirubin up to 340 μmol/l and slightly higher are considered safe, but the shorter the gestation and the more ill the baby, the lower is the threshold for kernicterus. In our experience, a plasma bilirubin over 240 μmol/l in a sick infant below 1500 g carries a significant risk of sensorineural deafness. Thus all newborn infants must be scrutinised daily for jaundice in the first week and investigated if jaundice is marked. Phototherapy with white or blue light is usually effective in controlling hyperbilirubinaemia by altering the stereochemistry of the bilirubin molecule such that it becomes water soluble and secretable. However, exchange transfusion is still necessary in severe haemolytic disease and in very-low-birth-weight babies.

TEMPERATURE REGULATION

At birth, the baby emerges from a perfectly centrally heated environment to be exposed to cold

---

Table 13.3

Causes of Neonatal Unconjugated Hyperbilirubinaemia

Haemolysis	Rhesus, ABO and other blood group incompatibility
	Red cell defects, e.g. spherocytosis enzyme defects
	Bruising, e.g. cephalhaematoma
Short gestation	
Breast milk jaundice	
Infection	
Dehydration	
Hypothyroidism	

stress. Cooling by several degrees may occur within minutes if the wet neonate in the delivery room is not dried off, wrapped up and placed in a warm cot or against the mother's body. Cold stress can be a serious threat to newborns, especially preterm infants, and has been shown to increase mortality.

Children and adults may increase heat production by shivering, but newborns are unable to do this. Their principal source of heat production is from brown adipose tissue. These cells contain many fat vacuoles and numerous large mitochondria in the cytoplasm. In contrast, subcutaneous or white fat has a single fat vacuole with relatively few mitochondria. This metabolically active brown fat has a rich blood supply and is distributed around the main arteries, and has been called 'oil-fired central heating'. The cells can take up glucose, glycerol and fatty acids from the circulation, to be stored as triglyceride. Heat production is controlled by the sympathetic nervous system. When the temperature drops, sympathetic nerve endings release noradrenaline which activates the brown adipose cell, via cyclic adenosine monophosphate (cyclic AMP), to oxidise fatty acids. This oxidation is uncoupled from the generation of ATP and heat is produced which can be carried by the circulating blood to the rest of the body. A full-term infant may increase his metabolic rate from 6 ml of oxygen/kg/min to a maximum of 15 ml oxygen/kg/min. Thus hypoxia, hypothermia and hypoglycaemia are interrelated. Hypothermia increases the need for oxygen to fuel brown adipose tissue. Hypoxia and hypoglycaemia impair the ability of brown fat to respond by burning more fuel.

The lower the birth weight, the higher is the surface area to weight ratio and thus the greater is the surface for heat loss by convection, radiation and evaporation. In addition, small-for-gestational-age babies often have a relatively large head for the rest of the body, and thus have high metabolic requirements.

Sick and small babies who require intensive care procedures are most conveniently nursed under a radiant heater which can be servo-controlled to maintain the baby's skin temperature at 37°C. The side of the buttock is a good site for an 'average' skin temperature. The use of such radiant heaters increases the evaporation of water from the newborn skin and this is further increased in the more immature baby. However, the effects of this can be reduced by putting a thin layer of plastic sheeting over the baby between procedures and the increased water loss can be compensated by carefully increasing fluid intake.

Very-low-birth-weight infants who do not require frequent procedures are most conveniently nursed in a closed incubator in which the air temperature can be carefully controlled. The environmental temperatures for thermal neutrality (i.e. minimum metabolic requirement) have been determined, i.e. a 1000 g baby on the first day may require a temperature of 36°C.

Larger babies (over 1500 g) can be adequately maintained in a cot in a warm room (24°C or 75°F). In many countries, the best place is in bed with the mother and holding the baby naked against the mother's skin between the breasts has been successfully used for very-low-birth-weight infants in Colombia.

NEUROLOGICAL ADAPTATION TO EXTRAUTERINE LIFE

A full-term baby is able to open his eyes and fix visually on a face within minutes of birth. This is best demonstrated if the baby is wrapped up well, held upright or inclined and if the lighting is slightly subdued. He or she will also orientate to sound and show a number of postural reactions and neonatal responses. Neck flexion is usually slightly stronger than neck extension. Leg and arm recoil are brisk. The Moro and grasp reflexes are present. Within the first week, visual preference for a striped pattern to a grey background can be demonstrated and the baby becomes able to distinguish the smell of his mother's breast from that of other mothers.

The main threats to the neonatal brain are:

1. *Hypoxia/ischaemia during intrapartum asphyxia* with resulting cerebral oedema and convulsions.
2. Respiratory distress syndrome and asphyxia in preterm infants resulting in *haemorrhage in and around the cerebral ventricles* (Fig. 13.10).
3. Shock and hypotension giving ischaemic lesions, i.e. *periventricular leukomalacia* in preterm infants (Fig. 13.11) and *infarction of the cerebral cortex and basal ganglia* in term infants.
4. *Hypoglycaemia.*
5. *Meningitis.*

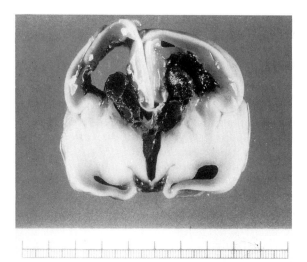

Fig. 13.10 *A coronal section of a preterm brain at autopsy. Massive intraventricular haemorrhage with ventricular dilatation.*

The potential problems of adaptation to extra-uterine life are usually successfully overcome by full-term infants. The more premature the baby, the more numerous are the potential problems.

FURTHER READING

Davis J.A., Dobbing J. eds. (1981). *Scientific Foundations of Paediatrics*. London: Heinemann Medical.

Roberton N.R.C. (1982). *A Manual of Neonatal Intensive Care*. London: Arnold.

Wigglesworth J. (1984). *Perinatal Pathology*. Philadelphia. W.B. Saunders.

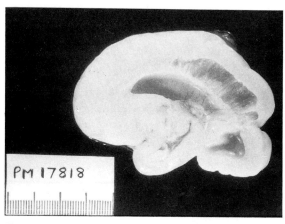

Fig. 13.11 *A parasagittal section of a preterm brain at autopsy. Massive cyst formation adjacent to the ventricle indicates periventricular leukomalacia.*

14

Maternal and Perinatal Mortality

MATERNAL MORTALITY

In developing countries the problems that Europe experienced in the first half of this century, causing most of the maternal mortality, namely haemorrhage, infection and shock, are unfortunately still very prevalent due to lack of facilities to treat these problems. The very long distances that women live

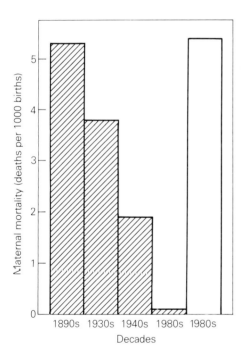

Fig. 14.1 *Maternal mortality rates during the last century in developed countries compared with an estimate of the current rates in developing countries.*

from primary help, the delay in making a diagnosis of, say, obstructed labour, and then the problems of travel to a hospital, apart from the deficiencies of services once there, mean that many women die in childbirth unnecessarily.

Accurate statistics from developing countries are impossible to obtain, but it is estimated that the maternal death rate in many such countries may be between 5 and 10 per 1000 births, or fifty to a hundred times that of the developed world. The improvement in developed countries during the last century is compared with the current position in developing countries in Fig. 14.1.

With the very major reduction in deaths from infection, haemorrhage and shock, the causes of maternal death which have now assumed an increased importance are thromboembolism, hypertension and the complications of general anaesthesia. Awareness that these are possible causes of maternal death, and constant vigilance for them, should enable the maternal mortality in developed countries to be reduced even further. Information compiled by the Confidential Enquiry into Maternal Deaths in the UK has shown that a major cause of problems is inexperienced staff dealing with situations with which they are unfamiliar. In developing countries, the wide-scale provision of even basic facilities will significantly improve maternal mortality rates.

PERINATAL MORTALITY

This is defined as the total number of stillbirths and first week neonatal deaths per 1000 total births. It reflects the standard of obstetric and neonatal care and facilities available. With improved neonatal resuscitation and intensive care, a number of babies survive the first week of life only to die within the first month from complications of pregnancy and delivery. A modification of the definition of perinatal mortality rate to include these late neonatal deaths (up to 28 days after delivery) should be considered.

Many of the causes of maternal mortality, such as fulminating infection, haemorrhage and shock also cause perinatal death. However, as the former were eliminated, the direct fetal causes of perinatal mortality became progressively more important, and the rate fell from 63 per 1000 births in 1933 to 11.8 per 1000 total births in 1981 in the UK.

Perinatal mortality rates in developed countries can vary considerably due to the availability and quality of care, the overall health of the population and, in some cases, the basis for the statistics. A sample of perinatal mortality rates in the late 1970s in Europe is shown in Table 14.1.

Some countries define a stillbirth or neonatal death on the basis of a baby weighing more than 500 g, while others adhere to a definition of 28 weeks from the last menstrual period. While the former (less than 0.5 kg) will inevitably include a number of potentially previable infants, it is a more accurate measurement than gestational age which, even with the increasing use of ultrasound, will always remain potentially unreliable. Again, reliable perinatal mortality statistics from developing countries which do not have birth registration, and in which most babies are born in the home, are impossible to obtain. It is reasonable to assume that they are between 10 and 20 times greater than those

in the developed countries. Factors such as poor social class, poor diet and poor housing and hygiene have a significant effect on perinatal mortality and morbidity. Initially, improvement of these will have as much impact on reducing the perinatal mortality as improvement in obstetric and neonatal services.

Stillbirths

The stillbirth rate in Western Europe is approximately 5–7 per 1000 total births at present. The major causes are antenatal and intrapartum hypoxia, infection and congenital abnormalities. Despite the low rate, many of these deaths are preventable and constant vigilance in labour, awareness of the dangers of infection, and better diagnosis of congenital abnormalities will continue the downward trend.

The stillbirth rate serves as an index of the standard of obstetric care and facilities.

Neonatal Deaths

The neonatal death rate in Western Europe is currently about 7/1000 live births. Congenital abnormalities are the most important cause, while respiratory problems, infection and intracranial haemorrhage are the main reasons for death in the otherwise normally formed infant. These are largely problems of the perterm and low-birth-weight infant and both neonatal mortality and, to a lesser extent, stillbirth rate are related to birth weight (Fig. 14.2). Some progress has been made towards reducing prematurity, such as the selective use of cervical cerclage, selected use of tocolytic drugs and better recognition of fetal hypoxia. An understanding of the biochemistry of labour and preterm labour in particular should improve the neonatal death rate in the future.

It is helpful to categorise perinatal deaths as follows:

1. Congenital abnormalities;
2. Deaths due to hypoxia, infection and other causes in immature infants;
3. The same as (2), but in mature infants.

A clustering of perinatal deaths in one category suggests a deficiency in the provision of the relevant facilities or care.

In developed countries, congenital abnormalities

Table 14.1

Perinatal Mortality Rates (per 1000 Live Births) in Some European Countries

Country	Year	Perinatal mortality rate
Czechoslovakia	1977	18.4
Denmark	1979	9.8
France	1981	12.3
Finland	1978	9.3
Hungary	1979	24.3
The Netherlands	1979	12.0
Norway	1979	11.9
Poland	1979	17.2
Sweden	1979	9.1
UK—England and Wales	1978	15.7
UK—Scotland	1979	14.2

(From World Health Statistics, 1981.)

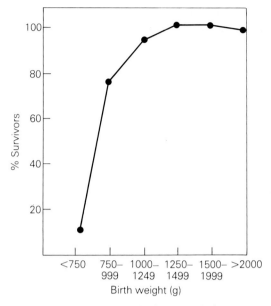

Fig. 14.2   *Survival of preterm babies.*

PERINATAL MORBIDITY

With more very-low-birth-weight babies surviving, is the pool of serious handicap increasing? The answer is probably not. Regional referral centres are providing obstetricians and neonatologists with the experience to allow them to change and improve clinical practice. A positive policy of delivery before a preterm fetus is significantly compromised by hypoxia or infection is resulting in more, but healthier, very-low-birth-weight babies, who require less neonatal intervention. Subsequently, they have fewer side-effects. However, this process requires a constant high level of medical and nursing skills, supported by expensive facilities.

FURTHER READING

are the most common single cause of neonatal death. Improved antenatal diagnosis allowing termination of pregnancy will reduce this figure. In developing countries, there will be an even spread of deaths throughout all categories. Collection of some reliable data, constant professional audit and thought concerning possible improvements, even in the worst situations, will bring about a reduction in perinatal mortality.

Chamberlain G., Philipp E., Howlett B., Masters K. (1978). *British Births 1970.* Vol. II: The Obstetric Case. London: Heinemann Medical.

Chamberlain R. (1975). *British Births 1970*, Vol. I: The First Week of Life. London: Heinemann Medical.

MacFarlane A., Mugford M. (1984). *Birth Counts. Statistics of Pregancy and Childbirth.* London: HMSO.

15

Psychological Aspects of Reproduction

> Birth, copulation, and death.
> That's all the facts, when you're down to brass tacks —
> Birth, copulation, and death.
>
> T.S. Eliot *Sweeney Agonistes*

Faced with the joys and sorrows, the achievements and travails, of pregnancy, labour, child-rearing, contraception, sterility, congenital deformity, miscarriage, and so on, it is only too easy for the doctor to stay insulated safely in technology — to behave like a vet when his patients are coping with some of the greatest psychosomatic happenings that set their destiny. Freud once remarked, about his discovery of the ubiquitous influence of sexual drives in illness and much else in life, that while his medical contemporaries might be outraged and incredulous, nothing he had unearthed was new either to poets or to nursery maids. The purpose of this chapter is to expand the clinician's consciousness in matters of reproduction, if not to the widsom of the poet, at least to compare respectably to Freud's nursery maids.

PREGNANCY AND PERSONAL VALIDATION

Nowadays, in modern society, we have so lost touch with natural things that simple truths, taken for granted about ourselves in the past, seem quaint or strange. With contraception the norm, sexual relationships and pregnancy have actually acquired an illusory separateness; while pregnancy, however beneficially, has been so medicalised and hospitalised that, like death and insanity, it is no longer part and parcel of everyday life.

We are far removed today from the ancient assumption that to be a man is to be potent and a father, to be a woman is to be a fertile and nurturing mother, and to be cursed is to be barren and childless. On the contrary, we can debate masculinity and femininity, question whether there exist any built-in or basic differences, and seriously wonder whether there is any virtue in fostering such differences, innate or acquired, if differences there be. Every store provides guidebooks to sexual fulfilment, in which the achievement of pregnancy is barely mentioned, although its prevention may get some space.

And yet, just below this surface, our nature remains the same, and that is what Freud, his nursery maids, and poets are all about. The man who is no use to his children remains of little use to women, nor often enough to himself or anyone else. The mother who cannot mother, or who is unable to conceive may still have an inner sense of futility and disaster that no capacity for multiple orgasms can counterbalance, even if that capacity survives her discovery of these handicaps.

Growth into manhood and womanhood proceeds from infancy and requires two or three decades. The formation, like that of psychosexual identity, is only part of the larger process by which the individual personality develops and changes, stage by stage, from the cradle to the grave, but it is the most prolonged and tortuous part and it easily goes wrong, with minor and major distortions, leading to trivial or crippling incapacities for masculine and feminine roles and tasks. For the mass of humanity, to make the grade as a man or woman is fundamental for happiness, peace of mind, and self-respect, and failure to do so is devastating. And there is the sense, deeply embedded, that to achieve this grade, success with the opposite sex is not sufficient. Certainly, in a woman, that sense is more obvious — this vital achievement is only secure, and only at last convincing, when her female body has borne and brought forth a perfect baby, and she has mothered good and sturdy children.

Therefore, in the attainment of personal and sexual validity, successful pregnancy and parenthood are of supreme consequence. In the ordinary way, this reality passes unnoticed, but should anything not go properly in the process, or even turn out to be just less than perfect, the personal threat can be vast. A delayed conception, an early miscarriage, a delivery needing artificial assistance, can unsettle the couple to a degree which, if the doctor is sharp enough both to observe it and spot the connection, seems disproportionate as far as the physical facts are concerned; while sterility, or a deformed baby, even if it dies at birth, can be endlessly undermining, with feelings of failure, blaming each other, or heaping it all onto the doctors and midwives ever afterwards.

Also, because pregnancy so powerfully, if tacitly, confers personal worth and validity in the normal healthy way, it is also readily pursued as a short cut to that validity, as an alternative to the long and difficult route of self-maturation. Among the distortions of psychosexual identity referred to before, spurious versions of masculinity and femininity abound — those who, after a fashion, can couple, traverse pregnancy, and give birth, but can only limp along, if they can manage at all, as parents to their ill-starred offspring.

CONCEPTION — AETIOLOGY AND SYNDROMES

The Pregnant Male

In antenatal clinics and doctors' surgeries, if it is not soon forgotten, little interest persists in the fact that the patient's pregnancy was caused by a man as well as by her own doing. As will emerge here, pregnancy is a state of mind and not only a state of body, and in that sense it is not peculiar to women. Likewise, clinical disturbances occur with this pregnant state of mind in men no less than women. It is well known that pregnancy can result in puerperal depression in women, but little known that it also commonly touches off breakdown in men — into

crime, alcoholism, infidelity, and other disorders. One purpose of antenatal care, surely, is to reduce the risk of these breakdowns in both sexes.

The doctor, therefore, should realise that, with every pregnancy, he has a duty to *two* psychologically gravid patients; and that besides aiming to deliver a healthy baby, there should be at the end *two* successfully prepared parents ready to receive their baby. Across the world, it was ordinary good sense in preindustrial societies to cater explicitly for the pregnant condition of men and to prepare them for the baby by the custom of couvade, whereby in a place with attendants, the husband experienced the pains of labour, while his wife gave birth. In fact, to this day in 20th century cities, if the doctor chooses to ask, he will find that, not so rarely, men can admit to some of the *physical* symptoms of the pregnancy that their partner displays openly.

Diagnosing the Pregnancy

The first task with pregnancy is a diagnostic one — to determine not only that it exists, but why. To neglect this can mean being left prognostically blind to dire emotional complications and sequelae, and to learn of them by surprise or, worse still, to miss them when they happen during its later course. It is pitifully insufficient merely to enquire whether the pregnancy was planned or unplanned, or to acknowledge perfunctorily that the seventh pregnancy of a housewife of 44 is a very different matter indeed from the first pregnancy of a lawyer of 34, or of a schoolgirl of 14, while treating them all in much the same way, with uniform antenatal clinic rituals, and no serious attention to their differences.

As with diagnosis in general, the task is made easier by knowing what to look for, and by having common syndromes in mind when assessing a pregnancy for its aetiology. For example, to recognise promptly that a pregnancy, planned or not, has been conceived in unconscious response to some undigested experience of loss, requires no esoteric clinical skills beyond the capacity to have this among other possibilities in mind, to be relevant, and not to forget that pregnancy is the work of a couple.

People can become peculiarly accessible with pregnancy, and it only needs a little time and an open ear to find out about the two people and their relationship; what relationship between their own parents they each experienced, and what had been the nature of the pregnancies in their respective families. Whether, at the start, the woman is present alone, or if her partner is there too, with a few leads of this simple kind, the information needed for a diagnostic orientation about the pregnancy and the couple will tumble forth. And, incidentally, because history does repeat itself, to learn how the couple's mothers dealt with their own pregnancies and babies is as good a guide as any to how it will go with this pregnancy and this baby.

'Planned', 'Accidental' and 'Unwanted' Pregnancy

'Planned' pregnancies — where the couple have an established and loving relationship, and want to start or add to their family — seem to need no further scrutiny. Many, perhaps most, such pregnancies are, of course, what they seem, but it is part of the human condition not to know what one really wants and for people not to be what they seem. Thus a percentage of long-hoped-for pregnancies, finally conceived after years of effort and medical treatment for sterility, will end deliberately aborted. Likewise, therapeutic termination of loudly unwanted pregnancies is followed sometimes at once, and not rarely in a year or two, by another pregnancy, which may again be unwanted and again be aborted, and even then be followed by a third pregnancy — and this in intelligent women who know all about contraception and passionately declare that their body is their property and they know what is best for it.

Therefore, the fact that the pregnancy was 'wanted' and 'planned' should not be an end to enquiry for other and perhaps worrying causative factors as well; nor should an insistence that the pregnancy was 'unwanted' and 'accidental' deter careful search for unrecognised purposes that it serves. The word 'accidental' has a place in particle physics, but in medicine it is unhelpful and overdue for discard. As for pregnancy, it is even less likely to be 'accidental' than those other conditions that occupy the so-called accident departments and teams of hospitals.

There are only two circumstances where pregnancy is convincingly accidental — the failure of a contraceptive coil or a tubal ligation; and rape by a stranger. And even then, having happened, it is not always unwanted whole-heartedly. Otherwise 'accidental' or 'unwanted' pregnancies can, as a rule, be

easily accounted for in one or more of the syndromes that follow. To terminate such a pregnancy without first accounting for it in this way, and evaluating its nature properly, may be a disastrous error, as this text will illustrate.

Pregnancy as a Response to Loss — General Considerations

The pregnancy instantly recognisable in this category is that which follows the death of a child — the 'replacement' pregnancy. Even so, the one that follows a stillbirth may not be spotted for what it is, and its psychological hazards may be overlooked. Indeed, it still happens after a perinatal death that it is the doctor of all people who blandly advises another pregnancy with all speed when, to embark on one without first healing the wound the loss has caused, can bring major emotional perils both for the couple and for the child so precipitately conceived.

Loss, in obvious, subtle, or symbolic forms is universally experienced — through deaths, separations, geographical moves, decaying relationships, changing status, fading beliefs, and disillusions. The encounter with loss at various developmental stages in life, and the psychological strategies for coping with it, are of central significance both for personal growth and for psychopathological vulnerability later. A failure to surmount loss may result in minor or major depression, with self-destructiveness or suicide; or it may lead to unconscious stratagems to counterbalance the loss rather than to feel, and work through, and get over it. Depression may then be evaded or, in the case of pregnancy which can be one such stratagem, postponed until after it finishes.

The prompt recognition that a pregnancy has this origin and latent purpose is important for two reasons, (1) to give warning of what lies ahead in the case of the woman, the man, or both; and (2) to allow the doctor an opportunity for simple psychotherapeutic work on unsettled emotional issues.

Pregnancy as a Response to Loss — Particular Examples

Bereavement — actual and threatened

Child-bearing age is also the age when the older generation begins to depart. The doctor can frequently elicit that, as if perchance and unconnected, the pregnancy commenced within a few weeks or months of the death of a grandparent or the life-threatening illness of a parent, and this should not too readily be dismissed as coincidence without first finding out if the task of mourning and recovery has been done, at least in some clear measure. This caution is especially necessary sometimes when pregnancy is related to what is really a train of illnesses and bereavements, often not easily seen as such, because they are interspersed between the families.

The link between bereavement and pregnancy should be kept in mind when any patient dies, or nearly dies. For example, the doctor attending the family when father has a coronary should remember the risk of the adolescent daughter shortly dismaying everyone with a pregnancy. To perceive the risk is half-way to preventing it — a little psychotherapeutic work may be enough to help the girl cope with her inner disturbance rather than act it out by pregnancy. By the same token, it is no help for the child with a grave illness or injury, when his mother responds with a pregnancy that the vigilant doctor, aware of the risk, could have prevented by timely discussion.

Separation

Partir, c'est mourir un peu — changes of abode, migration, departures of loved ones, while not literally bereavements, may psychologically be equivalent, and also be met not with grief and healthy recovery, but with 'accidental' pregnancy. With children, merely their symbolic separation — the youngest one starting school, the oldest one beginning to menstruate — can have the effect and quality of loss, and invisibly provoke the parents into a pregnancy which then is not necessarily welcome.

With 'unwanted' pregnancies, for which abortion is most pressingly requested, one or other of a cluster of these losses, which neither the woman nor the man seems to have in mind, may often be swiftly discovered. In fact, the patient disarmingly points them out sometimes: 'We've just moved away from my parents, at last, to a place of our own and I want a bit of freedom now, not another baby'; 'My daughter has just got engaged and we'll never be able to face people'; 'How can I cope with a baby now when my Dad's got cancer and needs me to look after him?'

Threatened separation of the couple

Just when a marriage or a love affair is breaking up, pregnancy seems to happen when neither party could have wanted it less. Or so it seems. And, popularly, it may also seem that this is a woman's unscrupulous way to hold on to a man. While this kind of pregnancy commonly presents with a request for an abortion, it always signifies a shared reluctance to separate, if not always shared in equal measure, so that abortion is sometimes not what the couple really need to help solve their difficulties.

Certainly, there is one variant where an abortion almost never should be performed. It can be suspected when a relationship, that is ending, existed steadily for a long time, and the woman explains that it just didn't seem to her that she would get pregnant, especially now when it was all over. A few questions will disclose that the pregnancy was truly unexpected, because the couple had originally taken risks and then 'forgotten' about contraception altogether, so that unbeknown to either, they had come to live with a relationship that more and more felt empty because it was literally sterile. An abortion in such circumstances neither rescues the woman nor relieves the departing man, but only leaves them sterile again and, worse still, without each other. Often, it suffices to bring the couple to a joint session in the clinic and to discuss their unrecognised experience and fears of sterility, which were expressed in prolonged 'carelessness' about contraception, for them to begin to regain contact with each other, and have doubts about the 'wanted' abortion, and soon enough, with one more session, to change their minds about it altogether. Far from being therapeutic, abortion here means destroying the baby they unwittingly longed for and finally despaired of having, and it can leave both parties bereft, guilty, angry, and separately licking a wound that will not heal. The request for abortion in cases like this illustrates that what people want and ask for may be very different from what they really need — a truth too often overlooked.

Pregnancy as a response to loss is commonly illustrated by its tendency to 'happen' very quickly in new and not very serious liaisons that follow the break-up of a marriage or a really important love affair.

Pregnancy as an antidepressant and as a suicidal equivalent

If pregnancy can be provoked by loss, to bypass the grief, fears, and depression that should be experienced and healthily overcome, it can also be unwittingly pursued as an antidote to depression. A common example nowadays is when an ill-judged abortion is quickly followed by another 'accidental' pregnancy — only seen as 'unwanted' if the relapse into depression that it has served to counter goes undetected. If this second pregnancy is also aborted, instead of a third, there may follow an overdose, though the surgeon and his social worker will never know, because some weeks have passed, their patient has gone elsewhere, and the abortion which the patient asked for will seem to have had no ill-effect.

If all this still seems doubtful, there are in fact cases, by no means rare, where pregnancy is pursued consciously and deliberately as an antidepressant. Many a woman with severe postnatal depression has observed that her symptoms magically fade if she falls pregnant — even when she has dreaded being so — only, alas, to return after the next childbirth. Some will apply this knowledge and deliberately conceive again — and, occasionally, again and again, even harbouring a phantasy of permanent pregnancy. Among simple-minded women with too many pregnancies, some are inarticulately like this. It can, therefore, happen that the kindly offer of sterilisation sometimes makes their domestic burdens disastrously worse — they are spared more children at the price of depressive paralysis and inability to mother those they already have. In other words, where the need for sterilisation seems so obvious, the case for circumspection is most serious.

Paradoxically, pregnancy can be pursued as an antidepressant manoeuvre, on the one hand, or for self-destructive purposes, on the other. Sometimes, both motives coexist latently, as in the example before where there is a trail of 'unwanted' pregnancies and 'wanted' abortions that leads finally to an overdose. It is easy to see that pregnancy can be socially self-destructive — for the clergyman and the parishioner entangled with each other; or for the recently widowed young mother, pregnant by the family man next door. Harder to see, but more important, is the fact that self-destructiveness is no less clinically sinister for being social than for being physical, and that pregnancies of this kind can serve hidden depressive processes as a suicidal equivalent. Whether terminated or not, the clinical care necessary is a long-term, psychologically sensitive exercise in the management of both depression and pregnancy.

Pregnancy in the service of aggression

There is a rough truth in saying that the counterpart of juvenile delinquency in boys is juvenile pregnancy in girls, and that the counterpart of crime in men is promiscuity or prostitution in women. Sex can be subverted for hostile ends, and pregnancy can be the expression of anger, destructiveness to oneself and others, and rivalry. This may be obvious with the schoolgirl who gets pregnant at her older sister's engagement party, or with the father who wrecks himself, his wife, and his family by impregnating his daughter, but more frequently it is not obvious, even in such gross cases when aggression is disclaimed and any injury regretted. Anger with parents, society, and the world in general, and jealousy of adults are common in adolescent pregnancies, and as often angrily denied. An example is the teenager who absolutely must have an abortion because the hospital said it was dangerous for her mother to have any shocks, and so now she would die if she found out about the pregnancy. The doctor may well raise an eyebrow about her motive in that case for getting pregnant in the first place; but if he does not, and if he fails to explore the girl's embattled relationship with her mother, she will 'accidentally' disclose the secret pregnancy anyway, along with his well-meant effort to arrange the abortion confidentially and spare the family an earthquake.

Pregnancy as a fast-train to womanhood and manhood

Adolescents with scant feelings of personal value, with sordid childhoods, rejected, or dumped, regularly become pregnant as soon as they leave the children's home, if not before, and in defiance of all good sense. If aborted, or if the baby is given away for adoption, they will become pregnant again. None of this is really difficult to understand; it punishes society which has never cared for them, it is heedless and punishing to the self which they do not esteem, and it offers a reborn and purified self in the new baby although, once it comes, it can be a further target too. But, over and above all these things, they are drawn, as if by instinct, by the alluring short cut to a sense of worth and feminine validation that, as was outlined before (p. 206) pregnancy seems to offer. The deprived youths who father these pregnancies are a male mirror image, with the same mix-up of buried and wordless motivations.

The same short cut is sometimes taken 'accidentally' by more ordinary youngsters, who unconsciously seek to gain some swift developmental reassurance from the experience of pregnancy. If they do need this, they are a long way from needing a baby as well, for the next phase of their personal development to proceed; and it may wreck their growth and their passage through life if the experience, and the pregnancy, are not terminated and they really do go on and produce a baby.

TERMINATION OF PREGNANCY

Some pregnancies are unwanted, or even abhorred and terrifying, and some should be terminated or else lives are ruined and futures blighted. Nevertheless, it should be clear now that, 'wanted' and 'planned', or 'accidental' and 'unwanted', pregnancy is commonly an outcome of significant circumstances that are overlooked, combined with emotional pressures that go undetected, which inveigle the couple unawares into pregnancy. While these causative factors have been grouped into convenient categories here, they seldom occur like that in pure culture — the motives are always mixed. Especially with pregnancies for which abortion is sought, the determinants to be discovered are usually multiple and, however intensely 'unwanted', the pregnancy is far from unmotivated. Indeed, in the course of bringing these determinants to light, both clinician and patient often may retrospectively grasp an inevitability about the pregnancy, and what was a futile calamity for the woman comes into focus as a meaningful, if poignant threat. Because the event is a life crisis, and life crises are particularly favourable for psychotherapeutic work, to render this pointless pregnancy intelligible is to release opportunities for personal maturation and healing.

In this way, as well, having understood the whys and wherefores of the pregnancy, a meaningful and panic-free agreement may be forged between doctor and patient as to whether it makes sense to terminate or not. Then, although the operation may be an abortion, the patient's whole experience will not have been in vain. On the contrary, it should be opposite in kind — promoting some growth, some learning, and some enhanced understanding of oneself and one's relationships with others.

Neither should the man in the case be forgotten and, ideally, the same exploratory work should be done with him. If husbands are normally consulted, it is seldom appreciated, for example, that, with a teenager, it can be violently disturbing that his girlfriend has been aborted and his baby extirpated without his knowledge, let alone his participation and consent. Even less is it known that his injury can have far-reaching effects.

In the end, the decision, whether to terminate a pregnancy may remain evenly balanced, and it is then helpful to remember that far more tragedies have been caused by wrongly refusing than by mistakenly performing an abortion. *To combine termination with sterilisation, however, even if requested, is misguided and dangerous.* The metamorphosis from pregnancy to instant sterility is not only shocking and demoralising, but it can lead to endless maladjustment and suffering and, given the emotional upheaval, the operative mortality not surprisingly is also unacceptably increased.

PSYCHOLOGICAL DEVELOPMENTS DURING PREGNANCY

As well as a state of physical development, pregnancy involves a state of mind which changes and evolves steadily over 40 weeks along with expansions in the partnership between the couple. This time is required for a woman to grow into a normal enough mother to greet and be so preoccupied with a newborn baby as to meet its needs. Consequently, a birth in any much shorter time, particularly in the first pregnancy, is a double hazard — there is a premature baby, frighteningly small to handle and rear, with a premature mother not yet arrived at readiness even for a normal baby. Worse still, where a woman cannot be seen to progress through the psychological evolution to be described here, and this can be suspected when she blithely disclaims any changes in emotion and feeling during pregnancy, the result is a mother in body, but not in soul, alienated from herself, from reality, and from her baby — a psychological catastrophe.

The psychological advances and transitions of pregnancy resemble and are in parallel with those in the body — there is a phase of establishing and consolidating a pregnant condition; an increasing definition of a baby within, and its otherness as a person; and a phase of separating from this new person within and preparing to meet and be preoccupied with it in the outside world. These phases are not clear-cut, but they are easily recognisable, and the clinician should be extremely concerned if any part of the sequence is not visible. It then behoves him to engage with the couple to discover the obstacles, and to work together to pass them by and go forward.

In pregnancy, but especially in their first, progress by the couple into new patterns in their relationship is a prerequisite to adequate parenthood. This advance comes about in two broad ways: (1) through exercising and building up capacities to mother and father each other, and (2) by a steady differentiation of maternal and paternal roles. These developments in the couple, which are crucial for the health and welfare of parents and babies, can be much fostered by psychologically attuned antenatal care, and by group and class methods.

The First Trimester: Establishing a Pregnant Condition

Is there a subjective sense of pregnancy, and how soon is it experienced? Certainly, even before a menstrual period is missed, the woman who has been pregnant before and tells the doctor she *knows* that she is so again, has a way of being correct. However, to be pregnant, to be convinced of this other than intellectually, and to be at one with it, takes weeks and, at first, despite the physical symptoms being a daily reminder in the background, there are moments when the pregnancy is forgotten and then remembered again as a novelty. It is a period when there are doubts of varying intensity at different times and in different persons, whether the pregnancy will survive and prosper or come to nothing, or even whether one is pregnant at all. At this stage, ambivalence about the pregnancy rises above the surface repeatedly, and the pregnancy is welcomed and feared, unwanted but at least, momentarily, longed for. The nidation in the mind is as insecure as in the womb.

Psychologically, the baby has little reality so far. It is a theoretical baby, the subject of phantasy, excitement and conversation, but the pregnancy is still a state of oneself, and not of oneself and another. The prevailing anxieties are to do with the pregnancy proceeding to any real baby whatever, rather than with anxieties as to what kind and quality of baby will emerge. For the man as well,

there is a long way to go before his pregnancy comes into being in earnest and with certitude.

The Second Trimester: Increasing Definition of the 'Baby Within' and its Otherness as a Person

In this phase, as the physical pregnancy becomes emergent and the alterations in the body conspicuous, the psychological pregnancy consolidates. The wavering quality of the first trimester fades, its anxieties diminish to be replaced by others or by some heightening of mood, and the subjective sense of a baby within begins to flicker and then take hold. Simultaneously, a lessening of nausea and other bodily discomforts in these weeks may greatly amplify this shift away from the first trimester to what then seems a transformed condition in the second.

Some women describe (if asked!) extreme alterations in their subjective state. There may be an intensification of ordinary experience, so that everything feels different or important, small events seem large, sensations more clear, and even colours, sounds and smells more vivid. There is an unthinking and unwise tendency not to question too closely pregnant women who say they feel very well. Not a few can reveal that they feel superbly well, or better than they ever remember in their lives, and while this is not necessarily ominous, the clinician, far from being reassured, should become more alert and enquiring as to the pregnancy and its antecedent circumstances, and more vigilant about the couple and their situation, as the pregnancy proceeds.

There is, among other reasons for this, the elementary consideration that, until pregnancy is safely over and a healthy baby delivered, it is realistic to have *some* anxieties about it, and only sane not to lose touch with the up and down tendency of life. Furthermore, it is women with troublesome postnatal depression who frequently report on its puzzling contrast with their remarkable well-being in pregnancy — a well-being which went unquestioned, if noted at all. Some will deliberately resort to pregnancy as an antidepressant to make them well again, as already mentioned in illustration of the links between pregnancy, loss and depression.

These changes in the second trimester in mood, in perception, in the day-to-day quality of being, which may be subtle or unmistakable, conveyed in words or only in body-language and behaviour, are conducive to a gradual focusing of oneself towards the, as yet, shadowy 'baby within'. The anxieties in the first trimester about the prospects of the pregnancy as such give way now to anxieties about the baby itself: will it be perfect, or flawed, or deformed?; is it being well-housed and provided for in the womb?; or are one's own health, habits and heredity spoiling that? Underlying this, of course, is the universal phantasy that negative feelings or normal ambivalence about the pregnancy have damaged the baby. An inevitable result later on is relentless guilt in *both* parents if, for whatever cause, a baby be malformed or injured at birth.

These advances in the pregnant state of mind, fortified through bodily affirmation all the time, take place much more automatically in women. By 20 weeks, they are being dramatically emphasised by the fluttering of fetal movements, although the moment is yet to come when the movements steadily belong to another organism and are not rumblings of one's own. However, parallel changes in the man, with realignments in the couple, are required for their partnership to prosper and to facilitate the increasing focus on the definition of the 'baby within'. Indeed, in order not to impede this progress, he must start to expand into impending fatherhood with an incipient sense of relationship to two likewise expanding people, each with special needs of him — that distant 'baby-within', and its mother, now profoundly gripped in an inexorable sequence of change.

This spontaneous process in the man, so vital for the couple, can be strengthened by favourable clinical methods, or deadened by unfavourable ones. The latter are still the rule — antenatal clinics where pregnancy is all a woman's business; where the nursing staff is entirely female; where fathers, if they turn up, are bystanders; where the couple are not received as such, and the case notes designate the mother alone; where, in fact, the couple belongs to no one in particular, its progress unmonitored, even if the mother is seen by the same doctor twice running.

The clinical procedures that foster the psychological advances of pregnancy, especially in the man, take shape from practices that are an antithesis of all this. In addition, ultrasound imaging can now be used in a way which deserves particular attention. Provided its employment is organised for this purpose no less than for others, and someone guides the parents in what to look for, the couple viewing the screen can share today, for the first time in human history, a direct experience of their tiny fetus with its beating heart, early in the second trimester. They can actually take away the first photo of their baby — the stranger journeying towards them from inner space, with most of its 40-week voyage still ahead, with their sense of parenthood, especially the man's, boosted by direct experience of their offspring.

By the end of the second trimester, the 'baby-within' has acquired some constant definition and the couple some decided extensions into parenting. There is a sense of being no longer quite the same couple, with traits of a threesome now, and with new needs and altered features to come to terms with and parent in each other and, to enable that, there are new capacities to be discovered. The theoretical baby of the first trimester has become a real one on the way now, although its 'otherness' as a separate person is still fluctuant and indistinct.

The Third Trimester: Separation and Preparing to Receive the Baby

Once the baby is viable and childbirth clearly beckons in the distance, the woman starts to mobilise with gaining pace for the great test ahead, and the couple gathers its forces for the life crisis of delivery and arrival of their new baby. These processes begin silently or modestly, but they should finally be loud and clear. If they are not, it is an alarm signal of the failure of antenatal care, of impending problems in labour, and a rotten start in life for the baby. Long before this point is reached, routine work has to be instituted with the couple to foster the developments to be made in the third trimester.

Life crises, whether joyful or sorrowful, make people singularly accessible to others and capable of growth and change, even to the point sometimes of religious conversion, and the last trimester of pregnancy is no exception. This fact should be used to intervene creatively with the couple, to sustain the psychological progress of pregnancy described here, to encourage personal and sexual maturation during its course into motherhood and fatherhood, and to assist the mustering of strengths for the confinement and the new family relationships to follow.

Because of their increased accessibility, pregnant couples take naturally to working for their common goals in groups. Antenatal 'classes' should, there- fore, be organised not merely as classes to instruct and inform about labour and baby care, but as task- oriented groups. These are made up of seven couples or so, working with mutual aid, self-help, education, and an abundance of physical exercises and touching (because childbirth and a baby are highly physical and tactile experiences!). Such groups, all starting at the same stage of pregnancy, meeting week by week, become cohesive, intense, morale raising and growth promoting. In fact, they can touch off an abiding, and sometimes quasi- religious enthusiasm for the better care of preg- nancy in society at large. The group's work is not done when the couples, one by one, drop out into their confinement, but re-emerges some weeks afterwards, when they assemble again to swap their stories and show their babies.

The tasks of the third trimester are to mobilise for the inevitable challenge of labour, to establish the 'otherness' and the separateness of the 'baby- within', and eventually to part with and meet it at one and the same moment. By their nature, these tasks are stressful, so that in this trimester, moods become less equable again, fresh anxieties easily appear about oneself, the confinement, and the baby, and sleep may be disturbed.

There are two diffuse disturbances to indicate that all is not well. The first arises from failure to carry through the appropriate psychological deve- lopments of the previous trimesters, and its severity depends on the degree of such failure. Now, when there is no turning back, one is being swept along into childbirth in a state of unreadiness. Sometimes, there is utter unreadiness and frank panic but, as a rule, the manifestations are discontents, bodily complaints, tension, and depression, and the fear has to be elicited. Commonly, the true state of affairs goes unrecognised until too late, when the woman is already in labour and an extremely poor candidate for it, and the confinement is a nightmare with physical complications very likely as well.

The second disturbance arises with failure in a major task of the third trimester — to separate off the 'baby-within' from oneself, and to accept its 'otherness' as a person. The task is more difficult than it seems to common sense, and this is because the eternally magical nature of pregnancy is too readily forgotten nowadays. It is forgotten although, no further back than our own childhood, pregnancy was an intriguing mystery, while across the ages and around the world, pregnant women were always revered or feared. Deep in the mind lie alluring phantasies of permanent pregnancy, divine pregnancy, demoniacal pregnancy, immaculate conception, virgin birth, and they existed there long before Christianity made so much of the latter. This undertone of magic can exalt the pregnant woman with a sense of importance, self-sufficiency, and completeness that often is only intensely felt by its disappearance when pregnancy ends and she is back to ordinariness again.

In these remaining weeks of pregnancy, the task of psychological separation from the 'baby-within' therefore serves vital purposes. It is a coming to terms in good time with the reality that the baby is another person and that one is, after all, only oneself and nothing more. Childbirth, which makes that physically so once again, will then not be a stunning disillusion and a depressing loss, even though moments of regret for the ending of pregnancy will still be normal enough amid the relief that follows. At the same time, the 'baby-within', already endowed with an external quality as another being, can be freely greeted with curiosity for its 'other- ness', its strangeness eagerly explored, when it turns into the 'real' or actual baby delivered. In other words, it will be welcomed as a person in its own right, with its own potential, and not grasped as an extension of oneself.

Because this task of establishing a separateness is of an uneasy and coming-down-to-earth kind, and coincidental with it is the knowledge that childbirth is closely to follow, it is accompanied by uneven moods, worries about the baby, and crops of other anxieties. Blandness and tranquillity suggest that this essential, if invisible, psychological work is perhaps not being done, that realities are being avoided, and that the couple need some urging and have some self-searching to do.

SOME PSYCHOLOGICAL CONCERNS IN LABOUR

For women, the challenge of pregnancy and its crowning achievement through labour, is the pro- duction of a healthy baby. It is an utterly personal responsibility and yet, in order to discharge it properly, she must allow her dependence on others to increase, in particular on her sexual partner and her womenfolk. By doing so, she, in turn, involves them in responsibilities and makes childbirth into a social action for receiving a new infant, and not just a solo *tour de force*. All this has been a primal task and fulfilment for her as a feminine being since time began, and like other primal tasks and fulfilments, such as breast feeding and making love, it is not at first glance most suitably pursued in hospital and among complete strangers.

In the modern age, the spectacular success of obstetrics in overcoming the physical hazards of pregnancy and labour has obscured the risks, and sometimes the high psychological cost it imposes, by interfering with and hospitalising a great natural process. The delivery, undamaged, of a healthy baby — this fulfilment of womankind — is now claimed by the obstetrician as his responsibility, and he takes on as well the protection and survival of the baby's mother, previously a responsibility shared out in the couple's social network. Paradoxically, the more efficient obstetrics becomes in the physical dimension, the greater the danger of it usurping, or diminishing and dulling, the sense of achievement of those primal tasks that make pregnancy and childbirth richly meaningful, enhancing the development of the couple, and igniting their receptivity for the newborn. The heightened dependence of the pregnant woman, surrounded by uniformed strangers in hospital (who quite outnumber the expectant father, if he is present), is only too easily switched on to nurses and doctors in place of those to whom it would naturally belong in the ordinary world, so that the social quality of labour is blunted and it becomes an individual endurance test in an impersonal setting.

The clinical management of labour, therefore, must aim for three goals. Two are familiar and traditional: the delivery of a healthy and unscathed baby; and the safety and survival of the mother. The third is not yet such an obstetric cliché: it is to safeguard and foster the struggle for personal achievement and fulfilment that are instinctive in pregnancy and labour. This means conducting the confinement not only to ensure physical safety, but to preserve its experience as a climactic finale to the couple's pregnancy, as an accomplishment of theirs which justifies every task and every developmental stride towards new parenthood during all three trimesters.

Of course, the work of conducting the confinement in this way properly begins with the couple in the antenatal period, with the monitoring of their personal development and progress through the trimesters, and with the educational and group methods already described. The least that can be done, and this is possible even when there has been no such preparation, is to encourage the woman to feel supported, but in possession of her own labour — that whatever artificial aid is given, it is her choice and her need. It is not evidence of her inadequacy, and certainly not the failure of her female body which vastly more proficient female midwives and doctors are remedying. Likewise, the man should have importance, space, and recognition, as the couple's other half; he should not be left to feel a bystander, his masculinity diminished by the potent technology of the obstetrician in the realm of his mate's pelvis.

By this juncture, it should be obvious why *any* obstetric intervention to facilitate labour can be a psychological threat — a humiliating take-over of one's proper task, a confirmation of one's body's inadequacy, of failure to make the grade, not having what it takes to do it oneself as a real woman would do. The severity of such threat varies with the degree of personal vulnerability and with the degree of intervention. For a person with deep insecurities, especially about her sexuality, a small episiotomy or last minute forceps can be more demoralising than a caesarean section for someone else who is confident of her womanhood and dwells in a loving marriage. However, it is only common sense to play safe in all cases and to keep these considerations in mind throughout labour, and whatever obstetric aid or intervention is to be offered, from simple analgesics or rupture of the membranes, to major surgery. There is never the reassurance that clinical interventions are innocent and non-injurious, if all that one observes is that the patient seems not to mind, or accepts everything, or in mindless tranquillity feels nothing with an epidural anaesthesia. This compliance may reflect no more than the intensified dependence of the woman in labour, and it may conceal a lame incapacity to believe in and assert herself, or some even worse prospect for her mental health in the puerperium.

PUERPERIUM: 'THE FOURTH TRIMESTER'

The end of pregnancy, like its start, provokes mixed feelings. There is the sense of accomplishment and of relief from burden, and there is the new arrival; but also, there is the return to ordinariness again and, at least, some sense of loss. A state of magic has disappeared and if moments of regret are normal, extreme cases of disillusion and collapse occur as well. Moreover, there is now the 'real' baby who can be more raw, red, animal-like, and demanding than was the romanticised 'baby-within'. A few tears will, therefore, be shed in the next few days by the healthiest mothers, and some, less sturdy, will slither from these 'baby blues' into depression — slowly in weeks or rapidly in days; brief or prolonged; bearable or unbearable; with overt unhappiness, or covert, and disguised in physical symptoms. Postnatal depression is never to be seen as a minor female malady and clinical vigilance, should be routine. Potentially, it is ruinous — of family life and marriage, of the baby's basic development and the mother's well-being in the months, if not years, to come. Commonly, it can lead to phobic distancing from the baby, or to a dread of touching it at all, so that infant rearing is joyless or a nightmare; and not so very uncommonly it can lead to emotional or physical neglect, shaking and battering, 'accidental' injury and occasionally a cot death.

The initial mixture of accomplishment, relief, gladness, and loss, in the days after delivery, is soon far outweighed by other developments that characterise the puerperium. They are so striking, and they bond mother and baby together as if the literal ending of pregnancy has not yet ended the containing relationship, that this period is aptly named 'the fourth trimester' by Sheila Kitzinger.

Like other mammals, mothers and babies are programmed, as if by magnetic force, to find each other, and the programme is vital for the future of both. No procedure which keeps them apart has ever convincingly been proven safe and harmless, while there is much evidence to the contrary. It is, therefore, no idle fad to insist that they be kept together from delivery — the baby held and handled at once by the couple, and 'rooming in' with the mother, cot by bedside afterwards. On the contrary, it is an insistence on a natural programme suffering as little interference as possible in the unnatural environment of a hospital. However, there are two unavoidable clinical circumstances which may interfere with or even disrupt the normal programme, which occur commonly, and sometimes occur together:

1. *When the neonate requires life support* for some period, physical separation from the mother is inevitable in some degree. It is actually the case that separation of the neonate in *special care baby units* is a factor regularly discovered in the background of child abuse, as well as in lesser, but serious, disorders of parent-child relationships. This eventuality, where the neonate's condition invokes exceptional medical care, is one where a really deliberate effort is required to maintain not just some formal contact between mother and baby, but the maximum togetherness possible. The effort is not simply one of overcoming practical difficulties; a steady effort is also needed as well to help the mother overcome some very mixed feelings towards the baby she has produced and who has turned out to be less than perfect. These feelings which may make her resistant, if unwittingly, to engaging with her baby are examined further below.

2. *Caesarean section* interferes more seriously with mother-baby contact than may be realised. As a surgical operation it is unique – the only one where the postoperative period is not convalescent; but requires new developments and new tasks to be set in train immediately. The mother has to take on a new baby and a great task in life when, in the normal way, after such surgery, the patient rests for a week or two. Now, when contact with the baby is so desirable, it is physically awkward, painful, and may depend on help from others. Having already failed to deliver her baby herself, the mother now may find she cannot attend to it herself, or nurse it herself. Again her feelings about the baby may become very mixed – not only has it, in a sense, been the cause of pain, injury, a permanent scar, and a sense of failure, but not rarely she will admit to such irrationally resentful thoughts about her baby if asked. And, if asked and understood, she will feel grateful, relieved, and supported in overcoming these troubled and frightening feelings.

In the first days of the puerperium, the mother discovers her baby, becomes occupied with it, and quickly preoccupied — Winnicott's state of *'primary maternal preoccupation'*. This crucial sequence must be watched and confirmed because, if it is not seen to take place, something is very gravely wrong and the management and care of the mother-baby duo needs urgently to be reconsidered and intensified. The process occurring is akin to falling in love and it has the same non-rational qualities, such as a disinterest for the time being in the rest of life and in activities and people other than the baby. The father's antenatal education, if not his own wisdom, helps him to understand and protect this arrangement, and to appreciate that it takes longer than the physical act of parturition to deliver the baby to himself and to others — that the baby has come home, but is not yet fully born.

Breast feeding symbolises this. It continues the baby's nutrition from the mother's body, as it was in pregnancy, and it repeatedly enacts and gives substance to their mutuality, inseparability, and closeness, the foundation on which security, stability, happiness, and effective social capacities can rise. The promotion of breast feeding is, therefore, far more than the promotion of breast milk as such, superior though it may be. If man shall not live by bread alone, babies certainly cannot live by milk alone.

FAILED PREGNANCY

Like every human enterprise, pregnancy can fail, and some people will cope with that resiliently, and some will fall apart. How they cope will depend on the severity of the failure on the one hand, and on their strength and vulnerability of mind and character, on the other. Some failures, such as an anencephalic stillbirth, are enormous and will flatten anybody, at least for a while; some, such as a miscarriage at 15 weeks, or the birth of a baby with a minor blemish, will decidedly upset most people, but only devastate a few.

Pregnancy can fail by coming to nothing through abortion, stillbirth, or neonatal death. It can also fail by producing a damaged or congenitally deformed baby, or by ending before its time, delivering a tiny premature baby (sometimes deformed as well, and always with a doubtful future) that needs extraordinary attention, to a premature mother not yet ready even for a normal baby. How should such disasters be met? There should be sufficient advance knowledge from proper diagnostic assessment of the couple and their pregnancy (*see* p. 207) to indicate what resources they may arouse, what fragilities they may tread upon, and what strategy of clinical assistance will be required.

Spontaneous Abortion

The later a pregnancy miscarries, the greater the shock and sense of failure. Although a standard medical response, it is no reassurance to explain that abortion is Nature's way of eliminating defective embryos and that the miscarriage may have been no great loss. When already down and inadequate, it is not helpful to hear that one's body might give forth a monster.

If one abortion may be fairly painless, a second is dispiriting or worse, and for women insecure in their femininity, every period a few days late can be suffered as a mini-abortion. *Recurrent abortion*, however, always touches off profound self-doubt, diffuse anxieties, and ultimately despair, usually kept veiled from society and from the doctor who does not look beyond the surface. Invariably, there are guilty phantasies gnawing away — about punishment for sexual misdeeds or a previous induced abortion; about the poverty of one's womb, or even images of it as a baby tomb or cemetery; about being to blame for the miscarriages through negative feelings and somehow mentally rejecting pregnancy. Of course, some ambivalence is normally there in early pregnancy, but as each pregnancy aborts, the next one is greeted with less and less trust, more negativity, and an increasingly persecutory aura of being weighed in the balance and found wanting. Recurrent abortion is a recurring grief and so demoralising for the couple as to make a psychotherapeutic programme of some kind essential.

Congenital Defect; Birth Injury; Prematurity

If a baby turns out to be less than perfect, let alone deformed, the parents' self-esteem and esteem of each other are instantly threatened, and in vulnerable cases, endlessly threatened. No matter how rational and well-informed, no couple, not even a medical couple, can give birth to a damaged or defective baby without a sense of failure, ruminative self-searching for faults and inadequacies, and an avalanche of guilt. They may not display this; or they may quickly absolve themselves and proclaim nothing beyond blaming others; but to take any such behaviour at its face value and to treat them accordingly, to make no allowance for their crushing sense of personal failure, and no clinical anticipation of its consequences, is not merely naive or unsophisticated, it is grossly negligent.

To complicate the issue, the medical and nursing staff, whether *they* realise it or not, get caught up emotionally, their own basic human fears being stirred, and find themselves in what is a failure for everybody. Their automatic and unthinking retreat is to be busy and distance themselves, to explain the event away with recondite theorising, and to be uncomprehending and defensive in face of the couple's emotional turbulence, should that be openly expressed and not politely subdued.

The couple must be confronted unhurriedly, in privacy, and in due ceremony for an awesome happening, with the candid recognition that their feelings are, or surely should be, tumultuous. 'You must want to cry and to scream; you must be angry; you must be blaming yourselves; you must be furious with us; you must be wondering *why me?* and *why us?* and *is it my fault? is it your fault?*, and *is it their fault?*' Moreover, a single session of this kind is only a start in the steady therapy of the crisis by the clinical team.

If the crisis is allowed to proceed mutely, by default, and with no deliberate plan of management, the pain that is there is amplified and can become chronic, and the disarray of the family that follows can become a wreckage. The parents may sink with remorse into depression, or dispose of guilt by recrimination and blaming each other, or collusively deny it and accuse the staff at the confinement, setting up legends about their actions then, and ever afterwards remembering them with curses to their dying day. Some of this is too enormous to prevent, but most couples will be responsive and grateful for the attempt, provided it shows an ability to share their feelings and to acknowledge the defeat, disappointment, and failure for *all* who were involved.

Stillbirth and Neonatal Death

Everything said above applies as forcibly to stillbirth and neonatal infant death. In the case of stillbirth, there are special features to consider, which cause confusion and can lead to clinical management that makes matters worse.

With stillbirth, the 'baby-within' — so momentous a figure in the pregnant state of mind of the couple (*see* p. 212) — never arrives to become the 'real' baby outside. Thus there is a death to be mourned, but no real person has been lost, and this is magnified and writ large if the stillborn infant is

whisked away, never seen, and vanishes in an unknown grave. The experience of stillbirth is, as a result, singularly bewildering and even if the baby only lives a few hours or days, a neonatal death does not have this quality.

Worse still, because there is no baby, the newly delivered mother has nothing to show for her pregnancy, nothing to share with other such mothers, no place in a maternity setting, and high eligibility for swift discharge home to lick her puzzling wounds in solitude. Traditionally, in hospital, the still (or silent) birth was followed by a still puerperium, with still (or silent) staff giving their attention elsewhere, to 'real' babies all around. The father could too readily identify with the staff as an onlooker, so that the mother was then left by herself to endure all this as a farrago of non-communication with others about a non-event. Not surprisingly, family doctors, who can instantly recall minor details of their patients' medical histories, commonly forget, or even deny, their ever having had a stillbirth.

The management of stillbirth must aim from the start to counteract this entire sequence of derealisation. Not in an artificial way, not by nervously seeking their agreement first, but simply because it is theirs, the parents should be given their dead baby in their arms and allowed plenty of time to hold it, examine it, and come back to it, and they should eventually be the ones to arrange its burial. It is no kindness to spare them this task and for hospital officials to dispose of the remains anonymously. Above all, there should be no 'stillness' but the very reverse — talking, listening, eliciting their feelings, accepting their anger, sensing their guilt, persuading them to grieve for the never-known child, easing them into the essential work of mourning and recovery. This work always takes months to complete, and they should be advised to postpone another pregnancy until then. Every member of the staff and any students should be given to understand that urging them, on the contrary, to forget the whole ghastly thing and get pregnant again as quickly as possible, violates their needs and their emotional condition. It should be noted that if they do become pregnant before properly mourning and successfully detaching themselves from the stillbirth, the person most at risk is the next baby. His unfortunate destiny is to be forever confused with the dead 'baby-within' that still remained undelivered in his parents' minds when he was conceived. In a shadowy sense, when he is born, he is received and reared as someone else by parents whose grief was never resolved, and he grows up a troubled child with a confused and blurred identity.

STERILITY AND CONTRACEPTION

It is frightening to be sterile. It can also be undermining or demoralising, bewildering or shattering, and many other things besides, and this is so whether sterility is involuntary or a matter of choice — by contraceptive agreement as a couple; by vasectomy or tubal ligation; or by lifestyle, such as homosexuality, celibacy, and so on. When it befalls an individual, especially a young and childless person, the discovery of sterility, or the experience of sterilisation by disease, injury or surgery, brings up a spectrum of hazards: frank depression, which can become a chronic handicap; self-devaluing and heedless risk-taking, one version of which is promiscuity, and another is addiction; and the expression of resentment, deprivation, and inferiority in hostile social conduct and in personal relationships.

For couples, infertility is, of course, a biblical and worldwide ground for divorce or polygamy, and a persistently childless couple is beset by divisive tensions, either obviously or latently, and they will only stay together if they can cope with and contain them. The doctor should be conversant with what these tensions are about, because they haunt every case of sterility and its treatment in his practice, and furthermore can arise with prolonged contraception in any couple without children. Also, there is some need here to examine the possibility that emotional factors may themselves obscurely influence fertility, impairing it altogether, or perhaps sometimes facilitating while inhibiting it at other times.

As with congenital deformities, it was assumed in the past, as it still is in unsophisticated societies, that when no baby ever came, the woman was to blame and barren. Nowadays, with the bets even, we know better and the sexes can blame each other. Assuredly, there is a primitive urge to flee the symbolic death of oneself that sterility can signify by laying it all at the other person's door, and certainly this is one source of tension for the couple. However, it is not the only one and often not the most unruly one. Especially with modern diagnosis, which will, at times, establish that one partner is sterile and the other is not, compassion and sadness will commonly well up to dissolve and dilute any

simple blame. More subtle blame is another matter and far hardier.

It is a blame more pervasive, more reciprocally destructive and, because it *is* surreptitious and subtle, less surmountable than simple accusations that *it's your sterility and not mine*. There arises with sterility a profound, if often subliminal, sense of rejection and worthlessness — an essence of oneself that could be a precious baby, from the intimate depths of one's own body, is offered but not received, not found good enough by one's partner to be given life. Because this suspicion is primordial and not rational, it easily seeps, mixed up with other intense anxieties as well, into the couple's perception of each other. Then illusions can develop that the partner *is* rejecting and unresponsive and that one *is* worthless and, therefore, unwanted, and the tensions this sets up can pollute the relationship with conflict, complaint, blame and guilt.

Now couples who, in the cold light of day, decide that they have no wish for children, or who, for whatever reason, choose contraception simply to remain childless for years, are each rejecting the other one's baby, not in phantasy, as with sterile couples, but in reality. Their doing so unwittingly does not eliminate that fact, or its implicit meaning, or its potentially subversive consequences for their relationship. All unaware of doing so, they make themselves prey to the same mutual suspicions and noxious interactions that waylay the sterile couple. As for male and female homosexual relationships, which are by definition sterile, they are even more exposed as couples to these dispiriting subterranean tensions.

Ultimately, because of these circular processes, the sterile couple's relationship can be so eroded, either visibly or below the waterline, that they are beset by illusions and bad feelings not only about themselves and each other, but also about any baby they might ever have. In their mental life, that baby becomes tainted by their own sense of badness and worthlessness and, to make matters worse, it is hated as well because of its hostile refusal to turn up and its eternal frustration of their wishes. Consequently, if a pregnancy eventually materialises, it may provoke powerful ambivalence more than delight, and occasionally there ensues the paradox that a baby on its way, after a decade in pursuit of cures for sterility, may be deliberately aborted.

Finally, an age-old topic of myth, phantasy, and folklore, there remains to be considered the influence on fertility of wishes, fears, feelings, personality, and states of mind. Certainly, if conception is determined by emotional factors among other things, it would in this respect be only like many other bodily functions. At present, since it is far from clearly understood how conception happens, or is inhibited, or facilitated, the possibility cannot be ruled out. On the contrary, there is circumstantial evidence in its favour, apart from the links, already mentioned, between pregnancy and preceding events such as loss and separation, which can be explained largely, if not perhaps entirely, by their effect on sexual behaviour rather than on fertility as such.

Thus, there is the perennial finding when a sterile couple adopts a baby that a pregnancy not only may follow, but may follow quickly. This is not so easy to explain away when, for example, after ten years of sterile marriage with gross oligospermia and failure of donor artificial insemination, a couple, three months after adopting in their mid-thirties, produced two babies of their own in twenty months. Not surprisingly, a common hope with adoption is that it will abolish sterility — and it seems to do so not so rarely.

Then, there are the travellers' tales of missionaries in the past among once-inaccessible tribes. In Samoa, they wondered how young people could have complete sexual freedom, while pregnancy hardly ever occurred except safely after marriage. This has some similarity to the popular belief that pregnancy is particularly unlikely to follow rape — this may or may not be true, but nobody really knows.

But as well as anecdote, there is the clinical impression of many observers that sterility often goes in tandem with a corresponding cast of perso-nality. There have been a number of studies that suggest this using series of couples, infertile with no discernible organic cause. The women in one such series were compared in their childhood background and life history to a neighbouring series of primigravidae, matched for age and social class, and they were unmistakably two groups of very different people. As opposed to the women at the antenatal clinic, those at the sterility clinic were more deprived in their upbringing, more subjected to family disasters, and more troubled in their sexual development.

Sterility is a baffling and tragic misfortune with which folk healers, religion, necromancy, and modern medicine have been endlessly caught up. In the end, it is but one in the range of disorders of sexuality and reproduction for the treatment of which disciplined and systematic psychotherapeutic procedures will always be relevant and often central.

FURTHER READING

Bibring Greta L. (1959). Psychological processes in pregnancy. *Psychoanal. Study Child*; **14**: 113–21.

Bibring Greta L. (1961). Psychological processes in pregnancy. *Psychoanal. Study Child*; **16**: 9–24.

Demmerstein L., Burrows G., eds. (1983). *Handbook of Psychosomatic Obstetrics and Gynaecology*. Amsterdam: Elsevier.

Deutsch Helene (1947). *The Psychology of Women*. London: Research Books.

Kissinger Sheila (1978). *The Experience of Childbirth*. London: Pelican Books.

16

The Breast

Although in most countries the management of breast disorders is undertaken by general surgeons, there are some in which this is done by gynaecologists. There is no doubt that the breast is very much concerned with reproduction and it is strongly under the influence of the sex steroids, oestrogen and progesterone. Breast changes, such as distension and discomfort, are commonly experienced during the luteal phase of the menstrual cycle; they are a very early sign of pregnancy and lactation is an important reproductive function described in Chapter 12. It seems appropriate, therefore, to consider breast pathology in this volume, as it can play such an important part in the life and health of women.

DEVELOPMENT OF THE FEMALE BREAST

During the 5th week of intrauterine life, the ectodermal primitive milk streaks (galactic bands) develop, consisting of two bands which extend along each side of the lateral embryonic trunk, from axilla to groin. These bands widen to form mammary ridges in the thoracic area and are the sites of the adult mammary glands. The distal parts of the bands regress.

At about 7 weeks, the ectodermal mammary anlage starts to invaginate the underlying mesenchyme. Epithelial cells continue to descend into the mesenchyme, so that by about the 12th week a definite nipple groove can be recognised. During the next few weeks mesenchymal cells then differentiate into smooth muscle fibres to form the musculature of the nipple and areola. Epithelial bands develop and branch to form a number of strips of epithelium. These represent the future secretory alveoli. With this branching, the stage of secondary mammary anlage is reached with subsequent differentiation of hair, sebaceous and sweat gland elements. Phylogenetically, the breast parenchyma

develops from sweat gland tissue and only the sweat glands in the secondary anlage continue to develop.

Later in the pregnancy, placental sex hormones enter the fetal circulation and induce canalisation of the branched epithelial elements. Near term, the final 20 to 25 mammary ducts are formed and parenchymal differentiation occurs, with development of recognisable lobular-alveoli elements. The mammary gland mass enlarges appreciably and colostrum secretion occurs in the neonate. This secretion is transient and diminishes after withdrawal of placental hormones.

During early childhood, there is further development of the secretory elements of the female breast. The terminal vesicles undergo further canalisation and form ducts, which grow and branch.

Puberty begins at about 11 years of age, under the influence of hypothalamic gonadotrophin-releasing hormones. Oestrogens stimulate elongation of the mammary ducts with reduplication of their epithelium. Proliferation of the terminal ductules occurs with formation of lobular buds. The volume and elasticity of the connective tissue increases, with deposition of fat and developing vascularity. Oestrogens are responsible for the first noticeable preadolescent changes, but further development of the adolescent breast occurs under the combined influence of oestrogens and progestogens. Other hormones, and especially prolactin, are necessary for the full maturation of the female breast. This evolution continues for about 5–6 years until maturity is reached.

ANATOMY OF THE MATURE FEMALE BREAST

Typically the mature breast is dome shaped, situated between the 2nd and 6th ribs vertically and extending horizontally from the border of the sternum to the midaxillary line. It lies predominantly on the large pectoralis major muscle, but overlaps parts of the serratus anterior, pectoralis minor, latissimus dorsi and rectus abdominus muscles. There is a projection of tissue into the axilla, known as the axillary tail of Spence, which can vary from a thin strip to an obvious wide band. The areola, a circular pigmented area of skin bearing the nipple, is located at the centre of the breast. The breast structure consists of skin, subcutaneous connective tissue and the main corpus mammae. The terminal milk ducts open on the surface through the nipple. Vestigial sebaceous gland elements, known as Montgomery's glands, open on the periphery of the areola through small elevations which are termed Morgagni's tubercles.

The breast is enveloped completely in pectoral fascia. Connecting strands of fibrous tissue, Cooper's suspensory ligaments, run from skin to the deep pectoral fascia. The corpus mammae consist of the breast parenchyma and intervening stroma, which contain loose connective tissue, fat, blood vessels, lymphatics and nerves. The functional part of the breast, the parenchyma, has ductal and lobular elements. Each lobule consists of up to 100 secretory units known as the alveoli. About 20 lobules combine to form a mammary lobe. There are about 20 lobes arranged in a circular fashion which converge on the nipple. The ducts draining a lobe are about 2 mm in diameter and their terminal subareolar portions are widened to form the lactiferous sinuses. The alveoli and smaller ductules are lined by a single layer of epithelial cells. Terminal portions of the main ducts are lined by squamous epithelium. Myoepithelial cells surround the ducts. These are contractile and move secretions along the duct system.

The blood supply of the breast is derived mainly from the internal mammary (medial/central), lateral thoracic (upper outer) and posterior intercostal (lower outer) arteries. The lymphatic drainage is very extensive, compatible with its dynamic state. The network of dermal lymphatics mostly collect in vessels that drain into the axillary lymph nodes. Some cutaneous drainage passes to lymphatics of the other breast and the abdomen.

A large subareolar plexus of lymphatics receives drainage from the nipple and areola and transmits lymph by major vessels, mainly to the axillary lymph nodes. The lymphatic drainage from the corpus mammae is predominantly to the axilla. A relatively small drainage occurs direct to the internal mammary lymph nodes, mostly, although not exclusively, from the medial half of the breast.

Much of the lymph drainage from the breast first passes to the anterior pectoral group of axillary nodes. These are situated under the anterior axillary fold along the lateral thoracic vein. From these nodes, lymphatics drain into the central, subscapular and thence onwards to the deep axillary groups of lymph nodes. Any of these groups can be bypassed, however, by lymphatics running direct from the breast.

The nerve supply to the breast is both somatic and autonomic. Somatic sensory nerves are derived from the 3rd or 4th branch of the cervical plexus (supraclavicular nerves) and from the intercostal nerves. These latter are especially concerned with sensory innervation of the areola and nipple. The autonomic nerve supply of the breast is also derived mainly from the 2nd to 6th intercostal nerves.

PHYSIOLOGY

With each menstrual cycle, the breast undergoes profound changes, with transient hyperaemia and proliferative activity of the secretory elements. The proliferative phase of the cycle is induced by ovarian oestrogens, with increased cellular mitosis and formation of epithelial tufts. This state persists into the secretory phase of the cycle. As progestogen activity increases, the mammary blood flow is increased and there is water retention in the connective tissue. Towards the end of menstruation, this activity regresses. Because the mammary proliferation induced by ovarian oestrogens never completely returns to the starting point of the previous cycle, slight progression of breast development continues up to the age of about 35 years. This may well be interrupted by pregnancy, of course, with all the added changes preparatory to full lactation. After the age of 35, there is a gradual tendency for the secretory elements of the breast to involute. As the menopause approaches, there is a gradual reduction of the glandular elements of the breast, with loss of elasticity and replacement by fibro-fatty tissue of varying amounts.

CONGENITAL ABNORMALITIES

Congenital absence of the breast, *amazia*, is a rare condition, which may be associated with other anomalies of the chest wall. Accessory breast tissue, and, in particular, the presence of supernumerary nipples, *polythelia*, is a common congenital abnormality. The accessory tissue is often situated in the line of the primitive mammary ridge. Accessory nipples are not uncommonly misdiagnosed as pigmented naevi.

Congenital nipple retraction may be responsible for difficult lactation. So long as the nipple itself is otherwise normal, the retraction can be corrected surgically by a V to Y plasty.

TRANSIENT MAMMARY NODULARITY

Prepubertal

Young girls occasionally develop tender nodularity beneath the nipple well before normal breast development is expected. The condition is self-limiting, disappearing within 6 months to 1 year. Normal breast formation occurs some years later. No treatment is indicated and, in particular, surgery should be avoided. This form of juvenile mammaplasia has to be distinguished from premature breast development which represents normal breast formation at an unusually early age in otherwise normal young girls.

Premenstrual

In this condition, there is an unusually prominent nodularity in one or both breasts during the premenstrual phase of the menstrual cycle. This is often associated with considerable discomfort and tenderness in the breasts.

Typically, the nodularity occurs in the upper outer quadrant, axillary tail and upper central area of the breast. The importance of the condition is recognition of its innocence and awareness of the anxiety it causes. The condition may be transient, lasting a few months only, or may persist for years. A full-term pregnancy often causes the condition to wane, the woman being free of the symptoms when normal menstruation resumes after the pregnancy.

Treatment depends very much on the severity of symptoms. Provision of adequate brassiere support, including at night, helps to reduce the discomfort. Simple analgesics may be sufficient to satisfy those

with less severe symptoms coupled with the reassurance that is always necessary for this condition. Administration of a diuretic may help, although my own belief is that this is of limited value. A more rational approach for the more severe forms of the condition is the administration of norethisterone at an appropriate stage of the menstrual cycle. If treatment starts two weeks before menstruation is anticipated, the premenstrual mastalgia is often reduced considerably.

MASTALGIA

The causes of painful breasts are legion. Premenstrual cyclical mastalgia has just been discussed. Pain in the breasts which is not related to menstruation occurs most frequently in older, premenopausal women and may or may not be associated with recognisable breast pathology. It assumes many forms, and varies from the trivial to extremely severe. Both breasts may be affected equally or the symptoms may be confined to one breast or part of one breast. Not infrequently, the pain is experienced in different parts of the breast at different times. Often, there appears to be a localised trigger point in the breast, where direct pressure consistently reproduces the pain. This occurs most often in the upper outer quadrant of the breast. In such patients, careful and repeated clinical examination is necessary to exclude an obvious lesion such as a cyst or duct ectasia. Early cancer of the breast occasionally causes localised pain. Mammography is often advisable and can be used quite safely in older, premenopausal women. When both clinical examination and mammography are normal, treatment then depends upon the severity of symptoms. Even in the presence of a reproducible trigger point, surgery is not the answer, however tempting it may be to excise the apparently offending segment. Many instances of apparent pain in the breast have a different origin, such as intercostal myalgia, costochondritis (Tietze's syndrome) and forms of neuralgia. These will be excluded by careful examination.

Effective treatment of primary mastalgia is difficult. Sensible advice about support for the breasts and reassurance that there is no serious disease will help. The severity of the pain may far exceed these simple measures, however, and more determined therapy may be necessary. The use of certain antigonadotrophic agents has achieved considerable success and Danazol (Danol) is popular. Because of the side-effects which may occur, notably weight gain, my own preference is to give relatively small doses of the agent, 200 or 300 mg daily, and persist for at least 6 weeks before deciding whether treatment is effective.

Occasionally, there will be a genuine psychological cause for apparent persistent disabling pain in the breasts. Such patients are few and not always easy to identify. Stress may aggravate primary mastalgia, but patients in whom there is a recognisable psychological cause of severe mastalgia are the exception.

BENIGN MAMMARY DYSPLASIA

Various terms have been used to describe this condition which is so common in the female breast, yet so difficult to understand. The World Health Organization has provided a definition which cannot be bettered, namely: 'a condition characterised by a spectrum of proliferative and regressive alterations of mammary tissue with an abnormal interplay of epithelial and connective tissue elements. The individual components almost never appear alone and, clinically, they combine variously and may produce a lump'.

The proportions of the various 'elements' vary

enormously. There may be almost pure glandular proliferation with little interstitial reaction, or there may be almost total replacement of normal breast architecture by dense fibrosis. Cystic changes frequently occur, ranging from a solitary large, thick-walled cyst to a multicystic state with numerous minute and small cysts diffusely scattered throughout the breast. These changes are summarised in Fig. 16.1.

Fibrocystic Disease

In many women more explicit pathology occurs in which there is a change in both the epithelial and connective tissue elements. In a typical case, there is a mixture of fibroadenotic and cystic elements. There is hyperplasia of the acini, often with marked interstitial fibrosis. Cyst formation appears to begin by dilatation of small ducts, although the acini also become involved. There may be abnormal secretion by the lining epithelial cells. Variations range from almost pure sclerosis (fibrosis) to widespread cystic change, with all manner of intermediate forms. The pathological significance of this spectrum of change lies in the recognition of non-proliferative or proliferative states. Non-proliferative disease includes fibrotic states, simple cysts, sclerosing duct adenosis and apocrine changes. The more worrying proliferative states include lobular hyperplasia, epitheliosis and duct papillomatosis. Proliferative and non-proliferative elements of fibrocystic disease can coexist within the same breast.

Clinically, fibrocystic disease of the breast can present in many ways.

Solitary cyst

Small solitary cysts occur most frequently in younger women, appearing as a tender, often painful, semimobile nodule. Many of these small cysts can remit spontaneously, often after menstruation. The likelihood of spontaneous remission means that a period of observation is fully justified. There are those who advocate the attempted needling of these small cysts, but generally this is an unrewarding exercise, frequently yielding no useful cytological information, bruising the patient and making subsequent clinical examination of the lesion difficult. Persistent small solitary cysts are best excised

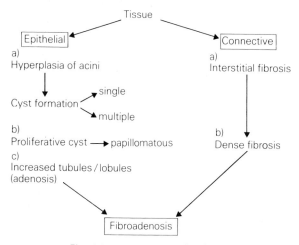

Fig. 16.1　*Mammary dysplasia.*

carefully and deliberately under general anaesthetic.

A particular variety of solitary cyst occurs in the areolar region of the breast, usually presenting as a small tender nodule at the margin of the areola. It occurs commonly in older, premenopausal women and may pose a diagnostic worry. These cysts are often thick-walled with a viscous inspissated content. Aspiration is unsatisfactory and they are best removed if early resolution does not occur. A periareolar incision provides a very acceptable cosmetic result.

A large variant of solitary cyst tends to occur in older, premenopausal women. Often, it appears rapidly as a large, painful mass in a previously normal breast, causing immediate anxiety to the patient because of the visibility of the bulge. Typically, the large solitary cyst feels hard, has a smooth spherical contour, with absence of skin tethering or deep attachment. Mobility may be limited, however. It is tempting to consider immediate aspiration of a large solitary cyst, which can be a satisfying experience for the patient and clinician. Occasionally, however, the rapid-onset, large solitary cyst either masks an associated carcinoma or may contain proliferative elements within its wall. It is preferable to admit such patients, so that the breast can be explored without delay if there are any remaining doubts, clinically, after aspiration. Exploration is indicated if there is (1) altered blood in the aspirate, (2) any residual lump after attempted aspiration, or (3) rapid recurrence after an apparently successful aspiration. Mammography is of limited help in these patients.

If aspiration is undertaken, it is customary to send the removed fluid for cytological examination. Patients should be asked to attend for result of the cytology and for re-examination of the breast clinically. Typically, the fluid from large solitary cysts is greenish in colour and turbid. Unfortunately cytology is often equivocal and its practical value is limited. Recent interest has centred around the chemical analysis of cyst fluid, as distinct from cytology. Variations in protein, electrolyte and enzyme content have been recorded and these may have some bearing upon the presence or absence of proliferative elements in the wall of the cyst.

If a cyst has to be removed because of genuine doubt, then every care must be taken not to rupture it during the procedure and to ensure that a generous margin of surrounding tissue is removed with the cyst. It goes without saying that counselling and reassurance form a very necessary part of the treatment.

Multicystic mastopathy

A condition of multiple cysts of varying size, from minute to large, frequently occurs alongside other dysplastic changes. The smaller cysts are often bluish in appearance due to the colour of their content. These are the traditional Bloodgood's blue-domed cysts. In multicystic mastopathy, one area only of a breast may be involved or the condition may be diffuse throughout both breasts. The condition may be associated with severe pain, which again varies from a very localised symptom to diffuse discomfort.

Multicystic mastopathy occurs most frequently in older, premenopausal women and difficulty occurs over the possibility of coexisting serious disease. Cystic disease is essentially a lesion of the breast lobules rather than the ducts, resulting from cellular activity and degeneration in the acinar regions, and not from the blockage of main ducts. Inflammation plays little part in the process, although occasionally a cyst may become secondarily infected. The condition varies in intensity, not necessarily related to cyclical activity, but does appear to lessen as the menopause approaches. Proliferative elements within or associated with individual cysts may increase the risk of subsequent malignant change within the affected breast, and for this reason the condition is not one to regard lightly.

Reasonably confident clinical absence of coexistent serious disease supported by a reassuring mammogram, justifies observation, so long as there is no severe associated pain. Surveillance must be meticulous and maintained while the condition persists. At intervals, a decision will have to be made regarding the aspiration of individual larger cysts or the need for selective representative biopsy to seek histological reassurance. As information accrues on the significance of proliferative states, there will undoubtedly be an increase in these procedures in this very common and difficult condition.

Another development in the management of persistent multicystic mastopathy is the use of antigonadotrophic agents. The true value of such agents still has to be decided, but they certainly can relieve associated pain and may cause genuine reduction in the degree of cystic change.

Absence of any proliferative element and a gradual reduction in the cystic change as the menopause nears are reassuring and allow a policy of observation to be adopted with greater confidence.

Proliferative cystic mastopathy

Occasionally, removal of an apparently innocent cyst will reveal worrying proliferation of the lining epithelium reaching papillomatosis proportions (Fig. 16.2). Treatment of intracystic papillomatosis is difficult. Information on the potential malignancy of the condition is scanty, but the appearances are sufficiently worrying to be cautious. If the condition is limited to one part of the breast, then segmental excision and careful follow-up are indicated. If the condition is more diffuse, then total removal of the breast must be considered. In this situation, the breast can be removed by a subcutaneous procedure, using an inframammary incision. The nipple and areola are left intact. The operation requires technical expertise to ensure that all breast tissue, including the tail, is removed. Breast contour can be restored subsequently by the insertion of a suitable synthetic mammary implant.

Fibroadenosis

The most common variant of dysplasia consists of changes affecting both glandular and connective tissue of the breast. There is a recognisable pattern of increased tubular and lobular elements (*adenosis*) combined with dense sclerotic change (*fibrosis*) in the interstitial tissue. The condition may be diffuse throughout the breast or may be confined to certain areas of one or both breasts. In some instances, there is actual replacement of glandular elements by fibrosis (*sclerosing adenosis*) and, in the most extreme form of sclerosis, there may be little, if any, remaining recognisable gland tissue. Cysts, large and small, may coexist with the fibroadenotic changes. Proliferative activity of the cells lining terminal ducts may be evident and in some instances papillomatous processes may develop within the ducts. A curious and not uncommon variant in the epithelium is 'pink-cell' change, in which the cells lining the ducts take on an eosinophilic quality, staining a characteristically pink colour.

Patients with fibroadenosis present in a variety of ways. The condition is most common in the 4th and 5th decades and is rare after the menopause. How-

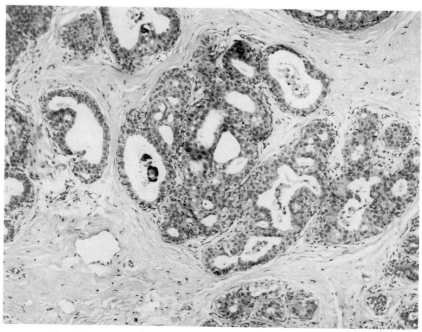

Fig. 16.2 *Example of intracyst hyperplasia and papillomatosis.*

ever, recently there does appear to be increasing incidence of the condition in younger women. Clinically, the condition causes a nodularity within the breasts which is more pronounced than that occurring naturally as a cyclical event. The condition is accompanied by varying degrees of pain. Presence of either a lump or pain, or both, is the reason for patients seeking advice. Common sites for apparently localised areas of fibroadenosis are the upper outer quadrant of the breast and the upper central area. In the latter position, nodules of fibroadenotic disease may feel particularly suspicious.

Fibroadenotic nodules tend to be firm in consistency with ill-defined margins, but with a smooth surface. They are often tender and hypersensitive. Although of limited mobility, there is no tethering of the skin or disruption of the surface anatomy of the breast and no attachment to deeper tissue. Despite these physical signs, however, there may be real concern about the diagnosis, and the decision whether or not to advise early biopsy is often difficult. Re-examination of the breasts at a different stage of the menstrual cycle may reveal marked variation, even though some nodularity persists throughout. Mammography may help in providing reassurance that there is no serious disease. Mammography is best avoided in women under 40 years, however, not just because of the radiation risk, but because the investigation is not particularly reliable in younger women. Results of attempted needle aspiration would suggest that sometimes it provides reassurance that the nodule is not malignant, but that it has very little influence on subsequent clinical management. Whether or not to recommend formal surgical excision of any particular nodule depends on a whole series of circumstances. The age of the patient, persistence of the nodule, mammographic uncertainty, or simple clinical anxiety, may all persuade the surgeon to operate. Previous history of excision of similar nodules, especially with proliferative histology, may be an important influencing factor. Recent developing interest in the histological identification of premalignant states in the breast is becoming increasingly important in this context.

Although it is convenient to separate cystic mastopathy and fibroadenosis for discussion purposes, it must be appreciated the both states coexist in differing proportions in many patients. What is important in assessing such patients is the degree of epithelial activity represented within the affected tissue, either in the form of intracyst or intraduct papillomatosis or as a more florid intraduct epitheliosis. Clinicians must be guided by the pathologist as to the degree of future risk represented by such changes.

INFLAMMATORY BREAST DISEASE

Benign Duct Ectasia

This condition appears to be occurring more frequently, especially in younger women. There is dilatation of the lactiferous ducts, most marked in their terminal portions, with periductal fibrosis and chronic inflammatory and foreign body changes. The dilated ducts may be distinguished from breast cysts under the microscope by the character of the lining epithelial cells. The inspissated material within the ducts has an amorphous appearance with minimal cell content. The frequent presence of plasma cells within the stroma has given rise to the term 'plasma cell mastitis', but the phrase has given way to the more descriptive 'duct ectasia' in recent years.

The most common age for the condition to present is in the 6th decade, during the years just after the menopause. However, the recent increased incidence among younger, premenopausal women is of interest. The most common symptom is pain in the central area of the breast, sometimes severe enough to require analgesics. Nipple discharge also occurs frequently. At first the discharge is trivial, but may become profuse and offensive as the condition worsens. Fibrotic changes around and between the ducts may cause the nipple to retract eventually.

On examination, the breast is often tender around the areola with an indurated texture. The nipple may be retracted and a greenish secretion may be expressed from many of the ducts. In older patients, the differential diagnosis of carcinoma has to be considered. The nature of the discharge and the absence of a palpable mass may suggest duct ectasia, as well as the often bilateral nature of the condition. Mammography is useful in such patients. Dilated ducts may be evident, as well as a distinctive linear calcification in the line of the ducts. In chronic cases, the calcification may be very extensive.

There is no effective medical treatment for established, symptomatic duct ectasia, although the occasional episode of acute inflammation will resolve with antibiotics and resting the breast with the arm in a sling. The only curative remedy is a full subareolar dissection with removal of all the terminal ducts within a single block of tissue.

The operation of subareolar dissection cannot be undertaken lightly, especially in younger women of childbearing age. After a prolonged period of conservative management, the decision to operate is made because of the frequency of painful episodes and progressive offensive discharge. Exploration must also be carried out if there is any real suspicion of malignancy, either clinically or on mammography. The operation is done through an infra-areolar incision situated at the margin of the areola and great care must be taken not to damage the blood supply to the nipple and areola. If done carefully, the ultimate result is very acceptable cosmetically, with complete relief of symptoms.

Mamillary Fistula

This condition is of considerable importance as it is often accompanied by a failure to recognise the true nature of the lesion. There is a communication between the surface and a blocked lactiferous sinus. The initial eruption occurs at the margin of the areola (Fig. 16.3a, b) and may easily be mistaken for a simple pustule or furuncle. The accumulated infected material in the sinus discharges intermittently through the fistulous surface opening. If the condition is not treated effectively, the infected area may extend and other fistulous openings may appear.

The treatment is surgical, the fistulous tract being laid open over a probe and the area saucerised. The affected area must be removed completely together with a segment of surrounding breast tissue. Although primary suture of the resulting wound may succeed, it is often wise to pack the cavity loosely and allow it to heal gradually from its base. A biopsy must always be taken at operation, because of the very occasional presence of an underlying causative intraduct carcinoma.

Acute Mastitis

Abscess

Most acute pyogenic abscesses of the breast occur in

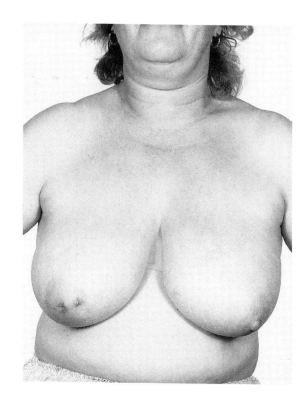

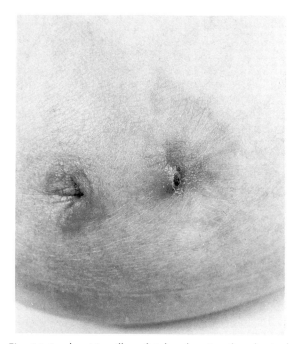

Fig. 16.3a, b *Mamillary fistula, showing the classical position of the fistula at the margin of the areola.*

the puerperium although, occasionally, one occurs in the middle-aged non-lactating woman. The staphylococcus and streptococcus are the usual infecting organisms. There is pain, swelling and tenderness in the affected breast, with fever and general malaise. A stage of acute infective mastitis precedes the abscess formation and the condition may be aborted by antibiotic therapy and suppression of lactation. The onset of abscess formation may be difficult to determine as fluctuation is a late sign.

With the formation of a true abscess, adequate drainage is required. An adequate incision is made over the area of softening and a preliminary guide needling may be helpful. Breast abscesses may be surprisingly large with a multilocular structure. All locules must be broken down by firm finger pressure and all contents evacuated. Drainage is established through a separate dependent incision. Healing must be encouraged to take place from the base of the cavity. The pus is examined bacteriologically and appropriate antibiotic therapy is advisable for a few days, especially if there is associated painful axillary lymphadenitis.

Chronic abscess

A chronic inflammatory mass with episodes of exacerbation may result when antibiotics are used to treat an acute abscess without adequate drainage. A chronic pyogenic abscess occasionally occurs in the non-lactating breast, the source of infection probably being an infected nipple. The treatment is drainage and curettage of the cavity which is then allowed to heal from within. Another source of a chronic well-encapsulated abscess is a clinically infected cyst. Sometimes these may be excised with a margin of normal breast tissue and safely closed by primary suture.

Whenever a chronic abscess occurs in a breast, the presence of an underlying carcinoma must always be excluded. Biopsies should always be taken from the wall of the abscess or from any associated suspect area.

Occasional causes of chronic breast abscess formation are tuberculosis, actinomycosis and hydatid disease. Tuberculous breast disease usually results from direct spread from either a tuberculous intercostal lymph node or a tuberculous rib. Cutaneous sinuses may occur and tuberculous axillary lymphadenitis coexist. The treatment is prolonged antituberculous drug therapy, although chronic

sinuses may be excised and abscess cavities curetted.

Fat Necrosis

Although areas of fat necrosis are often seen in association with other forms of breast disease, solitary traumatic fat necrosis is uncommon. It represents the slow aseptic saponification of damaged fat, the area becoming infiltrated by giant cells and young fibroblasts. The developed lesion presents as a firm, slightly tender mass which may give the appearance of tethering. It can be difficult to distinguish from carcinoma clinically, and usually the diagnosis is only revealed when the breast is explored and histology obtained.

Spontaneous fat necrosis occasionally occurs without history of trauma, especially in diabetic patients.

Mondor's Disease

This represents an apparently spontaneous thrombophlebitis of superficial veins in the periareolar region of the breast. It is important to ensure that there is no underlying lesion in the breast. The condition is self-limiting and heals in about 3 weeks.

BENIGN NEOPLASMS

Fibroadenoma

Fibroadenomas of the female breast are very common. Most are solitary, although multiple fibroadenomas are not unusual with extreme instances of diffuse fibroadenomas throughout the breast (fibroadenomatosis). The small intracanalicular fibroadenoma occurs typically in the young woman with otherwise completely normal breasts. The tumour has a well-defined capsule and has a characteristic histological appearance, being composed of connective tissue and glandular elements arranged so that the latter elements are stretched and distorted to give the clinical appearance of clefts. Although rare instances of secondary malignant change have been recorded, the tumour essentially may be regarded as totally innocent. Chronic fibroadenomas often undergo coarse calcification which produce a characteristic appearance on mammography. Clinically, the common small fibroadenoma presents as a hard, spherical, mobile lump, situated deep within the breast. Despite their innocence, the hardness of these tumours often gives cause for concern and they are best removed. It is unwise to attempt this under local anaesthetic due to the depth of the lesion, and the fact that incomplete removal may lead to recurrence. Removal under general anaesthetic is therefore advised.

Not all fibroadenomas are small and spherical. Larger varieties occur which often become lobulated. They tend to be less hard and have a mixed intracanalicular and pericanalicular structure. Microscopically, the latter appears as dense fibrous tissue arranged in whorls around the ductal and glandular elements. Once again, there is a well-defined capsule. The tumour is completely benign and occurs most commonly in older women. Rare giant fibroadenomas are rapidly growing tumours which cause marked enlargement of the breast and give rise to considerable concern clinically. These are also benign despite their size.

The curious *cystosarcoma phyllodes* may be considered here as it possibly represents a variety of giant fibroadenoma. It occurs typically in women of menopausal age and presents as a rapidly growing tumour which may occupy most of the breast and even cause pressure necrosis of the overlying skin. Although essentially benign, sarcomatous change may occur with subsequent metastases. Treatment of cystosarcoma phyllodes is simple total mastectomy with thorough histological examination to ensure that sarcomatous change has not occurred.

Intraduct Papilloma

Papillomatous change associated with cystic disease has already been discussed (p. 226). Benign papillary tumours also arise from the epithelium of the terminal ducts. Most are small, but occasionally the tumours may extend widely throughout the duct system. Typically, the small fragile pedunculated duct papilloma comes to light because of a nipple discharge emanating from a single duct orifice, which may be slightly dilated. The discharge may be clear or bloodstained and the diagnosis should always be considered if a younger woman complains of unilateral clear, nipple discharge occurring intermittently from the same duct orifice. Very occasionally a small nodule is palpable, but usually the breast appears to be comple-

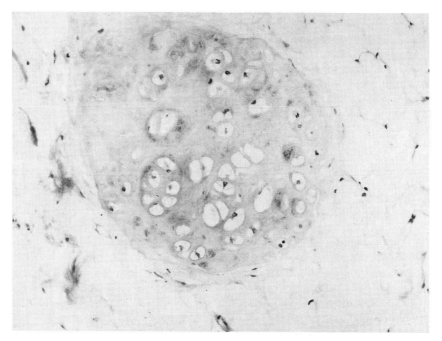

Fig. 16.4   *Benign chondroma of the breast. The cells are arranged irregularly in a hyaline matrix.*

tely normal clinically. Mammography is of limited value in the diagnosis of intraduct papillomas, which must usually be made, therefore, on the basis of the clinical history.

At operation, the affected duct is isolated by a fine probe and the duct with contained papilloma removed entirely (microdochectomy). Where more extensive papillomatosis exists, there is a rare risk of subsequent malignant change and wide examination of all affected tissue is required.

Other Benign Neoplasms

Numerous other benign neoplasms may occur occasionally in the breast. These include *adenomas* of the breast parenchyma or nipple, *angiomas*, *chondromas*, (Fig. 16.4), *leiomyomas* and *neurofibromas*. Special mention should be made of the *lipoma*. True encapsulated lipomas are not all that uncommon and can be removed quite simply when diagnosed. Care must be taken, however, not to confuse the true lipoma with the *pseudolipoma*, which represents fat distorted by the presence of an associated scirrhous carcinoma. The pseudolipoma has no capsule, although there may be difficulty in correctly recognising the lesion clinically.

GYNAECOMASTIA

Gynaecomastia is the term given to the enlargement of subareolar tissue in the male to give the appearance of a female breast. Its incidence has increased dramatically in recent years. True gynaecomastia should be distinguished clinically from mammaplasia in which nodules appear in the subareolar region. These nodules are often tender and occur most frequently in adolescent youth. This type of adolescent mammaplasia is usually self-limiting, lasting for some months and then disappearing spontaneously. Apart from reassurance, the only advice that need be given is to avoid trauma to the site. Very occasionally, adolescent mammaplasia is accompanied by a slight clear discharge, which is harmless and also disappears as the nodule regresses. The occasional case of persistent mammaplasia requires removal of the plaque through a small subareolar incision.

True gynaecomastia has to be taken seriously as it may be a reflection of some underlying and possibly dangerous disease elsewhere. Gynaecomastia may be unilateral or bilateral and, if unilateral, it may still be related to some underlying condition. Histologically, there is an increase in ductal and connective tissue elements without alveolar or tubule formation. The appearance is similar to that seen in the prepubertal female breast.

The condition occurs in all age groups and in about 50% some underlying cause will be found. In those patients without apparent underlying cause, spontaneous regression will take place in some, but others will require active treatment. Antigonadotrophic agents may cause regression, although there may be some anxiety over the effect of these agents on spermatogenesis. More usually, treatment consists of surgical excision of the breast tissue through a submammary incision.

Secondary Gynaecomastia

The search for an underlying cause of diagnosed gynaecomastia must be diligent, as there are many possibilities. Occasionally, gynaecomastia is recognised in young males in association with other evidence of generalised hormone imbalance, such as failure of proper development of penis and testes. Gynaecomastia occurring in association with the full Klinefelter syndrome is said to be associated with increased risk of subsequent malignancy in the female-type breast. Many drugs in use at present have been shown to cause gynaecomastia including oestrogen-like hormonal agents, certain antihypertensive drugs and some tranquillisers. Other conditions which should be excluded in men with unexplained gynaecomastia include hepatic and renal insufficiency, thyroid, pituitary, and adrenal disorders, and certain neoplasma known to be associated with ectopic hormone activity, such as testicular tumours and carcinoma of the lung.

MALIGNANT DISEASE OF THE BREAST

The management of breast cancer has changed profoundly over the past 25 years, but past achievements should not be forgotten. Before the recent intense interest in oncology, cancer of the breast was regarded as one of the few malignant diseases that could be cured, especially if diagnosed early.

Since the turn of the century, all reported series have shown a proportion of long-term survivors, living well beyond the time generally regarded as indicative of cure. It is true that, within the vagaries of this disease, even among the long-term survivors an occasional patient will develop further signs of the cancer many years after the original treatment. This is rare.

Carcinoma of the breast starts within a small duct or lobule and true *in-situ* stages of the disease can now be recognised. Intraduct carcinoma may persist for long periods before invasion occurs beyond the duct. In the majority of cases, the malignant cells are arranged in an irregular manner forming cell masses of various dimensions. In the better differentiated varieties, there are recognisable attempts at glandular formation. Once the tumour has broken through the walls of the ducts from which it arises, widespread cellular invasion of the connective tissue occurs. Not infrequently, there is a multifocal origin of the disease and it is probable that this is much more common than previously thought. Different grades of virulence of breast cancer occur, with the anaplastic poorly differentiated variety carrying the greater risk of early metastases. Fortunately this type is unusual, the

majority of breast cancers falling into the moderately well-differentiated range. As stated, most cancers of the breast are adenocarcinomas, although a number of different histological types occur with different behaviour patterns (Fig. 16.5). Connective tissue sarcomas are rare, but they do occur, as do angiosarcomas and lymphomas.

Endomammary lymphatic spread occurs at a variable stage of the life history of a developing breast cancer, the cells travelling to the peripheral sinuses of the regional lymph nodes. Some pass on to more proximal nodes and beyond, some are destroyed within the nodes and others will lodge where they are and reproduce metastatic tumour within the nodes. Cancers in all quadrants of the breast will metastasise to the axillary nodes, but internal mammary nodal disease occurs earlier and more frequently from tumours arising in the medial quadrants of the breast.

Clinical Aspects of Breast Cancer

Most cancers present as a lump in the breast, although recently an increasing number are being diagnosed radiologically before a palpable lump is

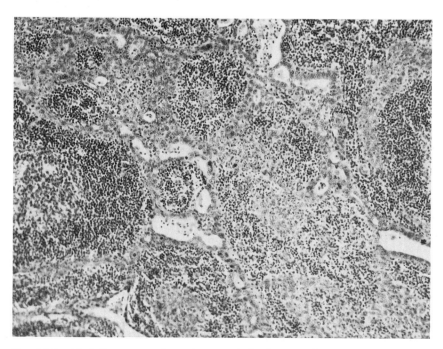

Fig. 16.5 *Medullary type of carcinoma of the breast, characterised by heavy lymphocytic infiltration of the tumour.*

apparent. The usual cancerous breast lump is hard, non-tender and has relatively ill-defined margins. The degree of mobility will depend upon the stage of the cancer, as will the presence of skin tethering or attachment to the underlying muscles. In advanced cases, the tumour is large and causes more profound changes in the breast due to its bulk and lymphatic spread. These changes include distortion or retraction of nipple and areola, shrinkage of surrounding breast tissue, oedema (peau d'orange) and light erythema of the skin, infiltration of the skin (en cuirrasse), or even satellite nodules and skin ulceration (Fig. 16.6a, b). With advanced cancers, the breast is often tender and painful.

The differential diagnosis of small cancers includes a tense cyst, a hard area of benign sclerosing adenosis, a nodule of fat necrosis, the occasional ill-defined deep fibroadenoma and a prominent benignly enlarged lymph node in the upper outer quadrant of the breast. Larger cancers may be confused with chronic breast abscess, giant fibroadenoma and even a large hard solitary cyst.

Clinical examination of the axillary lymph nodes reportedly is inaccurate in defining metastatic spread. Accuracy improves, however, the more effort is put into the examination. Modern staging of the disease demands not just an evaluation of involvement or non-involvement, but of the *degree*

of involvement. Interpretation can be improved further by examining the regional nodes under anaesthetic whenever the opportunity presents, during open biopsy of the breast, for example.

Establishing the Diagnosis

The role of needle aspiration cytology in patients suspected of having a cancer of the breast is debatable. If needle aspiration is practised, then it must be subservient to clinical judgement. Negative cytology must always be followed by further diagnostic effort if, clinically, the lesion remains suspicious. Equally, very few surgeons would be prepared to proceed on the strength of positive cytology alone; most require supplementary biopsy evidence. Two methods are available: *needle biopsy*, using instruments such as the tru-cut needle or a modified Desoutter drill, or *open biopsy* preferably under general anaesthesia. The advantages of needle biopsy are its immediacy and that it is done under local anaesthesia. Disadvantages are its lack of accuracy for smaller lumps, its impracticability for mammographic abnormalities, and the limited amount of tissue obtained for the pathologist. For smaller lesions, all the palpable lump or suspect area is removed. For larger lesions, a careful rep-

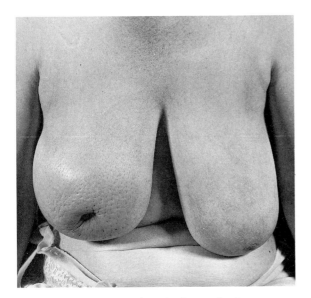 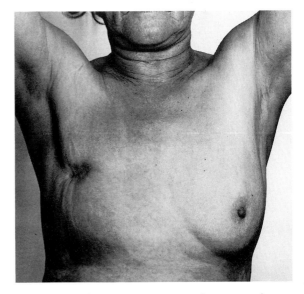

Fig. 16.6 *Examples of advanced primary cancer of the breast: (a) shows extensive peau d'orange and nipple retraction; (b) shows distortion of the breast and early ulceration.*

resentative incision biopsy is done. As there is no plan to proceed immediately, the pathologist is not required to give an opinion on a frozen section during the procedure, but is asked to give a detailed opinion as soon as possible.

Staging Breast Cancer

There are three good reasons for *not* proceeding at the time of biopsy on the evidence of an immediate frozen section histological report. First, with frozen section histology, false positive results occur and this is disastrous. Second, when the diagnosis is known, it is preferable to discuss the details of further treatment with the patient before proceeding. Third, there is now need to stage the disease accurately before deciding on definitive treatment.

Making the effort to stage breast cancer as accurately as possible is not generally popular, but it is logical if it is accepted that the treatment of adjudged early breast cancer is entirely different from that of advanced disease.

The TNM International system for classifying the stage of a cancer is particularly applicable to the breast (Table 16.1). It requires precise definition of the pretreatment state of the primary tumour, the regional lymph nodes and any distant metastases. This is achieved by careful clinical examination and

the use of such additional investigations as are relevant and readily available.

Clinical examination of a primary tumour of the breast includes its position and size (maximum diameter) and testing for any involvement of the surrounding tissues. Note is made of any skin tethering, infiltration or ulceration, of any oedema of breast or skin, of any distortion of nipple, areola or margin of the breast, of any secondary infection, inflammatory change or abscess formation, and of any attachment deeply to the pectoral muscles, ribs or costal cartilages. Occasionally, mammography may be used to support the clinical assessment. In particular, this may be valuable in confirming that the other breast is normal.

Preoperative evaluation of the regional lymph nodes essentially depends upon clinical acumen. Contrast lymphography and isotopic scanning of nodes have little practical value. The accuracy of staging of the regional lymph nodes can be improved by examination under general anaesthesia during diagnostic biopsy of the primary tumour.

If the patient has clinical evidence of distant metastases, this should be recorded and if symptoms point to a particular site, investigations appropriate to that site should be used to confirm spread. The search for occult metastases depends upon special investigations of the most likely sites, namely the lungs, bones and liver. Investigations basic to the search, therefore, are a chest x-ray, liver

---

Table 16.1

Essentials of TNM Classification for Breast Cancer

Tumour
- T_0 — No clinical evidence of primary tumour
- T_1 — Tumour of 2 cm or less in its greatest dimension
- T_2 — Tumour of more than 2 cm, but not more than 5 cm
- T_3 — Tumour of more than 5 cm
- T_4 — Tumour of any size with direct extension to chest wall or skin

Nodes
- N_0 — No palpable homolateral axillary lymph nodes
- N_1 — Mobile homolateral axillary nodes
  - N_{Ia} — thought not to be involved
  - N_{Ib} — nodes thought to be involved
- N_2 — Fixed involved homolateral axillary nodes
- N_3 — Involved supraclavicular nodes

Metastases
- M_0 — No evidence of distant metastases
- M_1 — Evidence of metastases

function tests and an isotopic bone scan. These can be supplemented by lung tomography, liver ultrasonography, and x-ray of specific suspect areas of the skeleton, according to the circumstances of the individual.

The result of this survey will provide as thorough and as accurate an assessment of the extent of the disease as possible. In particular, it will help to ensure that a patient with recognisable, advanced, incurable disease receives appropriate treatment.

Treatment of Early Breast Cancer

The definitive treatment of early breast cancer has been the subject of much debate in recent years. Ideas on the subject have changed profoundly and even now there is no clear consensus.

Radical mastectomy

The traditional use of radical mastectomy, whatever the true stage of the disease, was clearly wrong. Far too many patients were made worse by the procedure, usually due to the fact that the primary disease was too advanced at the time. Also, it was customary to combine the mastectomy with postoperative radiotherapy to the region, which certainly increased morbidity.

There is an argument to be made, however, for continuing to use the procedure for the treatment of genuine early breast cancer arising in the lateral half of the breast, where there is strong likelihood of early, curable involvement of the axillary lymph nodes. The Halsted radical mastectomy ensures complete removal of all possible affected axillary nodes, and there is no indication for any postoperative radiotherapy.

As well as the traditional Halsted operation, in which both pectoral muscles are removed and the whole specimen dissected as a single block, the alternative Patey operation is now widely used. In the Patey procedure, full axillary dissection is attempted, despite preserving the pectoralis major muscle. It is certain that some axillary nodes are missed in the Patey operation, which is not a true monobloc procedure.

Simple total mastectomy

Many surgeons now treat early breast cancer by removing the breast totally, but preserving the pectoral muscles. There is no attempt made to dissect the axilla fully, but nodes may be removed for sampling purposes. Proponents of the technique may (1) recommend immediate postoperative radiotherapy to the region routinely, (2) restrict radiotherapy to those in whom node sampling proves positive, or (3) use no radiotherapy at all, unless and until further local disease becomes clinically obvious.

Simple total mastectomy without postoperative radiotherapy probably is justified only for the clinically undetectable 'minimal' breast cancer diagosed on mammography, where the risk of existing nodal disease is truly very low.

Whether mastectomy is radical or simple, it is an operation which may have psychological effects on the woman. Breasts are strongly associated with femininity and sexuality. Loss of a breast may cause major damage to the woman's psyche unless there is adequate preoperative counselling with discussions of the potential problems and provision of adequate prosthesis.

Limited surgery

The most dramatic and possibly unjustified development in recent years has been the acceptance by some surgeons of the concept of limited surgery in the treatment of early breast cancer. Usually, although not always, this is followed by a course of radical radiotherapy to the breast and regional lymph nodes. Cure, therefore, really depends upon the ability of the radiotherapy to eliminate all tumour remaining after the limited surgical procedure. The long-term effectiveness of such treatment has yet to be proved.

Adjuvant therapy

With careful selection of patients with early breast cancer and adequate local treatment, the majority of such patients may be expected to survive their disease. The concept of supplementing the primary therapy with prolonged endocrine or cytotoxic chemotherapy poses the problem of treating the majority for the sake of the minority. It is doubtful whether such treatment ever converts incurable breast cancer to curable. For the present, adjuvant systemic therapy should be restricted to those patients in whom the risk of recurrent disease is genuinely high, as in those with an unexpected amount of nodal disease found by the pathologist.

Treatment of Advanced Breast Cancer

Included within this category are patients with advanced primary disease, recurrent local disease after primary treatment, and recognisable metastatic disease at one or many sites. None of these patients can be regarded as curable by any of the methods of treatment available at present. Remembering that the progression of breast cancer, especially the advanced primary tumour, may be a very slow process, evaluation of any improvement is not always easy. In particular, short-term remissions are of very little significance. The object of treatment of advanced breast cancer is to reduce the existing areas of disease as much as possible, and to control the disease in that reduced state for as long as possible.

Advanced primary breast cancer

There is no technical difficulty in removing the breast bearing an advanced primary breast cancer, but it has many disadvantages. First, it is almost certain that such patients will have occult metastatic disease, if not symptomatic. Second, there is high risk of existing major involvement of the regional nodes. Third, removal of such a breast carries a very high risk of early diffuse local recurrent disease.

One way of attempting to control an advanced primary tumour, without resorting to inappropriate surgery, is to rely upon high dosage radiotherapy. Because of the bulk of such tumours, this often fails. The problem of then dealing with advancing disease in an already heavily irradiated breast is formidable.

An alternative approach, and one that is gaining popularity, is to give the patient a trial of primary endocrine therapy. Not only is the response rate to endocrine therapy high in the previously untreated advanced primary tumour (Fig.16.7), but also such treatment may help control any existing metastatic disease. Even if the primary tumour has low receptor activity, it is still worth trying simple endocrine therapy, as an occasional response will occur. The only exceptions to this approach are those patients

with highly vascular ulcerative lesions or where the patient's compliance is doubtful.

The type of therapy varies according to the patient's age. In younger, menstruating women, the preferred method is surgical removal of the ovaries. For postmenopausal women, long-term use of the antioestrogen tamoxifen, 40 mg daily by mouth, is the treatment of choice. For the elderly woman with no evidence of cardiac instability, the use of stilboestrol 5 mg three times a day may produce dramatic regression of the tumour. If stilboestrol is thought inadvisable, then tamoxifen may be used as an alternative, remembering that the aim of all these treatments is to create a disturbance of the hormonal environment which surrounds the tumour.

Response to therapy may be very slow but, so long as the condition is not worsening, treatment may be continued safely. The decision to persist or not requires fine judgement and careful surveillance of these patients must be maintained. Ultimately, about 65% of all patients with advanced primary breast cancer will obtain some beneficial

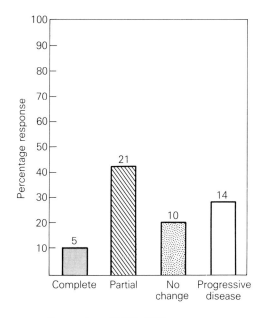

Responders   26/50=52%

Unchanged   10/50=20%

No response   14/50=28%

Fig. 16.7   *Response of advanced primary cancers of the breast to initial endocrine therapy in 50 consecutive patients.*

response, ranging from apparent complete disappearance of all the tumour to a condition of 'no change' in a previously deteriorating lesion. In some patients, such remission may last for years. When the disease recurs, a decision has to be made whether to continue with further endocrine therapy or to change to other treatment, either radiotherapy or cytotoxic chemotherapy.

Local recurrent disease

Local recurrent disease, either on the chest wall or in regional nodes, after previous definitive treatment of an apparently early breast cancer, must be regarded as therapeutic failure. Most patients who develop local recurrent disease will die subsequently from the disease. If the area has been irradiated previously, the situation is almost impossible.

When local recurrent disease is recognised, urgent treatment is needed. Occasionally, a single nodule may occur on the chest wall which can be dealt with effectively by wide local excision. Often the nodules are multiple and diffuse. If radiotherapy has not been used previously, this should be considered, although it may be reasonable to try endocrine therapy first.

Endocrine therapy for local recurrent disease is much less rewarding than for the advanced primary tumour, the response rate only being about 30%. The chance of a worthwhile response occurring after previous radiotherapy is minimal.

Often cytotoxic chemotherapy is recommended for diffuse and confluent local recurrent disease with some temporary success.

Distant metastatic disease

Distant metastatic spread from breast cancer cannot be cured. The best that can be achieved is to delay the inevitable for as long as possible and to alleviate the effects of the disease. Surgery, radiotherapy, endocrine therapy, cytotoxic chemotherapy and methods specific to the need, all have a role in treatment.

In many patients, there will be some immediate problem which requires specific attention. Localised areas of bone pain will usually respond to radiotherapy. Pathological fractures, near fractures and especially incipient paraplegia will require urgent orthopaedic attention. Pleural effusions will

often require aspiration or formal drainage. Unpleasant symptoms such as pain, nausea and anxiety will require specific medication and understanding. Metastatic breast cancer can afflict all systems and related symptoms occur which require specific attention. Other peripheral effects include hypercalcaemia, leucoerythroblastic anaemia and dermatomyositis (Fig. 16.8). These are very serious states which require appropriate treatment. They must not be mistaken for a natural deterioration of the patient due to the cancer or the chance of successful therapy will be missed. Acute hypercalcaemia, in particular, can manifest in many ways and should always be considered when a patient with metastatic breast cancer deteriorates suddenly.

Endocrine therapy

It is generally accepted that if a good response is achieved by endocrine therapy, this is likely to be more prolonged and more sympathetic than that obtained from cytotoxic chemotherapy. Endocrine therapy should always be considered first, therefore, although its scope is more limited in distant metastatic disease than in the advanced primary cancer.

Past experience of the use of endocrine therapy

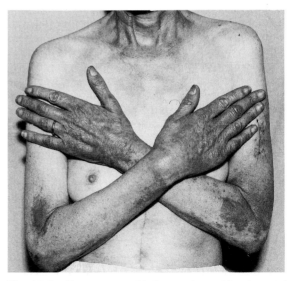

Fig. 16.8 *Dermatomyositis in a patient with advanced breast cancer.*

has provided information on the likelihood of beneficial response. Generally, patients with an interval of more than two years between previous mastectomy and recognition of distant metastases are more likely to respond than those with a short 'free' interval. Age has some effect; women around the menopause have a reduced chance of response. Also the sites of metastases have considerable influence. Skeletal and soft-tissue (cutaneous, lymph nodes) disease appears to respond more favourably than visceral (lung, liver, brain).

As well as these factors, there have been many attempts at assessing endocrine responsiveness by laboratory methods. Tumour enzyme activity, macrophage activity, elastin content of the tumour (elastosis), chromosome patterns (Barr Bodies) and distribution of urinary steroid metabolites (discriminant function), have all been the subject of investigation in this context. None have stood the test of time. The assessment of the tumour receptor activity appears to have much greater reliability, however, and measurement has now become routine in many centres.

Breast tumour steroid receptors are specific cytoplasmic protein molecules which have a high affinity for binding with oestrogens and progestogens. Tumours with high receptor activity generally have a good chance of responding to endocrine therapy and *vice versa*, particularly if the tumour contains oestrogen receptor in an activated form. Although there is now good evidence that receptor levels in metastases are generally lower than in the primary tumour, measurement of the receptor activity in the latter does give a good indication of subsequent endocrine responsiveness.

Patients with metastatic breast cancer, therefore, can be assessed individually according to a number of criteria. Unless the situation is highly unfavourable, it is usual to give the patient a trial of simple endocrine therapy before considering cytotoxics.

Simple endocrine therapy. In premenopausal women, ablation of ovarian function is the first procedure. This can be done either surgically or, in certain patients, by radiotherapy. Older women are treated with tamoxifen as for advanced primary disease. Frequent follow-up is maintained and response judged according to the patient's condition and objective regression of the disease. If genuine beneficial response occurs, treatment is maintained. Eventual relapse then requires further full evaluation to decide whether to continue with other endocrine therapy, such as progestogens, aminoglutethamide or even a major endocrine ablation. The drug aminoglutethamide, an aromatase inhibitor, has been introduced in recent years as a means of medically reducing the function of the adrenal glands. It is a valuable addition to the medical treatment of metastatic breast cancer.

Major endocrine ablation. This term includes surgical hypophysectomy by various routes, irradiation methods of pituitary ablation, and surgical removal of the adrenal glands. There is little justification for hypophysectomy or pituitary irradiation, as previous studies have shown that adrenalectomy is as effective. Adrenalectomy has a place in the treatment of advanced breast cancer, but it should only be used selectively. Patients to be considered for adrenalectomy are those in whom there appears to be no visceral disease, who have responded well to previous simple endocrine therapy. When a good response is obtained from adrenalectomy, this may be very prolonged, sometimes even exceeding a decade.

Cytotoxic chemotherapy

Candidates for cytotoxic chemotherapy are those in whom endocrine therapy is either contraindicated from the outset or has reached the end of its usefulness. Combination chemotherapy has become the routine. Popular combinations are adriamycin with cyclophosphamide and triple therapy of cyclophosphamide, methotrexate and 5-fluorouracil (CMF). Such treatment is usually given at intervals of 3–4 weeks and may require the patient to remain in hospital overnight. Unpleasant side-effects are common, but alleviation of these by appropriate medication is more effective than in the past.

There is no way of predicting response to cytotoxics. For this reason, patients must be watched carefully and treatment discontinued if no benefit is obvious after three or four courses. When response occurs, treatment is continued usually for one year and then reviewed. Cytotoxic chemotherapy will produce some evidence of response in about 60% of patients treated, but the duration of remission, unfortunately, is usually short.

Recent developments include attempts to correlate response to cytotoxics with receptor activity and combining with endocrine methods.

After-care of Breast Cancer

The effect of the diagnosis of cancer of the breast upon a woman is enormous. The fear of the disease and the impact of mastectomy are equally awful. No one should minimise the problems and giving adequate help is an integral part of the treatment of the patient and her disease. Fortunately, modern external breast prostheses have improved considerably.

A recent welcome introduction is the concept of surgical mammary reconstruction. Some surgeons advocate combining reconstruction with the mastectomy, but there are good arguments against this. Removing a breast for cancer is a major commitment which should command all of the cancer surgeon's concentration. To obtain the best result from reconstruction, separate plastic surgical skills are required. Also, the risk of masking local recurrent disease by an implanted prosthesis is considerable. It is sensible to delay reconstruction for at least two years. At that stage, patients who accept reconstruction will be more certain of their decision.

CANCER OF THE MALE BREAST

The increased risk of malignant change in certain types of gynaecomastia has been referred to previously (p. 231). There is also a small natural incidence of adenocarcinoma developing in the male breast, usually in the elderly.

If the disease is localised, radical mastectomy offers the chance of cure. Because of the small amount of breast tissue, such early cancers are few.

Cancers of the male breast may be endocrine responsive and, for the advanced disease, radiotherapy locally combined with orchidectomy may control the process temporarily. Tamoxifen therapy is now being advocated for advanced breast cancer in the male and adrenalectomy has a role in selected cases.

FURTHER READING

Burn I. (1985). The role of adrenalectomy in breast cancer. In *Seminars in Surgical Oncology*, Vol. 1, No. 3, pp. 132–38.

Dupont W.D., Page D.L. (1985). Risk factors for breast cancer in women with proliferative breast disease. *New Engl. J. Med*; **321** (3): 146–51.

Norton L.W., Davis J.R., Wiens J.L., Trego D.L. *et al.* (1984). Accuracy of aspiration cytology in detecting breast cancer. *Surgery*; **96** (4): 806–14.

Osborne M.P. (1983). Controversies in the management of primary breast cancer. A surgical analysis. *Cancer Invest*; **1** (3): 259–65.

Veronesi N., Saccozzi R., DelVecchio M. (1981). Comparing radical mastectomy with quadrantectomy axillary dissection and radiotherapy in patients with small cancers of the breast. *New Engl. J. Med*; **305**: 6–11.

17

Contraception

In comparison with economic trends or national crises, specific contraceptive measures have probably contributed little to population trends. Events such as the Depression of the 1920s and 1930s, followed by World War II in the 1940s have had much more profound effects on populations than the advent of the oral contraceptive pill or intrauterine devices. However, for the individual couple, the ability to control and space their family using one or several current methods as appropriate is very important to the well-being and happiness of parents and other children.

TRADITIONAL METHODS

Safe Period

This method depends on the avoidance of intercourse at a time when conception might take place. Despite an apparently regular 28 day cycle, the timing of ovulation is not precise and the duration of survival of ovum and sperm is variable. The ovum is likely to be capable of fertilisation for 24–36 h after ovulation, but sperm may survive in the female genital tract for up to 3 days. The preovulatory infertile period is difficult to recognise and is calculated on the basis of previous cycles and the date of the last menstrual period. If the cycles are irregular and short, then the preovulatory safe period is correspondingly short and unpredictable. Ovulation can be recognised in some women by a change in their cervical mucus, which becomes clear and copious, and/or by mild midcycle lower abdominal pain (mittelschmerz). A significant rise (0.5°C) in the basal body temperature occurs shortly after ovulation, but this is an imprecise method of detecting ovulation on a regular basis. The postovulatory safe period will commence 2 days after it is thought that ovulation has occurred.

The failure rate of this method is of the order of 30 per 100 woman years because of the difficulty of predicting the time of ovulation accurately. Attempts are being made to detect ovulation more precisely by means of recording temperature or pH changes in the vagina or by improving the ability of the woman to assess her own cervical mucus. It is not possible to say whether these techniques will be reliable in practice or whether they will reduce the failure rate significantly.

Coitus Interruptus (Male Withdrawal)

This has been an important method of limiting family size throughout the world for many centuries. Its use in developed countries has been, and still is, declining. There are no apparent side-effects of the method. However, if the female partner is to achieve orgasm and the male is to withdraw before any seminal fluid is expelled, he must exercise concentration and self-control. The frequency with which the method is used is difficult to assess, but it may be that the method is practised regularly or occasionally by 20% of social groups 3, 4 and 5, and somewhat less frequently by social classes 1 and 2. The failure rate is equally difficult to determine, but is probably of the order of 22 per 100 woman years. The main advantages of both these methods are that there are no health hazards and they do not require intervention from outside personnel, while the main disadvantage is a high pregnancy rate.

BARRIER METHODS

Condoms

These are latex rubber sheaths usually 0.04 mm in thickness. They are sometimes lubricated with spermicide, usually teat-ended to collect the ejaculate and are sold in a variety of colours. To be successful, they must be rolled onto the full length of the erect penis before penetration and after ejaculation the penis should be withdrawn before the erection is lost, lest the condom slip off or there is leakage of the seminal fluid from around its base. Care should be taken not to tear the condom during its application. Condoms are extremely strong and they are unlikely to burst during intercourse. Most claims of 'burst sheaths' probably reflect improper use or failure of use. Popularity of the condom varies considerably from country to country, its use being high in male dominated societies such as Japan, to being low in some South American countries and Australia. Use in Western Europe is about one-third of contraceptive users.

Advantages of the method are that it is good for people having casual relationships or couples having infrequent intercourse. The condom provides protection for either partner against acquiring gonorrhoea. The risks of acquiring AIDS (Autoimmune Deficiency Syndrome) through sexual intercourse is markedly reduced by the use of condoms. Their use in all casual sexual encounters is strongly advocated. Especially thick and stronger condoms are needed for use in anal intercourse.

Cervical epithelial neoplasia is a sexually transmitted disease possibly due to strains of 16 and 18 of the human papilloma virus and other constituents of seminal fluid. It is more common in women having intercourse at a young age and with multiple partners. The protective effect of condom use in these women could be significant, but remains to be proven. Condom use is advisable for about 6 weeks after cervical cautery when the epithelium undergoes metaplasia and is vulnerable to mitogens in seminal fluid.

The quoted failure rates vary greatly. Obviously, there is considerable scope for user failure, particularly if a condom is not used at every act of intercourse. In studies involving regular, well motivated users, the failure rate is about 4 per 100 woman years.

Diaphragms

These are made of latex and have a flat, circular spring edge or a coiled arcing spring which is more flexible and possibly more comfortable to wear. They are of variable size (45–100 mm) and have to be individually fitted. The diaphragm lies in the

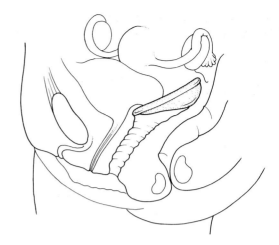

Fig. 17.1 *Diaphragm in position.*

posterior fornix behind the cervix posterosuperiorly and behind the pubic symphysis anteroinferiorly (Fig. 17.1). The cervix is thus covered by the dome of the diaphragm. Before insertion, the diaphragm must have spermicide applied to both of its surfaces, so that there is a layer of spermicide retained by the diaphragm over the external cervical os. This is as important as the actual barrier in the mode of action of the diaphragm. Spermicidal pessaries should not be used as the fats contained in them can damage the rubber. The diaphragm can be left *in situ* for 6–8 h after first intercourse and will be effective for that time unless dislodged. It must then be removed, washed, dried and stored in a cool, dark place to prevent deterioration of the rubber. Use of the diaphragm is small, being about 4–5% of contraceptive users. It is more popular among higher social classes and in developed countries. Again, there is considerable scope for user failure, but if used regularly by well motivated women, the failure rate in some large scale studies in the UK is between 2 and 3 per 100 woman years. The advantages of this method are that it is free of health hazards and is suitable for occasional intercourse. Used regularly it can be reliable. The disadvantage is that the user must be happy with the idea and technique of insertion and this may not be aesthetically acceptable to many women.

Cervical Caps

These fit firmly over the cervix and act as a direct barrier, providing effective contraception for a small number of users. Their use is not sufficiently widespread to be able to quote a reliable use effectiveness rate, but it is probably similar to that of the diaphragm. They are made of rubber or plastic, require individual fitting and must be used with spermicide. They are unsuitable for women with abnormalities of the cervix.

Spermicides

The use of spermicide cream with the diaphragm is essential, while some condoms incorporate a spermicidal lubricant. Spermicidal pessaries, tablets or pastes used alone are not very effective. Results reported in the literature quote failure rates of from 2–25 per 100 woman years. Clinical impressions suggest that the higher figure is more likely. The most commonly used agent in spermicides is nonoxynol-9 (nonylphenoxypolyethoxyethanol). Other compounds are being investigated together with the use of devices such as vaginal rings which may slowly release the spermicide. Contraceptive sponges containing spermicide are available, but their efficacy has never been tested in large studies, and it is doubtful if they can provide anything other than some protection for occasional intercourse.

A variety of new spermicides are being studied in trials. These include chlorhexidine and propanolol, but at present their efficacy cannot be properly assessed.

INTRAUTERINE DEVICE (IUD)

Intrauterine devices can be either inert silastic or be medicated. These have copper wire wound round the stem or contain a progestogen. Common, currently used types of intrauterine device are shown in Fig. 17.2. The presence of the device in the uterine cavity does not alter endocrine function and ovulation takes place normally. A number of hypotheses have been put forward concerning their mode of action. Enhancement of tubal motility and alteration of cervical mucus have been suggested, but the evidence for these proposed modes of action is not strong. The IUD leads to a leukocytic infiltration of the endometrium, the so-called sterile inflammatory response, and the devices themselves have many macrophages adhering to them. These

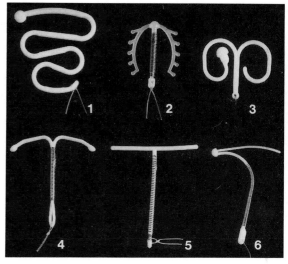

Fig. 17.2   *Some commonly used intrauterine devices. 1. Lippes loop; 2. Multiload; 3. Saf-T-Coil; 4. Novagard; 5. Ortho Gynae-T (Copper T); 6. Gravigard (Copper 7). Manufacture of devices 1. and 3. has recently ceased.*

can phagocytose spermatazoa and this may be why there are very few sperm which reach the fallopian tube in the presence of an intrauterine device. There is increased prostaglandin production from the endometrium with an IUD in situ, and this, in turn, may lead to enhanced myometral activity, particularly during the late luteal phase of the cycle. Uterine contractions of up to 100 mmHg in strength may interfere with implantation of the blastocyst. Subtle and, as yet, undocumented biochemical changes in the endometrium probably also occur which may affect implantation. The larger the inert device, the lower the pregnancy rate, but there will be higher rates of removal for pain and bleeding.

Copper in the form of wire has been added to the vertical stem of devices to reduce their size and to maintain a low pregnancy rate. The surface area of copper is 200–300 mm^2 and this allows copper at the rate of 50 μg per day to be released for up to 3 years. Copper enhances the endometrial 'inflammatory' response already described and allows the smaller device to give a lower pregnancy rate. Copper interferes with endometrial biochemistry, depressing oestrogen binding and thymidine uptake into DNA, impairs glycogen storage and inhibits metabolic enzymes such as lactate dehydrogenase. Despite this, if pregnancy does take place, there is no evidence that either the inert or copper containing device causes congenital abnormalities. The use effectiveness of IUDs varies from almost zero to about 8 per 100 woman years. Factors that affect the pregnancy rate are the ability of the fitter (a device placed improperly in the uterus will be more likely to fail or drop out unnoticed), the loss to follow-up rate and the duration of the study (long-term users tend to have a lower pregnancy rate than short-term users). In general, the pregnancy rate is accepted as being about 3 per 100 woman years and does not vary significantly from one device to another.

The advantages of the method are that it is not coitally related, it is simple, lasts for 3 years and has no effect on endocrine function, with few serious side-effects. Its disadvantages are that it may cause heavier periods or occasionally intermenstrual spotting. Its main disadvantage is an increased tendency to pelvic inflammatory disease. Although the incidence of pelvic inflammatory disease is increasing due to changing sexual habits, it is accepted that the IUD does further increase the risk due to bacteria ascending into the uterus. The method is not, therefore, the best for young, nulliparous, sexually very active women. Development of pelvic pain and dyspareunia in someone wearing

an IUD requires immediate attention to diagnose and if necessary treat pelvic inflammatory disease. Usually, the device would be removed during treatment and its replacement carefully considered afterwards. A history of recurrent pelvic inflammatory disease would be a contraindication to the use of an IUD. Valvular heart disease, because of the risks of bacteraemia and endocarditis, is a very strong contraindication to the use of an intrauterine device.

ORAL CONTRACEPTION

Oestrogen/Progestogen Containing Pills

These are taken daily for 21 days followed by 7 'pill free' days. Some brand packets contain 28 pills, the last 7 of which are inert, the reason for this being that pill-taking can be continuous. The dose of steroids used in the combined pill has declined considerably during the last 10 years. Few preparations contain 50 µg of ethinyl oestradiol, most containing between 20 and 35 µg. Doses of progestogens have also declined any many preparations

Table 17.1

Hormone Content of Combined Oral Contraceptives

Preparation	Progestogen	Preparation	Progestogen
Oestrogen: Ethinyloestradiol 20 µg		**Oestrogen: Ethinyloestradiol 30/40 µg**	
Loestrin 20	Norethisterone acetate 1 mg	Logynon	Levonorgestrel 50/75/125 µg
		Logynon ED	Levonorgestrel 50/75/125 µg
Oestrogen: Ethinyloestradiol 30 µg		Trinordiol	Levonorgestrel 50/75/125 µg
Conova 30	Ethynodiol diacetate 2 mg	**Oestrogen: Ethinyloestradiol 50 µg**	
Eugynon 30	Levonorgestrel 250 µg	Anovlar 21	Norethisterone acetate 4 mg
Loestrin 30	Norethisterone acetate 1.5 mg	Eugynon 50	Levonorgestrel 250 µg
Marvelon	Desogestrel 150 µg	Gynovlar 21	Norethisterone acetate 3 mg
Microgynon 30	Levonorgestrel 150 µg	Minilyn	Lynoestrenol 2.5 mg
Ovran 30	Levonorgestrel 250 µg	Minovlar ED	Norethisterone acetate 1 mg
Ovranette	Levonorgestrel 150 µg	Norlestrin	Norethisterone acetate 2.5 mg
Oestrogen: Ethinyloestradiol 35 µg		Orlest 21	Norethisterone acetate 1 mg
BiNovum	Norethisterone 0.5 and 1 mg	Ovran	Levonorgestrel 250 µg
Brevinor	Norethisterone 500 µg	Ovulen 50	Ethynodiol diacetate 1 mg
Neocon 1/35	Norethisterone 1 mg	**Oestrogen: Mestranol 50 µg**	
Norimin	Norethisterone 1 mg	Norinyl-1	Norethisterone 1 mg
Ovysmen	Norethisterone 500 µg	Ortho-novin 1/50	Norethisterone 1 mg
Synphase	Norethisterone 0.5 and 1 mg		
TriNovum	Norethisterone 0.5/0.75/1mg		

include 0.5 or 1.0 mg of norethisterone or 250 μg of levonorgestrel (current preparations are listed in Table 17.1). The concept of varying progestogenicity clearly applies to dose, but the relationship of one compound to another is more complex, as each compound affects different tissues in different ways. Whether there are differences in intracellular biochemistry caused by different progestogens remains to be evaluated. Until we know more about the intracellular changes caused by progestogens, it is prudent to use the smallest effective dose in the circumstances.

Mode of action

The combined pill acts by inhibiting the release of LHRH and so of gonadotrophins which, in turn, causes inactive ovaries and anovulation. This is the combined effect of both the oestrogen and progestogen components. The progestogen alters the cervical mucus so that it becomes thick and difficult for sperm to penetrate. There are alterations of endometrial biochemistry which could impair implantation, but these have not yet been fully determined. These three actions make the combined pill a highly effective contraceptive.

The method failure is less than 0.5 per 100 woman years and the overall failure rate is about 1.5 per 100 woman years. The ability to take tablets regularly is important in maintaining the efficacy, as forgetting even one or two tablets can allow ovulation to take place. Interaction with other drugs, such as some antibiotics, or failure of absorption due to gastroenteritis are also common reasons for failure of the method. The drugs listed in Table 17.2 may cause interaction with the pill's steroids.

Advantages of the method are its efficacy and that it is not coitally related, but there may be others, such as reduced menstrual loss or diminished dysmenorrhoea. Disadvantages are the need to take tablets daily, an increased vaginal discharge due either to increased cervical mucus or a tendency to candida infections, weight gain and headaches in some users. There are also wide ranging metabolic effects which have been extensively investigated during the past 20 years. The oestrogen component acting via hepatic oestrogen receptors alters protein synthesis. This is manifest by changes in enzymes, binding and transport proteins, and proteins involved in the coagulation mechanism. The pill causes increased risk of thrombosis, possibly through raised coagulation factors and fibrinogen and increased platelet adhesiveness. This may cause venous thromboembolism in susceptible individuals, namely those with a previous history of deep venous thrombosis or those with varicose veins and thrombophlebitis. In women with a family history of venous thromboembolic disease, antithrombin III deficiency in plasma should be excluded.

There are alterations in lipids, such as increased triglyceride levels as well as a reduction in the high

---

Table 17.2

Drugs Causing Interaction with Steroids in Oestrogen/Progestogen Pill

The following drugs may possibly reduce contraceptive efficacy, as measured by an increased incidence of breakthrough bleeding or pregnancy:
1.   amidopyrine; anti-inflammatory agents such as oxyphenbutazone and phenazone;
2.   phenacetin;
3.   anticonvulsants such as phenytoin, primidone and ethosuximide;
4.   antibiotics such as ampicillin, chloramphenicol, rifampicin, sulphamethoxypyridazine and nitrofurantoin;
5.   barbiturates such as hexobarbitone, phenobarbitone and methylphenobarbitone;
6.   sedatives such as chlordiazepoxide, chlorpromazine and meprobromate and chloral hydrate derivatives used as hypnotics;
7.   vasoconstrictors, such as dihydroergotamine;

Oral contraceptives may alter the dose required of the following groups of drugs:
1.   anticoagulants;
2.   tricyclic antidepressants such as imipramine;
3.   corticosteroids;
4.   insulin or oral hypoglycaemic agents.

(HDL) and an increase in the low density (LDL) lipoprotein fractions of cholesterol, the latter being caused by the progestogen component. Arterial thrombosis may result in susceptible women — those who already have abnormal lipids, obese women, and those who smoke heavily, particularly over the age of 35. There is debate as to whether or not pill steroids cause impairment of glucose tolerance. Many of the relevant studies were carried out on the higher dose pills used 10 years ago. The current pills probably have no significant effect on carbohydrate metabolism, except in susceptible women such as latent diabetics, i.e. those with a history of abnormal carbohydrate metabolism in a previous pregnancy.

Carcinogenesis and the pill is a controversial issue. Pill use early in the reproductive era has been associated with a higher incidence of breast cancer in some studies, but not in others. This has been attributed to the progestogen component. An association between pill use and carcinoma of the cervix has also been suggested. While the former may be a genuine anxiety, the latter is more likely to be due to the acquisition of sexually transmitted carcinogens, although the effect of the sex steroids on the cervical epithelial cells cannot be entirely disregarded. Multicentre case control studies involving several countries have not shown any positive association between oral contraceptive use and either breast or cervical cancer, but have suggested a protective effect against endometrial cancer.

Hypertension may be caused or exacerbated by the combined pill in about 1% of users. Biochemical mechanisms are not clear, but may involve altered renin-angiotensin or aldosterone production. Regular checks of blood pressure in pill users is mandatory. The combined pill may reduce milk volume and is not the contraceptive of first choice for lactating mothers.

Triphasic Pills

These contain oestrogen and progestogen in varying amounts rather than constant amounts. The active tablets are taken for 21 days followed by 7 placebo pills. The dose of progestogen is less during the first 10 days of the 21 day tablet cycle, and more during the second 10 days, thereby reducing the total dose of steroid ingested. Their efficacy and side-effects are similar to those of the combined pill.

Progestogen Only Pills

These contain small doses of norethisterone (0.35 mg), levonorgestrel (0.03 mg) or ethynodiol diacetate (0.5 mg) and are taken daily on a continuous basis. They alter ovarian function, but do not inhibit ovulation in more than 50% of cycles. Persistent follicular cysts with relatively high circulating oestrogen levels may occur in a proportion of users. The mode of action is on the ovary, on the endometrium and on cervical mucus. Failure rates have varied widely from one trial to another. It is generally accepted that the true failure rate is about 4–6 per 100 woman years. The main advantage of the method is the relative absence of metabolic side-effects due to the low dose of progestogen used and the absence of oestrogen. There is no effect on milk volume or composition and so this is a method of choice for the lactating woman. The disadvantages are: (1) that the tablets must be taken daily and preferably at a constant time of day to maintain adequate blood levels, and (2) irregular menstrual bleeding, caused by all progestogen only contraceptives.

INJECTABLE HORMONAL CONTRACEPTIVES

These consist of intramuscular injections of either medroxyprogesterone acetate 150 mg given every 12 weeks or norethisterone oenanthate 200 mg given either every 8 or 10 weeks. Their use has been surrounded by much unwarranted controversy, but gradually scientific facts are being accepted and these two injectables are now licensed for use in a large and increasing number of countries including the UK. They act by inhibiting ovulation as well as by exerting the other progestogenic contraceptive effects on the endometrium and cervical mucus already described. Consequently, they are very effective contraceptives with failure rates of about 0.5 per 100 woman years and it is easy to differentiate user from method failure. The advantages of the method are: (1) its efficacy; (2) it is a non-coitally related method; (3) despite irregular bleeding, there may be increased haemoglobin levels and increased weight gain, both of which may be of value in developing countries. A disadvantage of the method is the irregular bleeding similar to that seen with other progestogen only methods, the cause of which is still uncertain. The high plasma levels of progestogen, particularly during the first 4–6 weeks of the injection interval, lead to suppression of the hypothalamic-pituitary-ovarian axis and endometrial atrophy causing variable periods of amenorrhoea in a number of users. Compared with the combined pill, there is a relative absence of metabolic changes. Synthetic progestogens do not significantly alter the coagulation factors, and while there is an increase in plasma insulin, this is compensated for by insulin antagonism in the tissues, so that carbohydrate tolerance is not altered. Liver function tests are not altered. Milk volume and composition are not altered by injectable progestogens and so the method is a suitable one for lactating women, provided it is started 6 weeks after delivery. Transfer to the infant of tiny amounts of progestogen in breast milk should be avoided during the first 6 weeks of life.

Plasma lipids are altered by progestogens, particularly by the 19 nortestosterone derivatives. High density lipoprotein cholesterol is reduced by about 25% in users of norethisterone oenanthate. There is a slight, but inconsistent and insignificant elevation of low density lipoprotein cholesterol. High density lipoprotein cholesterol (HDLC) is a transport form of lipid and so its reduction will increase the deposition of cholesterol and atheroma formation. Although there is no epidemiological evidence to suggest that injectable progestogens increase the risks of myocardial infarction, these data suggest that, if they are used for long enough in a Western country, this may happen, and infarction could occur. Their long-term use has been largely of medroxy progesterone acetate in Asia where the natural incidence of myocardial infarction is very low. Until there is more information, they should not be used in high risk patients, namely those with a strong family history of heart attacks, hyperlipidaemia, obese women or those who smoke heavily. Existing compounds in smaller doses, with or without oestrogens, are being tried as monthly injectables, as are new compounds such as esters of levonorgestrel.

STERILISATION

This is becoming increasingly common as the method of fertility control in developed countries. Counselling is very important, so that women realise the irreversibility of the procedure as well as the failure rate which, for the Pomeroy operation, is 3–5 per 1000 cases, and for the clip and silicone ring application is a little higher. It is very important that the operation is not carried out in relation to an acute domestic crisis or at the time of termination of pregnancy. The stress of these situations can often lead to wrong decisions being made with subsequent long-term regrets and recriminations.

The Pomeroy operation has been the most widely used sterilisation procedure throughout the world. The principles are shown in Fig. 17.3 The essential features are: (1) the use of absorbable suture material for the tying of the fallopian tubes, (2) the tubes should not be crushed beforehand and (3) the removal of a segment of tube greater than 1 cm in length. The cut ends of the tube should be divergent at the end of the procedure reducing the risk of reuniting.

Other procedures requiring laparotomy involve burying the medial end of the tube in the uterus (Irving's operation); separating the two ends of the cut tube by peritoneum from the broad ligament (Uchida's operation); and fimbriectomy.

Laparoscopic sterilisation has become increasingly popular. The application of spring loaded clips which occlude the tube and cause ischaemic necrosis, but for only 1 mm lateral to each side of the

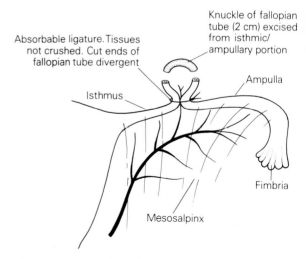

Fig. 17.3   *Principles of the Pomeroy sterilisation procedure.*

clip, is a commonly used method. This procedure does not alter the vasculature of the salpinx and destroys the shortest length of tube, making reversal easier.

Another laparoscopic method is the application of a silastic ring around a loop of mesosalpinx. This is the equivalent of the Pomeroy procedure without excision of the knuckle of tube (Madlener's operation). It will cause ischaemic necrosis and occlusion of the tube. The advantages of these operations are the absence of an open laparotomy and, consequently, a reduced length of stay in hospital. The disadvantages are the risks of laparoscopy which, in experienced hands, are minimal and those of occasional difficulty in identifying the tube due to adhesions. Finally, there is a risk of haemorrhage from the mesosalpinx if it is torn during application of the ring.

Electrocoagulation of the tube has fallen in popularity due to possible complications such as burns to the bowel, and also to the extensive destruction of the tube required if sterilisation is to be effective, which makes reversibility virtually impossible.

Long-term follow-up of all these methods is crucial in determining accurate failure rates.

Most requests for reversal of sterilisation come from women who were sterilised before the age of 30 or from those who were in an unstable relationship at the time of operation. Reversibility is easier if a short segment (less than 2 cm) of isthmus/ampulla is occluded or removed and, if this is the case, successful restoration of fertility can be predicted in 75% of cases.

Vasectomy

The identification of the vas deferens, excision of a 2 cm segment of it and the separation of the cut ends by doubling them back on each other, is usually a simple operation performed under local anaesthetic. It prevents access of sperm from the testes into the ejaculate, but about 30 ejaculations are required to empty the seminal vesicles of live sperm. At least one sample with azoospermia is necessary before the method can be deemed to be effective. The failure rate is low. The incidence of circulating antibodies to sperm increases from 2% to over 50% after vasectomy. Even though reversibility can be accomplished anatomically, fertility is markedly reduced because of these antibodies.

NEW METHODS

Four approaches to alternative methods of contraception are currently being investigated. These are (1) release of existing steroids or variations of them from different vehicles; (2) alteration of the hypothalamic-pituitary axis inhibiting ovulation; (3) chemical methods of inhibiting spermatogenesis; and (4) immunological interference with implantation.

The two methods of releasing existing steroids, in this case levonorgestrel, are the subcutaneous implant releasing 40–45 µg per day (Norplant) and the intravaginal ring, releasing 20 µg per day. Both methods will be available in an increasing number of countries within the next few years.

Implant

This consists of six silastic tubes, each 2.5 cm long and 3 mm in diameter, containing levonorgestrel crystals. They are inserted subcutaneously in the upper arm using a trochar and cannula after a small skin incision is made under local anaesthetic. The failure rate is about 1 per 100 woman years and protection can be given for up to 6 years (Norplant 6). Removal is not difficult. Single devices of the same dimensions releasing levonorgestrel from sesame oil, contained within a polymer shell, and double devices releasing levonorgestrel from crystals within a silastic tube (Norplant 2) are being tried.

The advantages are the provision of an effective method of contraception for a long time without patient involvement. The disadvantages are irregularity of the menstrual cycle, which diminishes with duration of use, and those of an invasive procedure for insertion and removal.

Vaginal Ring

This is made up of a silastic core impregnated with levonorgestrel and covered by an outer, inert layer of silastic. The ring is 60 mm in diameter, pliable and easily inserted into the posterior fornix of the vagina. Levonorgestrel is released at the rate of 20 µg per day. The current rings last for 3 months and should not be removed except for short periods of time (less than 30 min). Ovulation is inhibited in about 40% of cycles and ovarian function is altered in 25%. In the remainder, ovarian function is entirely normal. The device exerts its main contraceptive action on cervical mucus and endometrial biochemistry. The failure rate is 3.6 per 100 woman years. The main problem, as with all progestogen only devices, is irregular cycles and, in a few women, frequent expulsions of the ring usually occurring at defaecation. A major advantage is its absence of metabolic effects. There are no effects on lipids, because of the very low dose of steroid used. A further advantage is that it is controlled by the woman herself and is extremely simple to use and understand.

Alterations of the Hypothalamic Pituitary Axis

This has been carried out using synthetic peptides which are analogues of GnRH and which act either as antagonists or as agonists of this compound. The antagonistic analogues act by competitive binding to pituitary receptor sites, abolishing the LH surge and so inhibiting ovulation. Administration is intranasally or by injection and only small scale studies have been carried out. Long-term effects and contraceptive efficacy have not been investigated. GnRH agonists, such as buserelin or nafarelin, given intranasally, have been investigated more fully and found to inhibit ovulation regularly. These compounds act by desensitising the pituitary so that it fails to respond to oestradiol, thereby abolishing the LH surge required for ovulation. Oestradiol levels are reduced as a result of ovarian suppression, the endometrium becomes inactive and there are bleeding irregularities. Alternative routes of administration, such as implants or injectables, will be tried in the future, as well as the possibility of combined therapy with an agonist given intermittently together with a progestogen to improve cycle control.

Chemical Methods of Inhibiting Spermatogenesis

A number of compounds are being investigated that may inhibit spermatogenesis. The most widely known of these is gossypol, found as a trace contaminant of cotton seed oil in China. Its efficacy in preventing sperm maturation and reducing motility and capacity for fertilisation is being assessed. Certain side-effects have been reported after large doses, including hyperkalaemia and subsequent cardiac arrthymias.

Immunological Methods

The concept of inducing antibodies to HCG by vaccination, thereby preventing implantation, is an attractive one. However, the difficulties must not be underestimated. These are: (1) variability of antibody titre induced and (2) the variability from person to person of its duration of action. Successful animal studies have led to preliminary studies in humans. However, at this stage the approach must be considered as very much an experimental one.

FURTHER READING

Fraser I.S., Wiesberg E.A. (1981). A comprehensive review of injectable contraception with special emphasis on depomedtoxyprogesterone acetate. *Med. J. Aust*; Vol. 1, Suppl. **1**: 1–19.
Hafez E.S.E., ed. (1979). *Human Reproduction, Conception and Contraception*, 2nd edn. Hagerstown, Maryland: Harper and Row.
Harper M.J.K. (1983). *Birth Control Technologies*. London: Heinemann Medical.
Hawkins D.F., Elder M.G. (1979). *Human Fertility Control*. London: Butterworth.
Snowdon R., Williams M.Z., Hawkins D. *The IUD. A Practical Guide*. London: Croom Helm.

18

Cessation of Reproduction

THE MENOPAUSE

Definition

The menopause is the final cessation of menstruation, i.e. the last period. However, a woman's reproductive ability declines over a period of two to three years and is called *the climacteric*, 'a period of life specially liable to a change of health' (*Shorter Oxford English Dictionary*). It usually occurs in the late 40s or early 50s and may be characterised by menstrual disturbance associated with anovular cycles, vasomotor and psychological symptoms. The latter may be associated with psychosexual problems.

Physiology

The menopause occurs because of progressive ovarian failure.

The ovary develops from primordial germ cells, which have migrated into the genital (gonadal) ridge from the endoderm of the yolk sac. At birth, the ovary contains all the potential germ cells that are likely to mature during the woman's reproductive life (about one million), but by the time the girl reaches puberty only 40 000 primary oocytes remain.

Each primary oocyte is found within an ovarian primordial follicle surrounded by follicular cells. After puberty, during each menstrual cycle follicles attempt to mature, but only one succeeds and ovulates to form the corpus luteum which then degenerates to form the corpus albicans. The others degenerate to form atretic follicles. The ovary of the menopausal woman is small and relatively devoid of follicles. However, at the ovarian hilus, groups of hilar cells become more prominent. These are actively secreting endocrine cells resembling Leydig cells of the testis. Tumours of these cells cause masculinisation, and it is this observation plus the similarity to Leydig cells which suggest that they secrete androgens.

As time passes, the ovaries become increasingly small until they consist mainly of fibrous tissue. However, depletion of oocytes cannot be the whole story. In a breed of rat which has a menopause, menopausal ovaries have been grafted into ovulating rats with a return of ovulation in those ovaries.

A consequence of ovarian failure at the menopause is a fall in the level of circulating oestrogen so that, by means of the negative feed-back mechanism between ovarian oestrogen and the anterior pituitary, large amounts of FSH are produced (up to ten times the levels in premenopausal women, Fig. 18.1). The hormone appears in the urine and forms the basis of a biochemical test to confirm the onset of the climacteric/menopause. LH levels also rise up to threefold, and both levels may rise in the year before the menopause. It must be stressed that levels of oestrogen and gonadotrophins fluctuate during the climacteric, and therefore the biochemical tests may be of little value, but they are of value in the patient who presents with psychological symptoms, which may be due to the menopause or to psychiatric disturbance. Normal gonadotrophin and oestrogen levels in such a patient would indicate referral to a psychiatrist rather than an attempt to manage symptoms with hormone replacement therapy (HRT).

Oestrogen may continue to be produced by theca cells in the ovary, and postmenopausal bleeding secondary to endometrial hyperplasia or endometrial carcinoma may be the presenting symptom in a patient with a tumour of theca cells (thecoma).

The menopause may be iatrogenic. Bilateral salpingo-oöphorectomy (usually performed at the same time as total abdominal hysterectomy) is performed for endometriosis, chronic pelvic inflammatory disease, uterine, cervical and ovarian cancer.

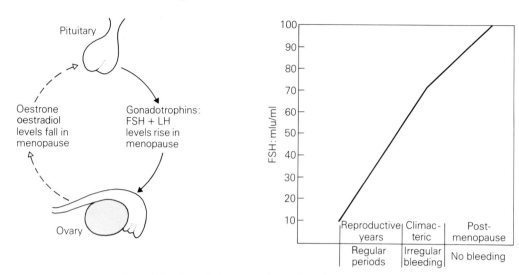

Fig. 18.1   *The pituitary ovarian axis at the menopause.*

However the menopause comes about, it is accompanied by a great fall in oestrogen production, as the ovarian follicle and the corpus luteum are the major scources of oestradiol. This produces local and systemic effects of such variety that many organs can be considered as target organs for the hormone.

Symptoms

Vasomotor symptoms

The patient will complain of 'hot flushes' and sweats which may occur in the climacteric or after the menopause, mainly at night. A woman's ability to cope with these symptoms depends on the frequency and severity of the attacks. They may be accompanied by palpitations, and may be severe enough to disturb her sleep. Although self-limiting, about 25% of women may experience such symptoms for more than 5 years.

The exact cause of 'hot flushes' is not known, but the fall in oestrogen may be associated with vasomotor instability, although it is suggested that an hypothalamic disturbance or high levels of circulating FSH and LH may also be responsible.

Emotional and psychological problems

The woman may complain of anxiety and depression, loss of libido, which may accompany structural changes in the genital tract, rapid mood changes, irritability and poor memory. Classical psychiatric disorders seldom, if ever, result from ovarian failure, but a complaint of insomnia must be further investigated to exclude genuine psychological disturbance. A woman's attitude to her menopause or climacteric depends upon her own psychological background and her experience of her mother's menopause and that of other female relatives. The patient will require sympathy and reassurance from the doctor as well as appropriate medical treatment. More specific counselling from psychotherapists or psychiatrists may be necessary in a few severe cases.

Skeleton

Bone is constantly turning over. Osteoclasts are multinucleated cells responsible for bone resorption while osteoblasts synthesise new bone by forming a collagen matrix which is subsequently mineralised to make the bone hard. Cortical bone forms most of the skeleton (80%) but trabecular bone is the major constituent of vertebral bodies and forms quite a large part (approximately 25%) of bone in the femur and radius. Trabecular bone turns over much faster than cortical bone and after the menopause the trabecular bone loss is about 1% per annum.

Plasma calcium levels are unchanged during the menopause. Lack of oestrogen results in increased bone resorption, reflected by increased calcium and hydroxyproline excretion, which reflects loss of calcium and collagen from bone. Collagen is lost from other sites of the body as well as bone, namely skin and joints. It is this loss of collagen that contributes to the overall ageing appearance and loss of bone, particularly from the vertebra that causes reduction in height with bent stature and kyphosis in extreme cases (Fig. 18.2). There is an increased incidence of fractures, particularly of the neck of femur and distal end of radius. Ligaments lose their elasticity and loss of collagen leads to degenerative changes in the joints.

Exogenous oestrogens and progestogens have a bone sparing effect. Calcitonin reduces bone resorption by reducing the effects of parathyroid hormone and of dihydroxycolecalciferol.

Cardiovascular problems

Distinct from the vasomotor problems, but also associated with the lower menopausal oestrogen

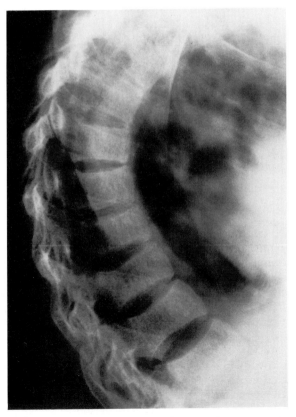

Fig. 18.2 *X-ray to illustrate kyphosis and osteoporosis.*

levels, is atherosclerosis, due to a progressive increase in the plasma concentration of cholesterol, triglycerides and low and very low density lipoproteins, with a reduction in high density lipoproteins. The increase may be as much as 20%. The protection against coronary artery disease found in premenopausal women declines, and the mortality rate from coronary thrombosis gradually comes to equal that of men.

Target organs of the genital tract

The target organs of the genital tract are the uterus and its appendages, the cervix, the vagina and vulva, the urethra and the bladder.

Shrinkage of the uterus as the myometrium becomes converted to fibrous tissue causes no problems. Atrophic changes in the epithelium of the cervix and vagina result in thinning and dryness. The pH rises to about 7.2, compared with 4.5 in the reproductive years, because as opposed to the premenopausal years, there is no glycogen present for Döderleins bacilli to convert to lactic acid. This produces a susceptibility to infection plus atrophic vaginitis. The latter may be a cause of postmenopausal bleeding, a symptom requiring urgent investigation and treatment. Atrophic vaginal skin has a reduced number of superficial cells and an increased number of basal cells. These changes can be demonstrated cytologically on a lateral vaginal wall smear. The karyopyknotic index (KI), which is the proportion of superficial cells to basal cells, provides useful and reliable information about oestrogen effects as oestrogen increases the number of superficial cells and, therefore, if a woman with postmenopausal bleeding has a high KI, the gynaecologist should look for an oestrogen secreting granulosa cell ovarian tumour (Figs. 18.3 and 18.4).

The external genitalia decrease in size and there is loss of pubic hair. The transitional epithelium of the bladder trigone undergoes atrophy, and, at cystoscopy, it is not uncommon to see atrophic changes resembling those in the vagina over the whole bladder epithelium. The urethra arising from the same ectoderm as the vaginal vestibule also appears to be under the influence of oestrogen. This sensitivity to oestrogen is of clinical use in the management of an urethral caruncle, a condition most commonly seen in menopausal women. After excision, recurrence may be prevented by the use of local oestrogen cream.

Atrophic changes in the bladder may cause

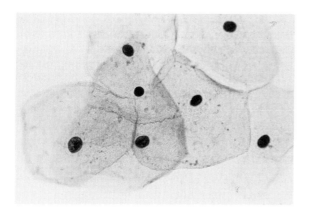

Fig. 18.3 *Mature squamous epithelial cells from normal vaginal epithelium (x 125). (Courtesy of Dr E. Hudson, Northwick Park Hospital, London.)*

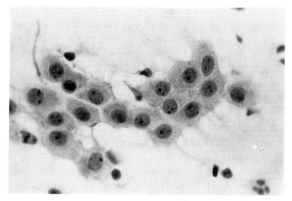

Fig. 18.4 *Squamous cells from atrophic vaginal epithelium (x 125). (Courtesy of Dr E. Hudson, Northwick Park Hospital, London.)*

detrusor instability with urgency and urge incontinence. Atrophic vaginitis may give rise to sensations resembling those of prolapse.

Diagnosis

A diagnosis is based on the history, examination and special tests.

History

Symptoms of the menopause are characteristic, although it is sometimes difficult to determine whether psychological symptoms are primarily due to lack of oestrogen.

Symptoms are detailed above, but they can be usefully listed at this point:

1. *Hot flushes:* as antigonadotrophins do not produce an improvement in this symptom, it is unlikely that raised FSH/LH levels are solely responsible.
2. *Insomnia:* flushes and sweats occurring mainly at night.
3. *Palpitations and dizziness::* these occur in less than 50% of patients.
4. *Gastrointestinal symptoms.*
5. *Mood changes and depression:* anxiety with irritability may accompany depression, as may loss of memory and concentration.
6. *Discomfort in the vagina:* bacterial or fungal infection.
7. *Dyspareunia:* this leads to loss of libido and apareunia.
8. *Postmenopausal bleeding:* this comes from the atrophic epithelium.
9. *Detrusor instability:* as a result of atrophic trigonitis, this leads to a higher resting intravesical pressure, which produces symptoms of urgency and urge incontinence and apparent stress incontinence.
10. *Atrophic urethritis:* this may mimic cystitis with bladder instability, a condition referred to as 'the urethral syndrome'. An urethral caruncle may present as haematuria or postmenopausal bleeding.
11. *Angina or myocardial infarction.*
12. *Arthritis and fractures.*

Examination

A sensitive, but thorough physical examination should be performed, i.e. the blood pressure taken, the urine tested, the breasts examined, a cervical smear taken and a pelvic examination performed. The cervical smear is important, because the peak incidence of carcinoma of the cervix occurs in women in the 6th decade, while that for endometrial cancer peaks in the 7th decade. A high vaginal swab should be taken if there is evidence of infection, and a rectal examination should be performed, because carcinoma of the rectum and colon is the most common cancer, with the main incidence between 50 and 80 years. As in all examinations the woman must be put at ease and constantly reassured.

Special tests

Raised serum FSH and LH estimations will confirm the diagnosis. High levels of circulating oestrogens will exclude the diagnosis.

Differential Diagnosis

As a major presenting symptom of the menopause is flushing, the differential diagnosis should include other conditions that have the same effect. These include hyperactive thyroid, phaeochromocytoma, and carcinoid syndrome.

Treatment

The patient should be treated sympathetically. She must be advised that her symptoms are understood to be physical symptoms and that there is a good physiological basis for them. She should be encouraged to adopt an optimistic attitude to this period of her life, especially as hormone replacement therapy (HRT) can offer symptomatic relief and continued well-being. The mainstay of treatment is oestrogen replacement, which may be given locally or systemically.

Local oestrogens

The usual preparations are creams containing either Dienoestrol or conjugated oestrogens. Atrophic vaginitis responds well to these, although they are more effective in preventing atrophy than in reversing it. Pruritis of the vulva (kraurosis vulvae) may be helped by local oestrogens, but it is important to investigate a vulval dystrophy, as the hypertrophic dystrophy will respond to local corticosteroids, and the atrophic dystrophy may benefit from local testosterone ointment. It is very important to remember that, although applied locally, oestrogens are in general readily absorbed through the skin and mucous membranes, and because of this, their use is contraindicated in patients with carcinoma of the endometrium or breast.

The daily dose of Dienoestrol, which is supplied with a vaginal applicator, is 1–2 full applications daily for 2 weeks, then half the dose for a further 2 weeks. Conjugated oestrogens come in a non-liquefying base, 0.625 mg/g; the daily dose is 2–4 g using the calibrated vaginal applicator.

Systemic oestrogens

Absolute contraindications to the use of systemic oestrogens are:

Carcinoma of the breast
Carcinoma of the endometrium
Endometrial hyperplasia.

Relative contraindications are:

Liver disease
Previous thromboembolism
Hypertension.

Systemic hormones can, of course, be used to treat atrophic conditions of the genital tract but, because of concern about possible minor and major complications of their systemic administration, (nausea, vomiting, diarrhoea, carcinogenic action, water retention, hypertension and altered glucose tolerance), local preparations are preferred. Systemic therapy is required for systemic symptoms, and can be delivered in several ways:

Implants. Oestradiol BPC pellets are manufactured in three sizes: 25, 50 and 100 mg. They may be inserted at the time of surgery, unless castration has been performed as part of the treatment for endometriosis, endometrial cancer or other hormone dependent cancer, and if there is no abnormality of the liver function tests. The pellet is usually placed under the rectus sheath, but replacements may be inserted, using a trocar and cannula under local anaesthetic, into the fat of the anterior abdominal wall. Pellets of 25 mg can last up to 32–36 weeks, and 100 mg may last for up to one year. Testosterone implants may be inserted at the same time to promote a sense of well-being and improve libido.

Oral preparations. Many oral preparations are available, singly or in combination with a progestogen. Because of the adverse effect on clotting factors, ethinyl oestradiol is contraindicated. The woman with a uterus should be given at least 12 days of progestogen in each cycle to protect the endometrium from malignant change and to induce withdrawal bleeding. Regular withdrawal bleeding with this therapy is almost always associated with normal endometrium and, therefore, endometrial biopsy is only required if there is unscheduled bleeding. The patient receiving unopposed oestrogen therapy, i.e. without a progestogen, should undergo annual biopsy, as endometrial hyperplasia (a precursor of endometrial cancer) has been found to occur even with regular withdrawal bleeding. Recently dermal patches releasing oestrogen, thereby avoiding passage through the liver, have become available. At present, they are changed every few days and oral progestogen therapy is necessary to effect a withdrawal bleed.

Treatment is usually continued for at least 2 years, although the view has been expressed that in view of the protection afforded by HRT against osteoporosis and, therefore, against fractures, usually of the wrist or neck of femur, reason for *not* carrying on with the treatment should be sought. Long-term treatment requires regular assessment of weight, blood pressure, lipid profiles and liver function tests, plus thorough breast and pelvic examinations and 2-yearly cervical cytology. Ideally, two smears should be taken, the first from the posterior fornix to detect endometrial cells and blood, the second from the cervix. A positive smear from the posterior fornix should be followed by curettage to exclude endometrial pathology. Equipment such as the Vabra curette and the Accurette can enable the gynaecologist to obtain endometrial samples for cytology and histopathology in the outpatient clinic.

When there is an absolute contraindication to oestrogen therapy, vasomotor symptoms may be treated with Clonidine hydrochloride, an anti-hypertensive agent, in a dosage of 25–50 mg twice daily, rising to 75 mg twice daily after 2 weeks. Norethisterone 5 mg daily may also be tried.

POSTMENOPAUSAL BLEEDING (PMB)

Definition

Any bleeding after the menopause, but in practice any bleeding 6 months or more after the last period. PMB may originate from anywhere in the genital tract, and the cause may be benign or malignant (Table 18.1).

Trauma in the form of intercourse should not be forgotten as a possible cause of PMB. It is very important to realise that sometimes the woman does not know from where the bleeding has come, and has assumed the source to be the vagina as was the case with her periods. A detailed history is required to elucidate the symptom. Cystoscopy and sigmoidoscopy may be required.

Benign

Senile endometritis may explain bleeding from the uterus in those cases in which a totally inactive endometrium is obtained at curettage for PMB. Genital tuberculosis is rare, but known to mimic many gynaecological symptoms.

Table 18.1

Aetiology of Postmenopausal Bleeding

Benign	Malignant
Uterine	Cervical carcinoma
Senile endometritis	Endometrial carcinoma/sarcoma
Polyp: endometrial; fibroid	Vulval carcinoma
HRT	Vaginal carcinoma ⎫ rare
Influence of functional granulosa/	Fallopian tube carcinoma ⎭
thecoma cells	
Tuberculosis	
Cervix	
Atrophic cervicitis	
Polyp	
Vagina	
Atrophic vaginitis	
Infection	
Urethral caruncle	

It is common to see petechial haemorrhages and large friable blood vessels on the atrophic cervix and easy to understand how these can bleed. Similar changes occur in the vagina; infection may be the common precipitating factor.

An urethral caruncle is a small, red, fleshy outgrowth at the urethral meatus, usually of the posterior wall, which may be just a localised prolapse of the urethral epithelium, or a granuloma, resulting from infection. They are usually benign and most common in menopausal women.

Malignant

Cervical and endometrial carcinoma are well recognised causes of PMB. After the age of 60, the ratio of endometrial to cervical cancer is about 4:1. Later, uterine sarcoma becomes a possibility. Vulval carcinoma usually presents as PMB on cleaning or drying the vulvoperineal region although, of course, the tumour may present as just a lump. Vaginal and fallopian tube carcinoma are very rare. The former is of current interest, because of its association with vaginal adenosis which is associated with the administration of diethyl stilboestrol (DES) during pregnancy to the mothers of the affected women. The latter more characteristically present with a watery discharge, which may be sudden and heavy and mistaken by the patient for incontinence of urine.

Management

Diagnosis depends upon history, examination and special tests.

History

Bleeding is the essential feature, but a detailed history is required to determine accurately the source of the bleeding:

When did the bleeding occur?
How much bleeding was there?
How many episodes have there been?
Was it related to micturition or defaecation?
Was the urine itself coloured?
Was the blood mixed with the motions? Was there any slime?
Was the blood bright or dark?
Is there any alteration in bowel habit?
Is there any weight loss?
Any other symptoms?

A full gynaecological history should include the following questions:
Age of the menarche (although there is no consistent evidence that the age of the menarche is related to the onset of the menopause)
Age at the menopause
Any postcoital bleeding?
Any dyspareunia?
Any abnormal vaginal discharge?
Parity (endometrial carcinoma is three times more common in nulliparous women).

The history should exclude ingestion of oestrogen containing drugs (HRT) and also the use of face and body creams which may contain oestrogen.

Examination

A general examination is performed with particular reference to detection of lymphodenopathy, the breasts and abdomen, and evidence of oestrogen deficiency: kyphosis, atrophic changes in the genital tract, or of oestrogen stimulation such as copious cervical mucus, or a well oestrogenised vagina.

Special tests

The essential investigation in PMB is endometrial biopsy/uterine curettage. This should be preceded in the clinic by cytology of the lateral vaginal wall, to detect abnormal oestrogen stimulation, and of the cervix. Endometrial samples can be obtained with the Accurette or Vabra, but the focus of carcinoma may be so small that it is missed unless formal curettage is performed. If the cervical smear is abnormal (i.e. it shows evidence of cervical intraepithelial neoplasia), the woman should be referred for colposcopy, when colposcopically orientated biopsies will be taken. Colposcopy provides direct magnified visualisation of the patterns of cervical epithelial cells. In elderly patients, the squamocolumnar junction is usually well up the endocervical canal and, therefore, not visible. Specimens may be obtained by endocervical curettage, but this may miss the endocervical lesion. Cone biopsy of the cervix is a more logical procedure. In the presence of an obvious invasive lesion, an incision/wedge biopsy will provide sufficient tissue for histopathological diagnosis and will not delay surgery (Wertheim-Meigs hysterectomy) if this is chosen as the treatment of choice. At one time, it was held that cone biopsy caused the dissemination of cancer, but logically any biopsy procedure has the same chance of opening blood vessels and tissue spaces for the spread of cancer.

Should carcinoma of the cervix, vagina or endometrium be discovered, the lesion is staged, and the appropriate treatment/management planned with all relevant colleagues.

Cystoscopy and sigmoidoscopy should not be forgotten. Colonoscopy may be required. Tests for faecal occult blood provide a useful screening test.

Treatment

Lesions of the bowel or bladder will require referral to the appropriate specialist. Carcinoma of the uterus and cervix will be discussed in Chapter 20.

Massive postmenopausal vaginal bleeding rarely occurs unless it is due to malignancy, in which case transfusion and emergency curettage may be required. Curettage is of limited use except to establish a diagnosis. Emergency radiotherapy is of value in controlling bleeding from genital carcinomas.

Atrophic changes causing PMB are best treated by local oestrogens (p. 253). Excision of prolapsed urethral epithelium and caruncles is standard treatment. Local oestrogens may prevent recurrence.

FURTHER READING

Cooke I.D. ed. (1978). *The Role of Estrogen/Progestogen in the Management of the Menopause*. Lancaster: MTP Press.

Coope J. (1984). Menopause, diagnosis and treatment. *Brit. Med. J*; **iii**: 888–90.

19

Benign Disorders of the Reproductive Organs and Bladder

VAGINAL INFECTIONS

Physiology

The squamous epithelium of the vagina and vulva is thin and undifferentiated in the child and the postmenopausal woman because of the lack of oestrogen. Oestrogen causes a thickening of the epithelium and differentiation into the well recognised, basal, intermediate and superficial cell layers, characteristic of the reproductive years. The percentage of flattened superficial cells with a high nuclear-cytoplasmic ratio indicates the degree of oestrogenic activity. Progesterone causes a decrease in the number of superficial cells, while the intermediate cells increase (Fig. 19.1).

The vaginal epithelial cells contain much glycogen. The formation of glycogen, abundant within the superficial cells, is another oestrogenic effect, thus providing a dense protective epithelium. Glycogen is easily fermented or broken down to produce lactic acid and, therefore, increases the acidity of the vagina, which is toxic to many

pathogenic organisms and saprophytes. The healthy vagina of the woman of reproductive age contains lactobacilli and acidogenic corynbacteria. Fungi, which would otherwise grow, are restricted by this acid pH (pH 3.5–4.1). The acidity of the vagina can be changed by other factors: drugs, intercourse and cervical erosions. The columnar cells of the endocervix produce an alkaline cervical mucus, so, if there is an excess of these, as in an ectropion or large cervical erosion, then the vaginal pH will rise. Intercourse provokes an increase in the vaginal pH as the vaginal lubricant secreted by the vaginal epithelium increases the pH to 6 or 7 as will the seminal fluid. This pH will persist for hours after intercourse. Frequent intercourse causes the vagina to be alkaline, toxic to the lactobacilli and corynbacteria, but suitable for pathogens.

Descriptions of vaginal infection with *candida albicans, trichomonas vaginalis, neisseria gonorrhoea, chlamydia trachomatis, herpes vaginalis* and *gardnerella vaginalis* follow.

Vaginitis in children is uncommon. It may be due to trichomonal or other pathogenic organisms acquired by non-sexual contact in the home, or secondary to an intravaginal foreign body.

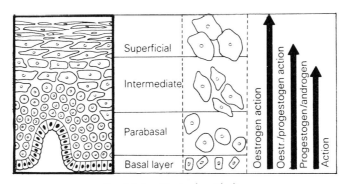

Fig. 19.1 *Vaginal epithelium.*

Candida Albicans (C. Albicans)

Candida albicans is the most virulent of the candida species of yeast. It possesses hyphae, pseudohyphae and spores, which are recognised easily on a wet preparation slide. The hyphae and buds of the fungus are seen clearly when 10% potassium hydroxide (KOH) solution, which lyses epithelial cells, inflammatory leucocytes and debris, is added to the wet preparation slide. When blastospores predominate, it is a pathogenic infection, while predominantly pseudohyphae suggest a saprophytic infection. *C. albicans* is a low grade opportunistic organism and is often present in the vagina without causing clinical symptoms or signs. An overgrowth commonly occurs in pregnancy, diabetes, long-term corticosteroid and immunosuppressive therapy as well as treatment with broad spectrum antibiotics. The widespread use of antibiotics and the fashion of nylon knickers, tights and jeans, which produce a warm moist culture for candida, has contributed to the recent dramatic rise in the incidence of candidal vaginal infections. Indiscriminate antibiotic treatment of similar infections has also contributed to this increased incidence.

Symptoms and signs

Candidal vaginitis is easy to diagnose. There is an intense vulval pruritis, exacerbated at night with a thick discharge likened to 'curdled milk'. Erythema of the labia minora is an unusual presentation. A blood sugar should be performed when glycosuria and a candidal infection is encountered in the young child or postmenopausal woman. Any patient complaining of dysuria should be examined for vaginal discharge.

Diagnosis

A wet preparation is crucial, and as previously mentioned hyphae and spores are identified easily if a drop of 10% KOH is added. A vaginal swab, conveyed in Stuart's or Sabouraud's transport medium, should be taken and sent for culture.

Treatment

All fungal infections will respond to topical 1% aqueous solution of gentian violet, but this is messy and often produces an allergic reaction (15%). There is, however, a 95% cure rate if applied properly and allowed to dry. It is rarely used now, but is useful in the resistant case.

Polyene antifungal drugs such as nystatin are effective. These cause increased permeability of the fungal membrane and leakage of cellular components. They can be applied by cream or pessary. Creams are more effective than pessaries, because the cream is evenly spread across the vaginal membrane, but patient compliance is poor. Imidazole derivatives such as clotrimazole are also effective in the one dose pessary, which dissolves over 3 days.

Systemic ketoconazole is effective in resistant cases where there may be gastrointestinal involvement. It should be used with care, as cases of hepatotoxicity have recently been described.

The male sexual partner of any woman with a fungal vaginitis requires treatment. The male can carry the fungus and is often symptomless, thereby reinfecting the woman. Treatment is by using antifungal cream applied to the glans penis and prepuce twice daily for 5–7 days.

Trichomonas Vaginalis (T. Vaginalis)

Trichomonas (T) vaginalis infection is the second most common vaginal infection (Fig. 19.2). It is caused by a flagellated protozoa which inhabits female and male paraurethral glands from whence it can autoinfect susceptible vaginae. *T. vaginalis* has been known to survive for up to 25 h in chlorinated swimming pools, but usually is sexually transferred when an inoculum is transported in the buffered alkaline medium of semen.

Symptoms and signs

Patients complain of a profuse discharge with pruritis, which is less severe than a candidal pruritis. On examination, the vagina will be reddened and inflamed. The discharge is classically described as 'greenish, effervescent and frothy' but this is, in fact, rarely seen. Indeed, a frothy vaginal discharge is more likely to be caused by *Gardnerella vaginalis*. This trichomonal discharge is usually a grey-white opaque colour with an occasional bubble with a pH between 5 and 7. *Trichomonas* is found rarely in a discharge with a low pH. Occasionally the classic 'strawberry' appearance of the vagina and cervix is seen.

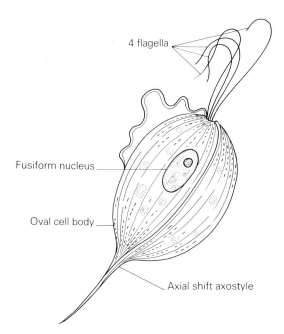

4 flagella

Fusiform nucleus

Oval cell body

Axial shift axostyle

Fig. 19.2 *Trichomonas vaginalis.*

Diagnosis

T. vaginalis has a characteristic swirling movement under the microscope where the flagella seem to move independently from the oval body. Colposcopy shows the characteristic Y-shaped blood vessels on the cervix.

Treatment

Metronidazole, 200 mg tds for 7 days is specific treatment for *T. vaginalis*. This organism is sexually transmitted, so the partner must also be treated. The drug is contraindicated in early pregnancy and when breast feeding. It is also associated with nausea which is aggravated by alcohol.

Genital Herpes

Publicity given to the dramatic increase of this condition has caused alarm and confusion. Herpes is caused by herpes simplex virus II (HSV II), although HSV I is increasingly found in vaginal herpes, because of oral sexual habits. Vaginal herpes is often asymptomatic, but primary vulval herpes is a distressing and painful condition.

Symptoms and signs

Primary herpes causes malaise, low grade fever, inguinal lymphadenopathy and thin watery discharge. Single herpetic vesicles appear or coalesce to form clusters, which then ulcerate. The intense pain of primary herpetic urethritis sometimes causes urinary retention. A latent infection follows the primary infection when this virus inhabits the sacral ganglia, but it reappears periodically causing mild recurrent infection.

Diagnosis

This is difficult, although culture is preferred to high antibody titres which reflect pre-existing latent infection.

Treatment

Treatment of the distressingly painful primary infection has, until recently, been confined to antibiotics to prevent bacterial secondary infection, and analgesia for the pain. Local treatment consists of virucidal chemotherapy with pyrimidine or purine derivatives such as idoxuridine. The new purine derivative, acyclovir, is effective i.v. for the treatment of primary herpes. Oral acyclovir may reduce the shedding of virus particles in recurrent episodes, and topical treatment will speed up the healing of vesicles.

Genital Warts

Condylomata acuminata result from infection with human papovavirus (HPV) and are sexually transmitted. They are extremely infectious, infecting 65% of the patients' consorts. Invasive cervical cancers are associated with human papovavirus (HPV) types 16 and 18, while cervical dysplasia which is associated with types 6 and 11 rarely progress to malignancy.

Treatment

The application of 25% podophyllin cream twice weekly has been the traditional treatment, but this can be awkward and causes local ulceration. Treatment with electrocautery, cryocautery or laser coagulation is effective.

Gardnerella Vaginalis (G. Vaginalis)

There has been confusion about classification of this Gram-negative bacillus and its pathogenicity has been questioned. It was previously known as *Haemophilus vaginalis* and may occur in 33% of asymptomatic patients and approximately 98% of patients with a non-specific symptomatic vaginitis. Concurrent infection with other organisms is common.

Symptoms and signs

G. vaginalis vaginitis causes a thin, watery, opaque vaginal discharge with a disagreeable smell, especially after intercourse. This smell is accentuated when a drop of 10% KOH is added to the wet preparation slide. Clue cells are seen on wet preparation. These are granular vaginal, epithelial cells with an irregular outline which have huge numbers of *G. vaginalis* bacilli attached to the surface. They can be seen on Papanicolaou smears. Over 90% of women with a vaginal discharge and a vaginal pH of 5 or greater will have either *T. vaginalis* or *G. vaginalis* vaginitis. Culture of this organism is difficult, which accounts for the confusion about its pathogenicity.

Treatment

Metronidazole 200 mg 8-hourly for patient and consort for 7 days is effective. Topical sulphonamide creams are ineffective.

Neisseria Gonorrhoeae (N. Gonorrhoea)

The majority of women are asymptomatic with vaginal infection caused by this Gram-negative diplococcus. The main sites of infection are the endocervix and urethra. Swabs should be taken from these sites in all cases of suspected gonorrhoea.

Symptoms and signs

Some patients, however, may complain of painful vulval oedema several days after sexual transmission, caused by an inflammation of the vulval mucous membranes, inflamed Skene's ducts and congested Bartholin's glands, which are found in the vestibule and fourchette, respectively. Both may form an extremely painful and tender Skene's or Bartholin's abscess. Surgical drainage under general anaesthetic is required and Bartholin's abscesses are traditionally marsupialised. This means excising the skin over the abscess and suturing it back in four segments, so that the abscess cavity is opened up completely. Healing is by granulation and re-epithelialisation. Antibiotic treatment alone encourages a chronic infection.

Diagnosis

Gram stains should be prepared in Outpatients. Swabs for culture must be taken from the cervix, urethra, perirectal areas and, if possible, around Skene's and Bartholin's glands. These should be plated immediately or kept in Stuart's medium for 24–28 h. It is important to remember that concurrent infection with other organisms, particularly *C. trachomatis*, *T. vaginalis* and genital warts, is common with gonococcal infection and syphilis must not be forgotten.

Treatment

Procaine penicillin 2.4 mg i.m. into each buttock is compulsory with 1 g of oral probenicid to delay excretion of penicillin. If a β lactamase producing gonococcus is diagnosed, or the patient is sensitive to penicillin, then spectinomycin 4 gm, i.m. is given.

Chlamydia Trachomatis

Chlamydia trachomatis is an important cause of non-specific infection of the genital tract. These organisms are frequently the cause of non-specific urethritis and cervicitis. Chlamydiae are intracellular organisms that are difficult to culture. Their presence is determined by visualising intracellular inclusion bodies, but more recently immunofluorescent staining of smear has been used.

PELVIC INFLAMMATORY DISEASE

In the past ten years there has been renewed interest in pelvic inflammatory disease. The central role of *Neisseria gonorrhoea* as the initiator of most cases of sexually transmitted pelvic inflammatory disease has been questioned, and it is now apparent that various anaerobic bacteria or *Chlamydia trachomatis* (*C. trachomatis*) are major causes of this condition.

The terminology of pelvic infection is confusing and there is no recent definition suitable to cover all causes. The term 'pelvic inflammatory disease' is increasingly used and is synonymous with salpingitis and pelvic sepsis. The acronym ESP (Endometritis — Salpingitis — Peritonitis) is commonly used in the United States. It can be defined as a microbial inflammatory process involving the endocervix, endometrium and tubal epithelium with subsequent inflammation of the parametrium and spill of tubal exudate into the peritoneal cavity. It is usually associated with ascending genital infection in sexually active women of childbearing age.

Epidemiology

The promiscuity of the permissive society has provoked a dramatic increase of this condition over the past ten years.

Aetiology

The causes are listed in Table 19.1.

N. Gonorrhoea

N. gonorrhoea remains a major cause of pelvic inflammatory disease throughout the world. It causes a bilateral endosalpingitis leading to destruction of ciliated endothelial cells within the fallopian tube. These specialised cells are necessary for sperm and ovum transport. Moderate infection causes pyosalpinx formation and severe infection, tubo-ovarian abscess with formation of adhesions. A resolved pyosalpinx forms a hydrosalpinx causing permanent occlusion of the fimbrial ostia.

Chlamydia trachomatis

Chlamydia trachomatis (*C. trachomatis*) is another major cause of pelvic infection. The chlamydiae were formerly classified as Rickettsia, being very small, immobile, spherical or rodlike parasitic organisms, which resemble bacteria but which, like viruses, cannot reproduce outside the cells of their hosts.

Table 19.1

Causes of Pelvic Sepsis

1 PRIMARY PELVIC SEPSIS
(Ascending genital infection)

Exogenous agents

Sexually transmitted:
  N.gonorrhoea
  C. trachomatis
  Mycoplasma hominis
  U. urealyticum
  Viruses

Endogenous agents

  Bacteroides
  Peptococcus
  Anaerobic streptococci
  E. coli
  Actinomyces

Iatrogenic

D & C
Termination of pregnancy
Hysterosalpingogram
Insertion of IUCD
Postoperative

2 SECONDARY PELVIC SEPSIS
  Pelvic peritonitis
  Mycobacterium tuberculosis
    (blood borne).

They have a complicated life cycle and the infectious particle, the elementary body, is small and metabolically inactive. It has a rigid hard envelope and is similar to Gram-negative organisms. It is taken into the host cell by phagocytosis, reorganising to form, within 12 h, the reticulate body, which is intracellular and metabolically active. This reticulate body divides repeatedly by binary fission, so that within 20 h, the cytoplasm of the host cell contains many reticulate bodies. These eventually reorganise into inclusions; namely, the elementary bodies. Latency, or the persistence of the organism in an inapparent infection, is characteristic of chlamydial infections. They may prove difficult to isolate or observe in chronic infections and persist in the genital tract as subclinical salpingitis which is reactivated when host resistance is low. They may cause a considerable degree of permanent fallopian tubal endothelial cell destruction despite appearing to be such a mild infection. Chlamydiae are difficult to diagnose by culture, but the development of monoclonal antichlamydial antibody techniques offer a rapid, more reliable diagnosis.

Ureaplasma urealyticum

Mycoplasma was first isolated from a Bartholin's abscess in 1937. A tiny mycoplasma was later described — hence *T. mycoplasma*, now known as *Ureaplasma urealyticum*. This is a very small organism which is sexually transmitted, difficult to isolate and is responsible for less than 10% of cases of pelvic inflammatory disease. *C. trachomatis* and *U. urealyticum* are both sensitive to tetracyclines. Iatrogenic causes of pelvic inflammatory disease are listed in Table 19.1.

Other causes

Severe pelvic infection commonly follows illegal abortion. Today, some pelvic infections can develop after therapeutic abortions, but it is debatable whether these patients require prophylactic antibiotics. Hysterosalpingograms are an unusual cause of pelvic infection, but this procedure can cause a recrudescence of chronic pelvic inflammatory disease. The intrauterine device is not a direct cause of pelvic inflammatory disease, but can facilitate ascending infection by sexually transmitted organisms via the threads. They should, therefore, not be offered as a first choice contraceptive to young nulliparous women who have not yet formed a stable monogamous relationship. Postoperative

pelvic infection can occur and prophylactic antibiotics are commonly given to hysterectomy patients.

Endogenous agents which cause pelvic infections are listed in Table 19.1. These are of low pathogenicity and some may be classified as secondary invaders. Pelvic inflammatory disease is known to be polymicrobial and these agents (especially anaerobes) cause a superimposed infection after tissue destruction, initially caused by a sexually transmitted organism. Bacteroides and actinomycetes may be found in tubo-ovarian abscesses. Anaerobic streptococci are a common cause of ascending puerperal pelvic infection. Today, blood borne secondary pelvic infection by *Mycobacterium tuberculosis* causing an obliterative endosalpingitis is rare in the UK, but it is a possible cause of infertility in immigrants.

Diagnosis

The classic criteria for diagnosis are listed in Table 19.2. Unfortunately, these signs and symptoms may be based on unconfirmed observations. The clinical diagnosis may only be correct in 65% of women with laparoscopically verified pelvic inflammatory disease.

The differential diagnosis includes appendicitis, endometriosis, ectopic pregnancy and bleeding or ruptured ovarian cysts. Fever may be present in only 30% of cases of pelvic inflammatory disease. Chlamydial salpingitis is a mild insidious relapsing condition with few signs, so liberal use of these classic criteria leads to overdiagnosis; conversely, too strict an adherence leads to underdiagnosis. Revised clinical criteria are set out in Table 19.3 and liberal use of the laparoscope is recommended, especially where there is any doubt of the diagnosis. All patients with suspected PID, not responding to adequate and appropriate therapy, should be laparoscoped. The liver should be routinely examined at every diagnostic laparoscopy for 'violin-string' adhesions typical of the Curtis-Fitzhugh syndrome. This is a result of chlamydial hepatic and perihepatic infection, which may follow pelvic chlamydial infection.

Treatment

Before commencing treatment, any in situ intrauterine contraceptive device (IUCD) should be removed immediately.

Table 19.2

Classic Clinical Criteria for Diagnosis of Pelvic Sepsis

---

1. Lower abdominal pain
2. Purulent endocervical discharge
3. Cervical excitation tenderness
4. Adnexal tenderness
5. Fever
6. Leucocytosis

Table 19.3

Referral Criteria for the Diagnosis of Pelvic Sepsis

---

1. Abdominal tenderness with or without rebound tenderness	All three
2. Cervical excitation tenderness	necessary for
3. Adnexal tenderness	diagnosis

Plus one or more of the following:

1. Positive endocervical swab showing Gram negative intracellular diplicocci
2. Temperature of 38°C or greater
3. Leucocytosis of 10 000 or greater
4. Purulent material (with WBC present) from peritoneal cavity
5. Pelvic abscess or inflammatory mass demonstrated on ultrasound

---

Mild pelvic inflammatory disease

Mild pelvic inflammatory disease does not require admission to hospital — patients have localised symptoms, do not feel very ill and can go about their daily activities. Treatment should be with single large doses of penicillin G (4 mega units) or ampicillin (2 g orally) and probenecid 1 g (orally) if gonorrhoeae is suspected. After sampling from the endocervix, periurethra and perirectal areas, Gram smears should also be taken before treatment starts. Ampicillin is not very effective because of poor tissue penetration. Doxycycline has a longer half life and is known to achieve better tissue levels than oxytetracycline. Better patient compliance is achieved with doxycycline 100 mg daily, rather than oxytetracycline 250 mg 4 times daily. Metromidazole 400 mg tds should also be used in combination because of its efficacy against anaerobes and its low toxicity. Oral cephalosporins in doses of 500 mg four times daily may also be effective. All oral antibiotics should be given for 7–10 days, as shorter courses are more likely to lead to recurrence.

Moderate pelvic inflammatory disease

Patients are admitted to hospital for bed rest, as they usually feel unwell, some with pyrexia and all with marked pelvic and lower abdominal pain and tenderness. Laparoscopy is performed where possible and especially if the diagnosis is doubtful, or the pain persists for more than 24 h. Fimbrial sampling by laparoscopy or endometrial biopsy is performed for isolation of *N. gonorrhoeae, C. trachomalis* and bacteroides. Tetracyclines again are included in treatment regimens 24 h after initial i.m./i.v. penicillin and probenecid. If β-lactamase producing gonococci are detected, treatment regimens can be adjusted to include cefuroxime, cefoxitin, latomoxef or spectinomycin. Rectal or oral metronidazole is included, especially in patients with a previous history of pelvic infection, and gentamicin 60–80 mg i.m./i.v. is considered.

Severe pelvic inflammatory disease

These patients are obviously ill and require immediate admission and i.v. antibiotics, particularly, if a large tubo-ovarian abscess is suspected. Laparoscopy is contraindicated. Intravenous penicillin, rectal or i.v., or metronidazole and gentamicin should be included in treatment regimens. Severe sexually transmitted pelvic sepsis is unlikely to be associated with *C. trachomatis* and tetracyclines are not a prerequisite. Intravenous therapy should be commenced, electrolyte balance restored and urinary output closely observed. Treatment remains conservative and laparotomy is not advised unless a tubo-ovarian abscess has ruptured or requires draining. Peritoneal lavage and oophorectomy, not hysterectomy, can then be life saving.

Tubo-ovarian and pelvic abscesses

Large tubo-ovarian abscesses are an unusual event in the United Kingdom but relatively common in the United States and Africa. Again, treatment is conservative and overlaps with the medical treatment of severe sexually transmitted pelvic sepsis unless (1) clinical signs fail to show response to clinical management within 24 h; (2) generalised peritonitis persists beyond a 24 h period or (3) if there is no reduction in size of pelvic mass within 48 h.

Pelvic clearance is not recommended and only the adnexal mass is removed. Hysterectomy is not advised, but may be reluctantly considered in severe puerperal infection.

The use of posterior colpotomy is debatable as it may not resolve all cases. However, it can easily be performed when there is a large fluctuant mass bulging into the posterior vaginal fornix.

Sequelae

It has been estimated that one episode of pelvic inflammatory disease causes a 13% incidence of infertility; two episodes cause a 35% incidence and three episodes a rate of 78%. The exact incidence of ectopic pregnancy following pelvic inflammatory disease is uncertain, but is thought to be high. Reconstructive tubal microsurgery of hydrosalpinges offers a 20% chance of a successful pregnancy, but is less if extensive deciliation has occurred. Microsurgical correction of cornual disease offers approximately a 50% chance of successful pregnancy. There is, however, approximately a 10% risk of subsequent ectopic pregnancy. The degree of residual tubal damage often means that surgical correction is impossible, and that in vitro fertilisation offers the only hope of a successful pregnancy. The patient with chronic lower abdominal pain resulting from previous pelvic sepsis is well known to all medical practitioners, and pelvic clearance may not be the panacea. Early diagnosis, prompt treatment and adequate follow-up are necessary to prevent these tragic sequelae.

ECTOPIC PREGNANCY

This is defined as a pregnancy occurring outside the uterine cavity. The most common site is the fallopian tube with ovarian uterine cornua and intra-abdominal pregnancies being very rare (Fig. 19.3). Ovarian pregnancies present in a similar way to a tubal pregnancy. Cornual pregnancies cause severe pain while the uterine cornua is distending and then a very severe intra-abdominal emergency, with haemorrhage, when the uterus ruptures.

Abdominal pregnancies start from the expulsion of a viable conceptus from a tubal rupture. Placentation occurs in another site and the pregnancy can proceed to the 3rd trimester. The fetus is very easily felt and diagnosis is by ultrasound. Delivery is surgical and the placenta must be left *in situ* to involute as attempts to remove it cause intractable haemorrhage. The rest of this section deals with tubal pregnancy, which is a common but potentially life-threatening condition.

The clinical picture varies from a mild innocuous condition to a shocked, moribund patient. Awareness of the possibility of this condition is important so that diagnosis and life-saving operations can be undertaken. Two-thirds of women with an ectopic pregnancy will remain infertile and 10% will have a second ectopic. The incidence of this condition has risen dramatically in the Western world in the past 15 years. This can be attributed perhaps to better diagnosis, but increased promiscuity has resulted in a big rise in the incidence of pelvic inflammatory disease and hence ectopic pregnancy.

Clinical

The history and clinical signs are crucial to the diagnosis. Tubal pregnancies occur commonly between 20 and 25 years of age and their incidence appears to increase with age. It is common in women who have an IUCD *in situ*, or who have pelvic inflammatory disease, infertility, previous ectopic pregnancies or tubal surgery. Symptoms and signs vary, with abdominal pain being the most consistent symptom. The pain may be severe, but often eases and the intra-abdominal bleeding becomes significant. Vaginal bleeding characteristically follows the pain, although there may not be any bleeding at all. Dizziness and faintness follow the onset of severe pain. Shoulder tip pain from phrenic nerve stimulation results from blood under the diaphragm. It can be provoked by lifting the foot off the bed. Another symptom is painful defaecation. Only 10% will pass a uterine decidual cast.

The main clinical sign is lower abdominal tenderness with or without rebound tenderness. There are few clinical signs if it is a slow leaking ectopic. When there is a large haematoperitoneum, the abdomen is often soft with little tenderness, but has a 'doughy' consistency. Vaginal examination provokes cervical excitation and adnexal tenderness. Some gynaecologists argue that a vaginal examination should not be performed when an ectopic is suspected, in case profuse intraperitoneal bleeding is provoked by this bimanual palpation. Unilateral tenderness and possibly an adnexal mass may be felt at bimanual examination.

Diagnosis

Few cases of ectopic pregnancy will be missed if one suspects this condition. Laparoscopy, ultrasound and sensitive pregnancy tests have become import-ant diagnostic aids in the past ten years. There is a 25% false positive diagnostic rate at culdocentesis which is aspiration of the pouch of Douglas. A low haemoglobin and a low PCV are helpful blood indices. A positive pregnancy test is helpful, but it can be negative in 50% of cases of ectopic pregnancy. Laparoscopy is the absolute diagnostic tool and should be used whenever there is a suspicion of ectopic pregnancy. An in-patient with secondary amenorrhoea and undiagnosed lower abdominal pain persisting for more than 24 h requires a laparoscopy. Failure to see a gestation sac by ultrasound in a suspected ectopic strongly suggests a tubal pregnancy. An ectopic pregnancy is suspected when the β HCG level is above 6500 units/ml and an intrauterine sac is not seen on ultrasound. When an adnexal mass is also seen at ultrasound, laparoscopy or laparotomy is advised. The infertile patient on drugs such as clomiphene to induce ovulation may have one intrauterine pregnancy and one tubal pregnancy.

Treatment

Traditionally, immediate salpingectomy was the standard treatment for an ectopic pregnancy. Resuscitation of shocked patients should be commenced before operation, but surgery should not be delayed by prolonged attempts to restore the blood volume.

Conservative surgery has been recommended when a tubal abortion without tubal rupture is seen. Manual expression of an unruptured ampullary ectopic can be performed, but trophoblastic tissue can remain, causing delayed haemorrhage and often an increased risk of a further ectopic pregnancy. Microsurgical techniques such as linear salpingotomy and interval reanastomosis are advocated.

CERVICAL CONDITIONS

Cervix

Cervical polyps

These are usually mucous polyps arising from distended glands. They may be symptomless or they may cause postcoital or intermenstrual spot-

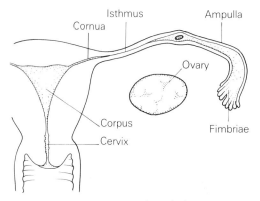

Fig. 19.3 *Common site for tubal pregnancy.*

ting. They can be avulsed easily, but it is better to perform a clinical dilatation and curettage to remove any associated endometrial polyps.

Cervical intraepithelial neoplasia (CIN)

This benign, but potentially malignant condition will be discussed in Chapter 20, p. 278.

Cervical erosion

This frequently diagnosed condition is a misnomer. The gross appearance of an erosion on the ectocervix is given by the red punctuate appearance of the columnar epithelium which has migrated from the endocervix onto the ectocervix. The reasons are obscure, but hormonal influences such as pregnancy and oral contraceptives are thought to be important. Columnar epithelium in the vagina is less resistant to infection than the normal stratified squamous epithelium. Chronic cervicitis with mucopurulent discharge and chronic pain may result. Postcoital bleeding may also occur from a large erosion. Vaginal pessaries of appropriate antibiotic or of antiseptic compounds, such as betadine, may give temporary relief. For recurring cases, treatment is by cervical cautery after checking that cervical cytology is normal. In the absence of symptoms such as discharge, pain or bleeding, no treatment is needed if the cytology is normal.

Ectropion

This defines the damaged cervix which gapes, allowing the normally situated columnar epithelium of the endocervix to be easily visible. Signs and symptoms are the same as for a cervical erosion. Treatment is rarely needed and involves cautery to the canal or repair of the cervix to restore its normal shape.

UTERINE CONDITIONS

Uterine Fibroids

Fibroids or leiomyomata are the most common tumours not only in the female genital tract, but in the human body. Approximately 20% of all women are thought to have them and the majority are

symptomless. They can be single or multiple, varying from the size of a pin to that of a football. The aetiology of these benign smooth muscle tumours is unknown but oestrogen is thought to play some part. They are more common in Negroes and nulliparous women. Symptoms are caused by increasing size and often occur around 30 years of age. They regress postmenopausally and, like the uterus, undergo atrophy.

Classification

This is shown in Fig. 19.4. Fibroids are divided into three groups: subserous, when they project from the peritoneal surface of the uterus; mural, when they are within the wall of the uterus; and submucous, when they project into the uterine cavity. They can develop long stalks and occasionally pedunculated submucous fibroids may be seen protruding through the cervix and even the introitus. Fibroids are characteristically firm, but may be soft and cystic due to degeneration, or rock hard due to calcification. When cut across, fibroids are seen to be contained in a false capsule of compressed uterine muscle and thus are easily enucleated. Red degeneration or necrobiosis of fibroids occurs in pregnancy. Fibroids rarely become infected and sarcomatous change is unusual (<1%).

Clinical

Fibroids are often silent and symptomless even whey they grow to a considerable size. They are

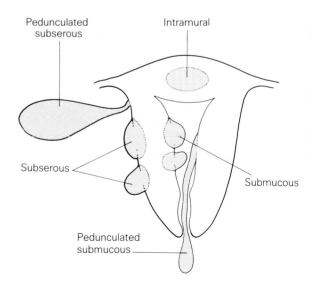

Fig. 19.4   *Types of uterine fibroids.*

discovered at vaginal or abdominal examination or the patient may notice a gradual increase in girth. Symptoms produced by fibroids are summarised in Table 19.4. Pressure effects on surrounding organs,

---

Table 19.4
Symptoms of Fibroids

Pressure effects	Urinary frequency
	Retention of urine
	Backache
	Constipation
Bleeding	Menorrhagia
	(enlarged uterine cavity)
	Intermenstrual
	Postcoital
	(pedunculated submucous fibroid)
Pain	Mild
	(hyaline degeneration)
	Moderate
	(red degeneration in pregnancy)
	Severe
	(torsion of pedunculated subserous)

---

such as constipation, is unusual, but introverted impacted fibroid uterus may cause acute urinary retention or occasionally urinary frequency. Dysfunctional uterine bleeding caused by the increased size and vascularity of the uterus may cause menorrhagia, especially if these are submucous fibroids. Pedunculated submucous fibroids protruding through the cervix present as intramenstrual, postcoital bleeding which may be heavy. Fibroids do not cause infertility: rather prolonged infertility is associated with the development of fibroids. Submucous cornual fibroids may occlude the proximal part of the fallopian tubes, but this is rarely encountered and should be confirmed either by hysterosalpingogram or hysteroscopy. Fibroids cause low backache, especially if large and the uterus is retroverted. Torsion of pedunculated fibroids is rare and causes acute pain.

Fibroids feel firm, smooth and rounded and the uterus is distorted. Differential diagnosis is from ovarian tumours and this sometimes is difficult, only being confirmed at laparotomy.

Treatment

The treatment of small fibroids, with the uterus only minimally enlarged, and without symptoms can be expectant. The patient should be seen regularly, say annually, to detect any possible increase in size. The woman should return at once if any pain develops, which could be caused by hyaline degeneration or infection.

If the fibroids cause menorrhagia and/or pain, medical treatment using non-steroidal anti-inflammatory drugs may be helpful in the short term, but surgical removal is usually needed. Abdominal hysterectomy is indicated in women who have completed their families and who complain of abnormal bleeding or pressure symptoms or in whom the fibroids are growing. Vaginal hysterectomy may be performed if the fibroids are not too large. The ovaries should be conserved if the woman is under 50, as they are usually normal.

Myomectomy. This involves removal of individual fibroids and then oversewing of the myometrium. The operation is not carried out very frequently because of the problems of haemostasis, infection, subsequent adhesion formation and the chance of recurrence. However, it is appropriate treatment in a patient with large fibroids causing symptoms, who wishes to retain her uterus either to have further children or for psychological reasons.

Treatment of fibroids in pregnancy is always conservative. Any surgical attempt to remove fibroids will provoke severe uncontrollable haemorrhage and surgery must be carried out after uterine involution has taken place. Red degeneration of fibroids can occur in pregnancy causing subacute pain, tenderness and occasionally signs of peritoneal irritation with guarding and rigidity. The treatment is conservative with bed rest, reassurrance and analgesia.

Hysterectomy. Hysterectomy is performed *abdominally* by a subumbilical midline incision for malignant conditions and for severe endometriosis in order to fully assess the extent of the disease and to allow for appropriate surgical treatment. It is also usually performed abdominally for menorrhagia via suprapubic transverse incision, especially if there is uterine enlargement due to fibroids. With a normal sized uterus, a *vaginal* hysterectomy is feasible. A history of infection or previous surgery suggesting possible adhesions makes vaginal hysterectomy risky. Vaginal hysterectomy is the operation of choice for uterovaginal prolapse with a normal or small sized uterus. The main risks of either operation are damage to the ureter and bladder. Details of these surgical procedures are outside the scope of this book. The reader should consult a specific gynaecological surgery book (p. 277).

Oophorectomy is not necessary unless the operation is being performed for malignant conditions. Some surgeons routinely remove the ovaries after a certain age, say 45 or 50, to eliminate the risks of developing subsequent ovarian carcinoma, although this risk is very small. Care must be taken during the operation to avoid damage to the ureters and bladder. The principal long-term complication is that of an enterocele.

Provided the patient has been fully counselled, there should be no psychological effects of hysterectomy such as loss of libido, depression, or increased weight. These problems are usually present before surgery and have become highlighted by the operation and the latter is blamed for them. Hence the need for adequate counselling beforehand. It is important to stress that, in general, hysterectomy causes no endocrine alterations.

Postoperatively there are no specific precautions. Heavy lifting should be avoided for 3 months and sexual intercourse can be resumed as soon as the patient feels comfortable.

ENDOMETRIOSIS

Endometriosis refers to ectopic foci of endometrium, either within the myometrium (adenomyosis), elsewhere on the peritoneal surface of other pelvic structures, or at distant sites. Its incidence is reported to be about 10% of menstruating women of whom 30–40% with endometriosis are infertile. The common sites within the pelvis are the ovaries, uterosacral ligaments, pouch of Douglas or, less commonly, fallopian tubes, or nodules on the peritoneum covering the pelvic side wall or bladder. The nodules are usually multiple and small, appearing as blue/black discrete raised areas, rarely more than 1 cm in diameter. If severe endometriosis is present, the nodules may be larger and associated with fibrosis around them. Severe chronic endometriosis can lead to many dense fibrous adhesions causing extensive pelvic damage. Endometriomata of the ovary (chocolate cysts) can present as moderately large ovarian cysts adherent to surrounding tissues. They contain thick chocolate-coloured fluid which can be irritant if allowed to leak into the peritoneal cavity.

More distant sites of endometriosis include the large or small bowel including the appendix, the umbilicus or operative scars, if surgery has involved opening the uterine cavity (hysterotomy, myomectomy).

The aetiology of endometriosis is uncertain, but the following hypotheses have been put forward:

1. Retrograde menstruation — viable fragments of endometrium are known to reach the pelvis via the fallopian tubes. These could then implant in certain susceptible individuals leading to foci of endometriosis. What determines a susceptible individual is not known.
2. Metaplasia and redifferentiation of coelomic epithelium covering the pelvic organs.
3. Implants of viable endometrium following surgery could account for endometriosis in surgical wounds following opening of the uterine cavity.
4. Lymphatic or blood borne 'metastases' or endometrial fragments.

Retrograde menstruation is likely to be the main cause, but other theories have their advocates.

Adenomyosis

This occurs when foci of active endometrium penetrate the myometrium. The uterus is usually externally uniform, but slightly enlarged. There are frequently heavy and painful periods. Histologically, a diagnosis is made on the basis of visualising endometrial stroma together with evidence of chronic haemorrhage, such as haemosiderin. Endometrial glands may or may not be seen. There is usually continuity between the glandular tissue of adenomyosis and the endometrium of the uterine cavity. The condition is benign, self-limiting and is not strongly associated with infertility.

Signs and Symptoms

The chief symptom of pelvic endometriosis is pelvic pain directly linked to the onset, maximum flow and duration of the menses. This is presumably due to the irritant action of blood from the endometrial foci on the peritoneum. The major effect of endometriosis is scarring, which leads to general fibrosis of pelvic tissues including the fallopian tubes. Other symptoms of endometriosis are dysmenorrhoea, dyspareunia and infertility. Infertility may be due to fibrosis and adhesions involving the fallopian tubes and ovaries. There is also an association between minor degrees of endometriosis and unexplained infertility. No definite cause has been demonstrated, but prostaglandins or other biochemical factors released by the ectopic endometrium may affect ovulation or tubal function. Endometriosis may induce an autoimmune response causing early embryo rejection and possibly accounting for the higher incidence of spontaneous abortion found in patients with endometriosis. None of these theories has been substantiated.

Diagnosis

Endometriosis is more common in nulliparous women and is diagnosed most frequently during the 3rd decade. The diagnosis may be suspected from the history by finding a fixed retroverted uterus, nodular scarring, often in the region of the uterosacral ligaments, and pelvic tenderness. A final diagnosis should be made at laparoscopy. The condition is a self-limiting one and, apart from the current symptoms and the possibility of infertility resulting from adhesions or rupture of a large endometrial cyst, it is a harmless condition, which should be borne in mind when treatment is being considered.

Treatment

There are two aspects of treatment: either prolonged inhibition of ovulation and subsequent endometrial suppression, or surgical ablation or removal of the endometriotic sites. Inhibition of ovulation and endometrial suppression can be achieved by use of the combined oral contraceptive pill, a high dose of progestogens such as dydrogesterone (20–30 mg daily), medroxyprogesterone acetate (5–15 mg daily) or danazol (200–600 mg daily), which is a competitive inhibitor of gonadotrophins. Side-effects include vaginal discharge, weight gain and acne and, very occasionally, serious androgenic side-effects such as voice change. For any significant effect to take place, treatment for up to 6 months is necessary. Treatment with gonadotrophin release hormone agonists, which inhibit ovulation, is being tried and early results are encouraging. Selective surgical ablation of isolated foci of endometriosis by excision or diathermy is an alternative to drug therapy. Patients with severe symptoms of extensive long-standing endometriosis may require total hysterectomy and bilateral salpingo-oophorectomy. This ensures the atrophy of other foci of endometriosis and so relief of symptoms.

GENITAL PROLAPSE

This can be defined as descent of adjacent organs through the fascial layers and into the vagina and sometimes beyond. Their definitions are shown in Table 19.5. Traditionally, uterine prolapse is defined as being of first, second or third degree. First degree means that the cervix just reaches the introitus on straining; second degree means that the cervix passes through the introitus on straining, while third degree or procidentia refers to passage of the entire uterus outside the vagina.

Most women who develop genital prolapse are multiparous. Cows and sheep characteristically have prolonged labours and develop prolapse, while horses and goats which tend to have rapid labours do not develop prolapse.

Contributing factors towards development of genital prolapse are listed in Table 19.6. Bearing down in labour before full cervical dilatation subjects the uterine supports to undue strain and, undoubtedly, contributes to the development of prolapse later in life when lack of oestrogen causes changes in collagen which weakens these uterovaginal supports.

An understanding of the functional anatomy of the pelvic floor shows why genital prolapse can occur. The bony pelvis is like a bowl with no base except that provided by the platform of the levator ani and coccygeus muscles, and by the pelvic fascia. The coccygeus muscle consists of the ischio-, ilio- and pubococcygeus muscles which blend together

Table 19.5

Descent of structure	Terminology used
Urethra	Urethrocele
Bladder	Cystocele
Small bowel	Enterocele
Rectum	Rectocele
Uterus	Uterovaginal prolapse

Table 19.6

Causes of Genital Prolapse

Weakened supports	Increased downward pressure
Congenital weakness (neuropathy, myopathy) e.g. spina bifida	Chronic cough
Multiparity	Constipation
Traumatic vaginal delivery	Abdominal masses
Large babies	Ascites
Inadequate perineal repairs	Uterine tumours
Failed postnatal exercises	
Poor nutrition	
Old age (hormone deficiency)	

on each side into a shelf that slopes medially downwards to produce a gutter effect in the midline pierced by the urethra, vagina and anal canal. These muscles arise from the ischial spines and pelvic bone to be inserted into the coccyx, and anococcygeal raphe and perineal body. These pelvic floor muscles normally contract to counteract any raised intra-abdominal pressure such as sneezing, laughing or coughing. A layer of fascia lies between these muscles and the peritoneal areolar tissue about the pelvic organs. Condensation of this fascia forms ligaments, such as the transverse cervical and uterosacral ligaments, which support the uterus, as well as the pubovesical fascia supporting the bladder and the rectovaginal fascia supporting the rectum.

Clinical Symptoms

Prolapse rarely starts during pregnancy, but symptoms may occur soon after delivery, stress incontinence being the most common. It is usually encountered in the middle-aged and elderly, who are often embarrassed and reluctant to visit the doctor until prolapse has been present for some time. Eighty per cent complain of a dragging sensation in the vagina or are aware of 'something coming down'. They may also complain of backache and urinary symptoms such as urgency, frequency, stress incontinence, or, rarely, urinary retention.

This occurs when there is a large cystocele with a well supported urethra leading to occlusion of the urethrovesical angle.

The sensation of the bowel being incompletely empty after defaecation occurs if there is an associated low rectocele. Sometimes the patient has to apply digital pressure on the rectocele from the vagina so that complete defaecation can occur. Keratinisation and decubitus ulceration of the exposed cervix occurs in procidentia caused by persistent exposure and rubbing of the epithelium which, in turn, results in bleeding and discharge, especially when infected.

Diagnosis

Genital prolapse is confirmed by careful examination and categorised into the three degrees mentioned on p. 269. The patient is first examined lying supine with legs abducted and drawn up. Third degree uterovaginal prolapse will be obvious. The vulva and introitus should be examined and the patient asked to cough, so demonstrating any stress incontinence. Second degree prolapse may also be seen. A double bladed speculum is then inserted, a cervical smear taken and any ulceration or keratinisation of the cervix or vagina noted. When this speculum is withdrawn slowly, enterocele and rectocele may be seen. A bimanual examination is then performed to identify any enlargement of the uterus or pelvic masses. The woman is then examined in the left lateral position with the right knee raised above the left one, with a single blade Sims speculum. This exposes the anterior and posterior vaginal walls and clearly reveals any cystocele and, when it is withdrawn, a rectocele or enterocele will be seen. Finally, a rectal examination will distinguish an enterocele from a high rectocele. The differential diagnosis includes any swelling at the introitus which, on superficial examination, may be mistaken for a true prolapse, but can consist of large cervical polyps, pedunculated fibroids, vaginal and Bartholin's cysts and, very rarely, chronic inversion of the uterus.

Treatment

Prophylactic

Ninety-five per cent of genital prolapse occurs in multiparous women, so prophylactic measures during and after labour are important. The second stage of labour should not be too long and patients must be prevented from bearing down before full dilatation. Postnatal exercises to tighten the perineal muscles, and drawing the anus forward are vital and every patient should continue these throughout the puerperium.

Ring or shelf pessaries are inserted in elderly patients who are unfit for surgery. Ring pessaries are also used for temporary relief of symptoms in prolapse occurring immediately after childbirth while awaiting the effects of involution and pelvic floor exercises. They are also used for relief of symptoms in those women awaiting surgery. Pessaries should be changed every 3 months to prevent impaction and vaginal ulceration. Application of local oestrogen creams improves the postmenopausal vaginal skin. In cases of procidentia, the uterus should be gently reinserted after moistening the dry uterus and a pessary inserted before proceeding to surgical repair at a later date. The use of local oestrogen cream will improve the condition of the vaginal mucosa before surgery.

Surgical

Today, fit patients with second or third degree uterovaginal prolapse, who are past childbearing age, undergo a vaginal hysterectomy (*see* p. 267) with anterior and posterior colporrhaphy, if there is associated cystocele and rectocele. If there is associated genuine stress incontinence, then widely placed urethral buttress sutures should be inserted. Others advocate a Burch colposuspension or a modified Peyera procedure to ensure permanent correction of the weak urethral sphincter. The Manchester operation consists of amputation of the cervix, tightening of the uterosacral ligaments and anteversion of the uterus by tightening the transverse cervical ligaments in front of the cervix, as well as anterior and posterior colporrhaphy. Most gynaecologists today perform a vaginal hysterectomy and colporrhaphies in preference to this procedure. However, it is sometimes performed in infirm patients who would not withstand a vaginal hysterectomy, or in younger women with a hypertrophied cervix without much uterine descent or in those wishing to keep the uterus. Vault prolapse can occur in up to 10% of patients following vaginal hysterectomy if care is not taken to excise any enterocele, or if a sufficiently high posterior colporrhaphy is not performed, or if the vaginal vault is not supported by suturing it to the transverse cervical ligaments. The middle-aged and elderly patient should be questioned about intercourse, and due care taken at operation to prevent removal of excessive vaginal skin leading to a narrowing of the introitus.

BLADDER PROBLEMS

Stress Incontinence

Stress incontinence denotes a symptom or a sign, but not a diagnosis. It commonly affects the middle-aged and elderly or the puerperal patient. About 5% of young nulliparous women have troublesome stress incontinence.

Stress incontinence was previously thought to be caused by the loss of the posterior urethrovesical angle as a result of increased intra-abdominal pressure such as coughing, or by a change in the angle of inclination of the urethral axis. Urinary continence depends upon a positive pressure gradient from the urethra to the bladder, thus ensuring that urethral pressure is always greater than the bladder pressure except during micturition. The urethral sphincter in women is weak and the urethral closing pressure is maintained by the effects of collagen, elastic tissue and urethral smooth and striated muscle. Incontinence does not occur in normal women because the proximal urethra and bladder neck lie above the pelvic floor. Coughing increases the intra-abdominal pressure, which is transmitted to this weak urethral sphincter increasing its closing power. Whenever the proximal urethra and bladder neck lie below the pelvic floor, as in a cystocoethrocele, the increased intra-abdominal pressure is not equally transmitted, so inefficient closure occurs, which cannot resist the increased intravesical pressure and incontinence results.

Stress incontinence may also be caused by a weakness of the urethral sphincter mechanism associated with multiparity, genital prolapse, menopausal atrophy or previous bladder neck surgery. Patients complaining of stress incontinence may or may not have associated frequency, urgency and urge incontinence. Demonstrable stress incontinence proves that the patient is incontinent, but does not diagnose the underlying condition.

Detrusor Instability

Detrusor instability or the unstable bladder presents with a history of frequency of micturition, sometimes as often as every 30–60 min, urgency of micturition, nocturia and urge and stress incontinence. It is a social problem, although it is perceived by the sufferer as possibly a serious organic problem. The detrusor muscle of the bladder contracts frequently and excessively, increasing the intravesical pressure markedly, and causing the frequent desire to micturate. Once urine reaches the proximal urethra, the micturition reflex is triggered and severe urgency and urge incontinence will follow.

The precise cause of detrusor instability is unknown in many cases, but it can follow pelvic surgery. Once the process starts, it can rapidly worsen as the woman responds to all the desires to micturate and temporarily loses the ability to suppress these, thereby establishing a vicious circle.

Overflow Incontinence

Overflow incontinence presents as constant dribbling, or voiding of small amounts of urine at frequent intervals, and stress incontinence. It can be caused by a lower motor neurone lesion, a pelvic mass, or inflammation of the urethra, vulva or vagina. Retention of urine can occur after pelvic surgery, epidural anaesthesia or following drugs such as ganglion blockers, anticholinergic drugs, β adrenergic stimulants and tricyclic antidepressants.

Fistulae

Vesicovaginal and uterovaginal fistulae occur after pelvic surgery and irradiation therapy for pelvic malignancies, but in developed countries they are very uncommon. In developing countries vesicovaginal fistulae commonly occur after prolonged labour which causes pressure necrosis of the bladder. These fistulae cause continuous incontinence, and can be seen on speculum examination.

Congenital abnormalities are rare and are normally diagnosed at birth or infancy, when the child does not become dry at the normal age. These include epispadias and ectopic ureters.

Functional incontinence is found in a small number of patients where there is no organic cause.

These anxious patients usually respond to reassurance or psychiatric counselling.

History and Examination

A detailed accurate history will yield clues as to the diagnosis. Urinary frequency may be caused by small bladder capacity or excessive drinking or the patient's inherent fear of wetting herself if she does not micturate often enough. Nocturia may be a symptom of detrusor instability, but is commonly caused by poor drinking habits and insomnia. Enuresis, past or present, is associated with detrusor instability.

Physical examination is usually unhelpful, but stress incontinence may be confirmed by asking the patient to cough with a full bladder. It does not, however, indicate the cause of the stress incontinence. Vaginal examination may reveal vaginitis, a pelvic mass or a uterovaginal prolapse, which may contribute to the stress incontinence. Neurological examination of the perineal branches of the sacral plexus must be performed to exclude a neurological cause in patients with mixed symptoms.

Diagnosis

Carefully history taking and careful examination will diagnose up to 90% of cases of genuine stress incontinence. However, a midstream specimen of urine must always be sent for culture to exclude a urinary tract infection. Urodynamic investigations such as cystometry — the measurement of bladder intraurethral or intra-abdominal pressures — will distinguish between genuine stress incontinence and detrusor instability in the majority of cases. Cystoscopy, micturating cystography and videocystourethrography are useful investigations in complicated cases with mixed symptoms.

Treatment

An accurate diagnosis must be made before proceeding to treatment, as genuine stress incontinence can be cured by surgery, but detrusor instability is not remedial to surgical repair.

There are numerous types of operation to elevate the bladder neck and proximal urethra to an intra-abdominal position to increase urethral sphincter closing pressure. Suprapubic procedures such as the Marshall-Marchetti-Krantz operation, Burch colposuspension and various sling procedures give better results than the traditional anterior colporrhaphy and bladder buttress sutures. The modified Peyera procedure combines both suprapubic sling and bladder buttress sutures and is used in the United States. Failure to cure genuine stress incontinence initially offers less chance of successful repair at successive operations, so choice of a suitable procedure is important.

The surgical principles of these operations are as follows:

Marshall-Marchetti-Krantz: paraurethral tissues are sutured to periosteum of posterior aspect of pubic symphysis.

Burch colposuspension: fascia overlying lateral vaginal fornices is sutured to pectineal ligaments. As vagina is suspended, so it raises the bladder and elongates the urethra.

Peyera procedure: thick fascia lateral to urethra is sutured bilaterally and tied to anterior rectus sheath giving a suspension and sling effect.

In all these three operations non-absorbable suture material is used.

Bladder support per vagina: bladder is mobilised and supported by plication of vesicovaginal fascia, using either absorbable or non-absorbable sutures (Kelly or Pacey sutures).

Detrusor instability is difficult to treat and patients are taught Frewen's regimen of bladder drill and exercises to improve the tone of the perineal muscles, so strengthening the pelvic floor. Frewen's regime involves (1) re-emphasising and retraining the ability to resist urge incontinence; (2) simultaneously reducing frequency of micturition by deliberately increasing the time between voiding. This has to be done gradually. If successful, not only is frequency improved, but also urgency nocturia and even stress incontinence will be reduced. This gives the patient more understanding of the problems and the realisation that self-treatment is important and usually successful. Frequent follow-up and reassurance leads to improvement in symptoms. An unstable bladder can be converted to a stable one in 80% of patients by these measures. The ganglion blocker, emepronium bromide, produces temporary relief of symptoms, and the tricyclic antidepressant imipramine helps those

with nocturia or enuresis as well as reducing urgency and urinary frequency.

BENIGN OVARIAN TUMOURS

The ovary is composed of epithelial cells derived from the coelomic epithelium, oocytes, which have differentiated from primitive germ cells, and medullary or mesenchymal elements. With such embryological cell lines being represented in the ovary, it is hardly surprising that no other organ in the body produces such a diversity and number of tumours. Classification of these tumours is difficult.

Tumour-like Conditions of the Ovary

Atretic cysts

When the graafian follicle or the corpus luteum are undergoing natural degeneration, they may become cystic. The cysts are small, often multiple and lined by granulosa cells, granulosa lutein cells, theca lutein cells or connective and hyaline tissue. Such cysts are invariably symptomless.

Distension or retention cysts

Cystic enlargement of a normal ovarian component is so common as to be considered physiological. It is of no pathological significance, although, if complicated by intracystic haemorrhage, the resultant tarry contents may be confused with endometriosis.

Follicular and theca lutein cysts

These cysts represent enlargements of unruptured graafian follicles. The ovum degenerates, but the granulosa and theca cells continue to secrete fluid. They rarely exceed 5 cm in size, are occasionally multiple and usually symptomless. Where granulosa cells predominate, enough oestrogen may be produced to cause menorrhagia. When oestrogen or progesterone production is continuous, short periods of amenorrhoea occur. Repeated cyst formation may cause iliac fossa pain. Treatment is rarely, if ever, required. The cysts often rupture spontaneously or during pelvic examination. Recurrent follicular cystic development can be suppressed by inhibiting ovulation with an oral contraceptive.

Corpus luteal cysts

A normal corpus luteum may become cystic, especially after haemorrhage into its cavity. Quite a large cyst can arise in the corpus luteum of pregnancy.

Occasionally, the corpus luteum becomes cystic and continues to produce progesterone. This causes short periods of amenorrhoea followed by heavier than usual menstruation, thus mimicking early pregnancy and spontaneous abortion or ectopic pregnancy.

Corpus luteum cysts require no treatment unless, exceptionally, excision to stop intraperitoneal bleeding.

Compound lutein cysts

In the presence of trophoblastic disease, large, multiple lutein cysts may arise in both ovaries. The excessive luteinisation is directly due to the production of human chorionic gonadotrophin (HCG) by the trophoblastic tissue. Once this tissue is removed, the hormonal stimulus disappears and the ovaries return to normal.

Solid luteoma of pregnancy

Solid foci, usually multiple, of luteal tissue may be found in the ovaries during pregnancy. They are caused by HCG stimulating theca or stromal cells. They are separate from the corpus luteum and may be up to 10 cm in diameter. Usually symptomless, they are found incidentally at caesarean section or laparotomy.

Benign Ovarian Pathology

Surface papilloma

This is a small, often multiple, pedunculated surface growth with a marked connective tissue core. It is usually an incidental finding at laparotomy.

Mucinous or pseudomucinous cystadenoma

This is the commonest primary neoplasm of the ovary, accounting for 30–40% of ovarian tumours (Fig. 19.5). It is unilateral in 90% of cases. Although

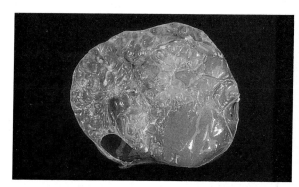

Fig. 19.5   *Benign mucinous multilocular cystadenoma. Small cystic spaces are present and some contain thick, glairy mucus.*

its growth is slow, it may attain huge proportions. It may develop at any time. It is a multilocular cyst, usually with a smooth, thick, fibrous wall. The lining membrane of the loculi is composed of tall, columnar, mucin-secreting cells with darkly staining nuclei situated near their base. Rarely, papillary ingrowths are present within the cyst and may reflect malignant degeneration to an adenocarcinoma, which occurs in 5–10% of cases.

The fluid within the cyst is mucinous, usually colourless and of variable consistency, containing a glycoprotein related to mucin. Although large in size, the cyst generally remains without adhesions and can be removed without difficulty. A rare complication of a cyst which ruptures and leaks its contents into the peritoneal cavity is pseudomyxoma peritonei. Cells from within the cyst implant in the parietal and visceral peritoneum and the omentum and continue to secrete mucin. Formidable multiple, intraperitoneal adhesions form, enclosing large masses of gelatinous material occupying loculi in all parts of the abdominal cavity. Even after removal at laparotomy, these gelatinous loculi tend to reform and the patient usually dies from cachexia after several operations. The condition may also be seen with mucocele of the appendix.

Serous cystadenoma (Fig. 19.6)

This cyst accounts for approximately 10% of ovarian tumours. It is usually smaller than its pseudomucinous counterpart, and is bilateral in 30–50% of cases. The outer surface is commonly smooth and thin walled and the entire cyst is unilocular. The contents are thin and watery, composed of various

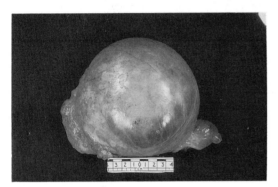

Fig. 19.6 *Benign serous cystadenoma of moderate size. Smooth outer surface with thin walls. The fallopian tube is stretched over the cyst.*

albumins and globulins, and are colourless, unless contaminated by blood pigments.

The inner surface of the cyst wall nearly always contains papilliferous projections, often warty or cauliflower-like in appearance. These papillae may range in number, being few and localised to one area, or fill the entire cyst, giving it a solid appearance, with all gradations in between. These papillae may occur on the outer surface and cause ascites. Although such a cyst may look malignant, the majority are histologically benign.

The lining cells are cuboidal or columnar and may be ciliated resembling the epithelium of the fallopian tube. Often small deposits of calcium are present in the stroma and are known as psammoma bodies. The epithelium may range from a well-differentiated benign pattern to the marked atypia and anaplasia of malignancy. In those cysts where the epithelium adopts a more intermediate pattern, it can be extremely difficult to allot the tumour into a benign or malignant category.

Fibroma

This tumour accounts for up to 5% of ovarian neoplasms. It is slow growing and rarely exceeds 12 cm in diameter. Usually spherical or ovoid in shape, it can be lobulated and is invariably mobile. It is solid and hard, and its cut surface is white and whorled. The tumour is bilateral in up to 10% of cases. It may replace the entire ovary or exist as a small surface nodule.

Histologically, it is composed of spindle cells of fibroblastic character. Plain muscle cells may or may not be present, but the tumour behaves in a similar fashion to a uterine fibroid. Hyaline change is common and most large fibromas show cystic changes caused by central necrosis due to poor blood supply.

A fibroma of the ovary may cause ascites in 20% of cases. Often associated is hydrothorax (usually right sided); Meig's syndrome is the triad of ovarian fibroma, ascites and hydrothorax. The origin of the fluid is variously ascribed to an exudate resulting from irritation of the peritoneum by the tumour or to an active secretion by the tumour.

Removal of the fibroma results in the spontaneous cure of the ascites and the hydrothorax. The findings always cause concern, since they impart a clinical impression of malignancy and therefore reassurance of the woman is important.

Adenofibroma

This is often a small fibropapillary nodule occurring on the surface of the ovary. It is solid and behaves similarly to the fibroma. Histologically, it contains both fibromatous and glandular tissues.

Benign cystic teratoma or dermoid cyst

These tumours are unique in that all three embryological layers — ectoderm, mesoderm and endoderm — may be represented. They probably arise from varied differentiation of totipotential cells within the ovary. Some suggest that they arise from parthenogenesis, where an ovum is stimulated to make a disorderly attempt to produce an embryo without first being fertilised.

Dermoid cysts account for 10–15% of ovarian tumours. They tend to occur at a relatively early age (18–30 years), and are usually symptomless. They are bilateral in 10% of cases. They rarely grow bigger than 12 cm in diameter and are usually unilocular with a thick, smooth capsule. They contain a thick, yellow, greasy sebaceous fluid, secreted by the glands within the wall, and often hair and teeth project into this fluid.

Histologically, the lining epithelium is typically stratified squamous-like skin, and contains the normal integuments of hair, sebaceous glands and sweat glands. Teeth and central nervous system tissues are not unusual, and cartilage and gastro-intestinal epithelium may be present. There is generally a nodal point in the cyst wall around which these tissues are distributed.

Although cystic teratomata are predominantly ectodermal in character, this is not always so, especially in the more solid variety. For example, when thyroid tissue predominates the cyst is called 'struma ovarii', and the glandular epithelium may be functional, capable of causing clinical hyperthyroidism. When other specialised tissues predominate, the cyst may be suffixed lipoma, myoma, chondroma or osteoma.

Once a teratoma is suspected clinically, the diagnosis is easily confirmed by the typical multiple echogeneity found at ultrasound scan, or the presence of teeth within the pelvis at x-ray. In most cases, benign cysts can be enucleated intact, but the contralateral ovary should be carefully inspected to exclude the presence of small cysts.

Other benign connective tissue tumours

Other solid tumours which may arise from the connective tissues of the ovary include myoma, lipoma, chondroma, osteoma, haemangioma and lymphangioma. All are extremely rare with no distinguishing clinical pattern. As mentioned earlier, some of these neoplasms may arise from a benign teratoma.

Clinical Features of Benign Ovarian Tumours

Benign primary ovarian neoplasms are most commonly found in women aged 40–60 years, the benign cystic teratoma being an exception.

Small tumours may be asymptomatic and found incidentally when the patient is examined for other reasons. When large, the patient may notice abdominal distension and the pressure effects of dyspepsia or frequency of micturition. Uterovaginal prolapse may be exacerbated by an ovarian cyst.

An innocent neoplasm is invariably painless unless an accident overtakes it (see below).

The physical signs are not difficult to elicit. When pelvic, the benign tumour is usually distinguishable from the uterus as a smooth, mobile adnexal swelling. Endometriomata may be irregular and fixed, features suggestive of malignancy. As the tumour rises into the abdomen, it may take up a central position, displacing the intestines above and to the sides. The tumour is dull to percussion centrally with areas of resonance laterally from displaced bowel allowing distinction from ascites.

The differential diagnosis and further investigations required are similar to those outlined under malignant epithelial tumours of the ovary.

Complications of Ovarian Cysts

These include:

1. Torsion of the pedicle;
2. Rupture of the cyst;
3. Haemorrhage into or from a cyst;
4. Infection.

All present with pain, swelling and tenderness over the cyst. Laporotomy is indicated.

Treatment

The management of benign ovarian tumours is to a large extent dictated by the age of the patient. In the young, it is important to preserve ovarian function and future fertility, and ovarian cystectomy is indicated. Where the adnexal tissues are unhealthy from ischaemic damage after torsion of the ovarian pedicle, salpingo-oophorectomy may be the only option. Total abdominal hysterectomy and bilateral salpingo-oophorectomy is generally accepted as the treatment of choice in those over 40 years, as the family is usually complete and there is the possibility of early malignant change within the cyst for which this operation would be the appropriate treatment.

Whichever procedure is performed, meticulous histological examination of the specimen is imperative to confirm the nature of the tumour. If totally benign, no further treatment will be required.

FURTHER READING

Fox H. (1984). Gynaecologic pathology: advances, perspectives and problems. In *Clinics in Obstetrics and Gynaecology*, Vol. 12, No. 1. London: W.B. Saunders.

Muse K.N., Wilson E.A. (1982). How does endometriosis cause infertility? *Fertil. Steril*; **38**: 145–52.

Monaghan J.M. (1987). *Gynaecological Surgery*. London: Ballière.

20

Malignant Disorders of the Reproductive Organs

CARCINOMA OF THE CERVIX

Carcinoma of the cervix is the second most common cancer in women in the UK after carcinoma of the breast. In the USA, it is the third most common cancer after the breast and endometrium. The peak incidence of cervical cancer occurs in the sixth decade, but it can occur as early as the second decade and it does seem that, increasingly, some aggressive tumours can affect women in their twenties.

Although the actual cause of the disease is not known, the following predisposing/associated factors are acknowledged:

Intercourse;
<20 years old at first intercourse or pregnancy;
Multiparity;
Non-barrier methods of contraception;.
Smoking;
Numerous sexual partners;

Human papovavirus: types 6 and 11 with CIN; types 16 and 18 with invasive carcinoma;
Possible association with *Herpes simplex 2* virus and other sexually transmitted diseases.

Cervical Intraepithelial Neoplasia

The term 'Cervical Intraepithelial Neoplasia' (CIN) has more recently been accepted to reflect the dynamic background of epithelial abnormalities. The degrees of abnormality merge imperceptibly and the distinguishing features of severe dysplasia and carcinoma-in-situ are artificial. CIN is graded 1 to 3 and how this relates to the old terminology is shown in Table 20.1. The more severe the CIN is, the more likely it is to progress both to a greater degree of CIN and to invasive carcinoma, while the less severe the CIN is, the more likely it is to regress.

Aetiology

The ectocervix is covered by stratified squamous

Table 20.1

Classification of CIN in Relation to the World Health Organization (WHO, 1975) Classification of Cervical Dysplasia

Normal	Squamous metaplasia	Probable low risk of early invasion		Probable high risk of early invasion	
Normal	Squamous metaplasia	CIN 1 Mild dysplasia	CIN 2 Moderate dysplasia	CIN 3–4 Severe dysplasia	Carcinoma in situ

(After M.C. Anderson, 1982. London: RCOG.)

epithelium. The endocervical canal is lined by columnar epithelium. These epithelial surfaces meet at the squamo-columnar junction (SCJ). Before puberty, the SCJ lies just within the endocervical canal at the external cervical os (Fig. 20.1).. During and soon after adolescence the ovarian hormones produce an increase in the volume of the cervix, resulting in the eversion of the lower portion of the endocervical canal. Columnar epithelium and the underlying glands and stroma come to lie on the vaginal portion of the cervix (Fig. 20.2). This newly exposed area is extremely important as not only may normal, physiological squamous metaplasia occur here, but also squamous intraepithelial or invasive neoplasia may arise. The area over which these changes are likely to occur is called the transformation zone.

The precise aetiology of CIN remains uncertain. The known associated factors such as age at first intercourse and multiple partners suggest that some factor transmitted at coitus may be important. Several causal agents have been suggested, four of which are noteworthy.

1. Smegma. Cervical neoplasia was noted to be less common in Jewish women. It was postulated that, since circumcised males did not have the collection of desquamated cells and secretions, known as smegma, which occurred under the foreskin of uncircumcised males, this substance was carcinogenic. There is no evidence to support this theory.

2. Spermatozoa. It has been proposed that the DNA of the sperm head becomes integrated with the subepithelial cell genome, and mutation of the cell occurs as a result. Whether such a stimulus is sufficient to induce neoplasia awaits proof.

3. Viral infection. *Herpes simplex* virus (type 2) is known to cause genital herpes, and following its isolation, some studies demonstrated that women with cervical dysplasia and carcinoma had a high titre of specific viral antibody. However, not all patients show a significant rise in titre and the previous findings are now thought simply to reflect promiscuity, as genital herpes is a very infectious venereal disease.

More recent evidence has shown that neoplasia may be induced by human papovavirus (HPV), or wart virus. Several types of HPV are known, and increasingly large numbers of women are found to have dysplastic changes in cervical smears along with cellular changes associated with wart infection. Also, warty infection of the cervix is increasingly recognised at colposcopic examination. HPV types 6 and 11 have been strongly implicated with CIN and types 16 and 18 with cervical carcinoma.

4. The high risk male. The subepithelial stromal cell is considered to be the cell from which new squamous metaplastic epithelium arises. These stromal cells are thought to contain surface DNA which induces protein synthesis. If interference occurs, the mechanism of protein synthesis is disrupted and a neoplastic cell is formed. Basic proteins, such as arginine rich proteins found in the sperm head, are capable of causing this disruption, and the sperm of some males is especially likely to do so.

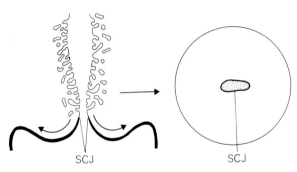

Fig. 20.1 *Prepubertal cervix. (After M.C. Anderson, 1982. London: RCOG.)*

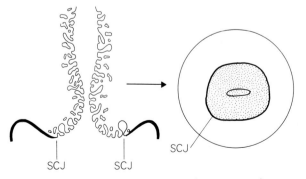

Fig. 20.2 *Postadolescent cervix. (After M.C. Anderson, 1982. London: RCOG.)*

Pathology

The diagnosis and grading of CIN is based on the histological criteria of maturation, differentiation and stratification of the cells, nuclear abnormalities and mitotic activity.

In CIN 1, loss of polarity and stratification are minimal. The nuclei are always enlarged, often irregular and darkly staining. Mitoses are often found, but are only occasionally abnormal and confined to the lower third of the epithelium. The cytoplasm is well preserved and keratinisation of the epithelial surface is common.

With CIN 2, the degree of epithelial abnormality is intermediate between CIN 1 and CIN 3. Atypia is pronounced in CIN 3. Polarity is lost, and the crowded cells have large, darkly staining nuclei. The abnormal cells are present throughout the entire thickness of the epithelium, but there is no invasion of the underlying stroma. Cytoplasm is scanty. Mitoses, both normal and abnormal, are scattered throughout the epithelium.

Diagnosis

CIN 3 has been reported at all ages from the early teens to the mid-eighties, with the most common age at diagnosis ranging from 30 to 45 years. It is characteristically asymptomatic, and while common gynaecological symptoms such as vaginal discharge, postcoital bleeding and intermenstrual bleeding may coexist with CIN, they are not the cause. Examination often reveals a normal cervix or, occasionally, a red patch, and colposcopy is required to fully appreciate the character and extent of the lesion.

Cervical screening. Exfoliative cytology is the most effective method of detecting cervical intra-epithelial neoplasia. The frequency of CIN in teen-agers is increasing, and most gynaecologists would recommend that any sexually active woman should have regular smears either at three- or five-year intervals. Promiscuous women in their teens or twenties should have annual smears.

CIN may be identified in smears, because the exfoliated cells show abnormal nuclei, increased nuclear : cytoplasmic ratio and immature cytoplasmic differentiation. Such a cell is termed dyskaryotic. The degree of dyskaryosis is determined from the size of the abnormal nucleus in relation to the amount of cytoplasm, the immaturity of the cyto-

plasm and the nuclear characteristics of malignancy. Detection of an abnormal smear should be followed by colposcopy.

Colposcopy. The colposcope (Fig. 20.3) provides an optical method for examining the illuminated cervix and lower genital tract at a magnification intermediate between the naked eye and lower power of the microscope.

The woman is placed in the lithotomy position and a Cusco speculum is introduced to expose the cervix. When the blades are separated, the cervix is everted and the lowermost parts of the endocervical canal are easily visualised. The cervix is gently wiped with a cotton wool, saline-soaked swab to remove any secretions or blood. The colour, pattern of blood vessels and surface contour of the cervix is noted. A 3% acetic acid solution is next applied. This coagulates the mucus, aiding its removal, and atypical epithelium becomes white. Usually, the

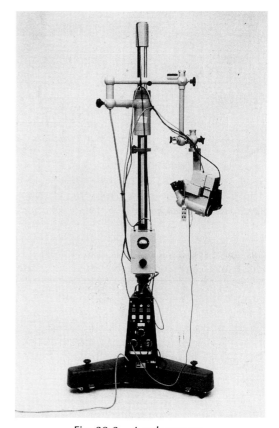

Fig. 20.3   *A colposcope.*

vascular pattern is accentuated, giving a mosaic or punctate pattern. If the endocervical limit of the transformation zone is not visualised, an endocervical speculum may be introduced into the cervical canal to allow further exposure. The upper limit of the transformation zone must be seen for the examination to be conclusive. Lugol's iodine may be applied to the cervix. The stain is taken up by the normal, glycogen-containing, squamous epithelium and areas of CIN fail to take up the stain as they are glycogen free.

Any abnormal areas may be biopsied, without significant discomfort, and submitted for histological examination.

Treatment

Local ablation. There are several techniques for local ablative therapy, but common to them all are the criteria for their use. These are extremely important and should never be ignored.

1. The most abnormal area should be sampled by biopsy before treatment.
2. The squamo-columnar junction must be fully visible.
3. There must be adequate follow-up.
4. The presence of invasive carcinoma is excluded.

The techniques for local ablation are listed below. They all eradicate the lesion by physical destruction, and they must be capable of destroying abnormal cells contained within the crypts of the cervical glands. These crypts have been shown to have a mean depth of 3.38 mm and, in order to ensure total destruction of any lesion, the tissue is treated to a depth of 6–7 mm.

Cryotherapy. Persistence of CIN occurs in about 10% of cases and retreatment achieves a cure rate of 96%.

Electrocoagulation diathermy. This method employs heat to destroy tissue. General anaesthesia is required and the remaining cervical tissue may undergo a degree of fibrosis.

CIN may be eradicated in up to 97.3% of patients by a single diathermy treatment.

Cold coagulation. A teflon probe is applied to the cervical tissue and heated to 100°C ('cold' in rela-

tion to diathermy). General anaesthesia is not required and side-effects are few. A 95% cure rate for CIN 3 may be achieved by this method.

Carbon dioxide laser therapy. This is accepted as one of the most effective modes of treatment for CIN. It is easy to use, the evaporation of the tissues is rapid, there is no damage to normal surrounding tissue and the endocervical canal after healing remains readily accessible for future screening. Cure rate after one treatment is 95%.

Cone biopsy. The main indications for cone biopsy are:

1. The lesion(s) or the transformation zone extend(s) into the endocervical canal, the upper limit remaining invisible.
2. Colposcopic suspicion of a microinvasive or invasive lesion.
3. Abnormal histology of endocervical curettings.
4. Repeated abnormal cervical cytology suggesting neoplasia without colposcopically visible abnormality.
5. The cervical smear suggests an invasive lesion not confirmed at colposcopy or by direct biopsy.

The aim of cone biopsy is to remove all the abnormal tissue with a small margin of normal tissue (Fig. 20.4). Incomplete excision of the lesion has been reported in from 5 to 40% of cases, and prior colposcopic assessment of the cervix may help in delineating the lesion accurately. The main complication after cone biopsy is haemorrhage. Packing of the vagina usually suffices, but secondary suturing is sometimes required. Cervical stenosis causing menstrual problems has been reported in 1–4% of cases. In subsequent pregnancy, there is a risk of spontaneous abortion and preterm labour, up to 22 and 10% respectively. The laser can be

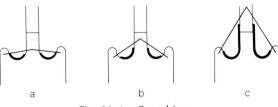

a   b   c

Fig. 20.4　*Cone biopsy.*

used to cut the cone, thereby minimising haemorrhage and allowing the operation to be done as an outpatient. At present this is experimental, but could become standard practice.

Hysterectomy. Hysterectomy is now only rarely used for the treatment of CIN. The indications are:

1. The presence of other gynaecological disorders requiring hysterectomy, such as fibroids, menorrhagia or uterovaginal prolapse. Cervical biopsy to confirm the intraepithelial nature of the lesion is worthwhile.
2. Sterilisation has been requested.
3. Remaining intraepithelial neoplasia at the excision lines of a cone biopsy. Local ablation or further cone biopsy may also be possible.
4. Persistent abnormal smears following local ablative techniques.
5. The lesion extends on to the vaginal vault. This may still be treatable with local measures, especially laser therapy, but hysterectomy may be appropriate. Colposcopic assessment is valuable in accurately determining the size of the vaginal cuff to be removed.
6. Occasionally, when CIN occurs in the postmenopausal patient, hysterectomy may be technically easier than cone biopsy, especially if the cervix is small.

The incidence of CIN continues to rise, reflecting the increased sexual freedom of the last 20 years. Frequent smears from the population most at risk, rather than from a low risk group who present at well-women clinics, followed by colposcopy and proper ablative treatment by well trained personnel should help to keep the increase from rising excessively.

Invasive Carcinoma of the Cervix

There are two types of epithelium found in the cervix: stratified squamous epithelium covering the vaginal portion and columnar epithelium which lines the cervical canal and its glands. There are therefore two types of tumour, 90% of these being squamous cell carcinoma arising from the squamous epithelium, usually at the squamo-columnar junction, and 10% of tumours arising from the columnar cells of the endocervix. Squamous cell carcinoma may extend upwards into the lower part of the cervical canal and, similarly, the columnar

cells may undergo squamous metaplasia and subsequent malignancy. A tumour involving both types of epithelium is termed an 'adenoacanthoma'.

The naked eye appearance of cervical carcinoma varies considerably. The lesion may be exophytic, forming a delicate polypoid mass which bleeds readily; it may arise within the endocervix and grow to distend the cervix, forming the barrel cervix; it may infiltrate the cervix, making it very hard and larger, without any external evidence of malignancy; it may form a malignant ulcer which extends off the cervix into the vaginal fornices.

Histopathology

The microscopical appearance of squamous cell carcinoma tumour will reveal large branching, solid epithelial columns of cells breaking through the basement membrane and penetrating into the fibromuscular tissue destroying it (Fig. 20.5). Peripheral cells from these invading columns are cubical and they become more irregular towards the centre. The nuclei are large, hyperchromatic and mitotic figures are frequent. The normal protoplasmic bridges which bind the cells together are usually clearly seen. Epithelial pearls, which are small areas of flattened cells arranged concentrically occur occasionally. If tumour growth is rapid, there will be multinucleated cells due to lack of cell body division. There will be areas of necrosis, as well as round cell infiltration and oedema of the stroma.

A well-differentiated Grade I tumour will show (1) keratin/epithelial pearls; (2) minimal variation in the size of tumour cells; (3) less than two mitoses per high power field.

A poorly differentiated Grade III tumour will show (1) hardly any resemblance to the tissue of origin; (2) no epithelial pearls and only slight keratin; (3) four mitoses or more per HPF. There is an intermediate group, Grade II. The degree of malignancy corresponds to the grade, thus well differentiated Grade I lesions do better than poorly differentiated Grade III lesions.

Adenocarcinoma of the cervix is composed of columnar secretory cells, which are tall and arranged in a glandular pattern with scant supporting stroma. Tubular formations project from the wall of the glands outwards invading the intravening stroma. These processes branch and elongate with the greater part of the spread being outwards in the cervix. Evidence of malignancy in these cases is based upon the invasion and destruction of the

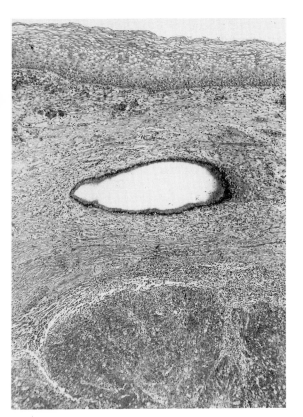

Fig. 20.5   *Carcinoma of the cervix. This section shows normal epithelium and endocervical gland. There is invasive tumour seen in the lower part of the section.*

the disease can be made (FIGO, International Federation of Gynaecology and Obstetrics), Table 20.2, but as no special investigations are involved a

Table 20.2

Staging of Carcinoma of the Cervix

Cervix		FIGO
Carcinoma in situ		0
Confined to cervix		I
Microinvasive		Ia
Invasive		Ib
Extension to	{ vagina (not lower ⅓) { parametrium (not pelvic wall)	II
Vagina (not lower ⅓)		IIa
Parametrium (not pelvic wall)		IIb
Extension to	{ lower ⅓ vagina { pelvic wall of parametrium	III
Lower ⅓ vagina		IIIa
Pelvic wall of parametrium		IIIb
Extension to bladder, rectum, beyond		
true pelvis		IVa
Distant organs		IVb

stroma by the proliferating tubules. Adenocarcinoma is not usually diagnosed until it is advanced.

Presentation

The patient usually presents with a history of PMB or postcoital bleeding (PCB), the latter being more common in younger women. Advanced cases may present with a foul blood-stained discharge. The diagnosis may be apparent clinically after taking the history and noting the findings on examination. The cervical tumour may be felt on vaginal and rectal examination to be involving the rectum, or uterosacral ligaments or pelvic side wall. The uterus may be enlarged by a pyometra. In these cases the carcinoma blocks the cervical canal causing retention of secretions, inflammation and often infection with anaerobes, although specific organisms may not be demonstrated. A clinical staging of

patient may be 'understaged' and could, as a result, be undertreated.

Accurate staging may avoid unnecessary treatments — especially surgery. Both surgery and radiotherapy carry a morbidity and the combination of both leads to greater morbidity. The majority of patients with cervical cancer are treated adequately by radiotherapy alone. There are reported reviews in which Stage I disease does as well with radiotherapy as with surgery. However, surgery offers the younger woman the chance of conserving ovarian and sexual function. Radiotherapy induces the menopause and fibrotic and atrophic changes in the vagina. Some surgeons limit radical surgery to Stage I lesions; others to Stage I and Stage IIa.

Carcinoma of the cervix spreads into the myometrium, the vaginal skin, the paracervical lymphatics and from there to the obturator, internal and external iliac nodes. It also directly invades the parametrial tissues, and can invade the rectum or bladder with fistual formation.

The inguinal, femoral common iliac and para-aortic nodes can be involved. The lymphatic spread of cervical carcinoma is illustrated in Fig. 20.6.

Surgery may still have a role to play in disease that has advanced beyond Stage I in those patients in whom the primary lesion is large and has expanded the cervix and possibly the lower uterus to give a barrel-shaped tumour. Hypoxia at the centre of such a tumour makes it less radiosensitive and, therefore, at the end of treatment viable tumour cells may be left amid the fibrous tissue resulting from the radiotherapy. No one can say looking at these cells whether they are active, dormant or dying, but a simple abdominal hysterectomy will remove them and possibly prevent central recurrence. In poorly differentiated lesions, chemotherapy may have a role to play, as adjuvant treatment to radiotherapy.

Management

History. The patient is usually referred with an abnormal cervical smear or postmenstrual bleeding, but may present through the casualty department with heavy abnormal bleeding or blood-stained discharge. Postcoital and abnormal intermenstrual bleeding may be features. Weight loss, bone pains and abdominal pains are all serious symptoms. Haematuria will suggest bladder involvement; tenesmus and rectal bleeding will infer rectal involvement. Neglected cases may present with small bowel obstruction, pelvic pain, abdominal gland masses or fistulae.

Examination. Thorough general examination is mandatory with especial reference to lymph nodes. Speculum examination plus cervical cytology should precede vaginal and rectal examination, which will form the basis for FIGO staging.

Special tests. Having reached the position of strongly suspecting a diagnosis of carcinoma of the cervix, special tests are required to confirm the diagnosis and 'stage' the disease (Table 20.3). The staging of carcinoma of the cervix is shown in Table 20.2, p. 283.

Treatment

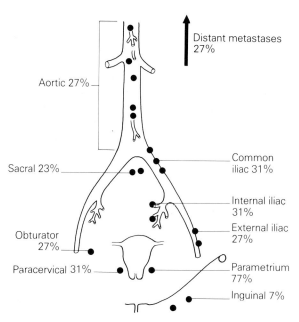

Fig. 20.6   *Nodes involved in spread of cervical carcinoma in untreated patients (After E. Henriksen, 1949. Amer. J. Obstet. Gynecol;* **58**:924.)

Table 20.3

Tests for Staging Carcinoma of the Cervix

Confirmation of the diagnosis
   Cervical cytology
   Punch/wedge/cone biopsy

Staging the lesion
   Colposcopy of the vagina and vulvo-perineal region
   Chest x-ray
   Intravenous urogram
   Urine cytology on an MSU
   Examination under anaesthetic
   Cystoscopy ± bladder biopsy
   Estimate bladder volume
   Biopsy of vaginal lesions (if any)
   Aspiration of connective tissue lateral to the uterus
      and within the broad ligament
   Parametrial aspiration
   Rectal examination ± sigmoidoscopy
   Lymphangiogram ± percutaneous lymph node
      aspiration
   Pelvic ultrasound scan
   Bone scan (in young patient with poorly
      differentiated/aggressive tumours)

Other investigations
   Full blood count
   Urea and electrolytes
   Creatinine and creatinine clearance
   Liver function tests
   Electrocardiogram

Stage 0 (CIN 3). Treatment is by complete destruction or removal of the affected area. If the dysplastic area is completely seen on the ectocervix and the squamo-columnar junction is completely visible, the choice of treatment lies between cone biopsy, simple hysterectomy or local ablation by laser, radical cautery, 'cold' coagulation or freezing. If the squamo-columnar junction is not seen, cone biopsy is required. Certain patients may be better treated by hysterectomy — those with menorrhagia, fibroids, a desire for sterilisation, etc. Where endo-cervical disease is present, cone biopsy or hysterectomy is performed.

Stage Ia (microinvasive disease). Treatment for Stage I disease is usually by surgical removal of the disease. If the lesion extends 2 mm or less into the stroma, cone biopsy or simple hysterectomy are currently considered to be adequate treatment.

Stage Ib. Wertheim-Meigs radical hysterectomy with pelvic lymphadenectomy. Preoperative staging should establish that the pelvic nodes are not involved. If they are, the disease is not curable by surgery. Wertheim himself removed the pelvic nodes to establish the prognosis, but only if they were enlarged. Surgery should be avoided if the lymph nodes are obviously involved with malignant disease. Technically such tumours are Stage IV, i.e. outside the reproductive tract.

Stages II, III, and IV. These receive radiotherapy with or without chemotherapy. Sometimes radiotherapy may be given preoperatively, although this increases the risks of operative and postoperative complications.

Radiotherapy. The undergraduate is not required to have a detailed knowledge of radiotherapy, but a brief outline of the treatment of cervical carcinoma follows.

External radiotherapy: 4500–5000 cGy are given to the pelvis, plus 2000–2500 cGy from an *intracavitary* source to Point A. (Point A is defined as lying 2 cm lateral to the central cervical canal and 2 cm above the lateral fornix in the axis of the uterus; approximately the point where the uterine artery crosses the ureter.) Intracavitary radiotherapy can be given using a radioactive material in ovoids which are placed at the vaginal vault under general anaesthesia together with a source in the uterus if present. A newer technique involves the use of an after-loading device, in which a mould is inserted into the vagina and then a radioactive source is mechanically inserted into the mould once the attendants have left the room.

If the para-aortic nodes are involved, 4000 cGy are given to this region and to the pelvis, followed by a further 1000 cGy to the pelvis and a further 2000 cGy is administered to Point A from an intracavitary source.

Chemotherapy. If chemotherapy is used, the usual drugs are cis-platinum, methotrexate and cyclophosphamide. Usually, two courses are given before radiotherapy, and some patients also receive chemotherapy after radiotherapy.

The prognosis for women with advanced cervical cancer is poor. At present, the benefits of chemotherapy are not well defined. In certain cases it may prolong survival, while in others it may cause shrinkage of a large proliferative lesion so that palliative surgical removal is feasible.

Follow-up

Ideally patients are followed up in a combined gynaecology/oncology clinic. At each visit the patient should be asked about normal discharge or bleeding, urinary problems, bowel habit and sexual activity. She should be weighed, and the breasts, abdomen, vagina and rectum examined. A vault or cervical smear should be taken. An annual chest x-ray should be performed. Intravenous urography, ultrasound scan and CAT scans of the pelvis can be requested as indicated. They are most helpful in those patients who are difficult to examine well. Nuclear Magnetic Resonance scans may be useful in distinguishing tumour from fibrous tissue in the woman who has had both surgery and radiotherapy.

The colposcope is a useful tool in the follow-up of these cases, as it allows close inspection of the genital tract from cervix/vault to vulva. There is a recognised association between cervical carcinoma and vulval carcinoma suggesting that there is a generalised change irrespective of cell type in such patients.

Throughout treatment, the gynaecologist should adopt an optimistic attitude towards the woman, and encourage a similar attitude in her. The disease and modes of treatment should be explained to her and to her relatives. Although in certain circumstances relatives may be given more details regarding prognosis than the patient, overall there should be no 'secrets' between doctor, patient and relatives. Such 'secrets' can cause tensions which lead to a deterioration in relationships.

CARCINOMA OF THE UTERUS/ ENDOMETRIUM

Endometrial carcinoma is the third most common malignancy among women in England and Wales after carcinoma of the breast and cervix. About 3800 cases occur annually. In the USA, it is the most common gynaecological malignancy with about 38 000 cases per annum. It is more common in nulliparous and obese women. An association with diabetes mellitus has not been confirmed, nor has an association with fibroids which are common anyway. Exogenous or endogenous oestrogens, from thecomas or granulosa cell tumours, have been associated with endometrial hyperplasia and carcinoma. The fact that some tumours are sensitive to progestogens does suggest that endometrial carcinoma is probably hormone sensitive/dependent. Oestrogen receptors can be demonstrated in most tumours.

Pathology

Cancer of the uterine body arises from the endometrium and has the typical structure of adenocarcinoma. This arises from the epithelium of the surface of the endometrium or from its glands. The upper part of the uterus is usually the first to be affected. Occasionally the tumour can descend as far as the cervical canal. The tumour is often slow growing and well localised with little invasion of the myometrium. It may form a friable polypoidal mass projecting into the uterine cavity. Adenocarcinoma may sometimes be diffuse, covering a large area of the uterine cavity. Pure squamous carcinoma of the endometrium, associated with polyps or pyometra, is very rare. Adenosquamous carcinoma, where the pattern is mixed, is not uncommon. The microscopic picture of endometrial adenocarcinoma is one of 'untidy' atypical glands with abnormal hyperactivity of the lining epithelial cells. Normally, the glands are uniform in appearance, and in the postmenopausal endometrium they are narrow and atrophic. The tumour can take the form of glandular proliferation with scanty stroma. The

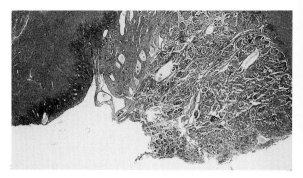

Fig. 20.7   *The focal nature of some cases of adenocarcinoma of the endometrium. A superficial cancer is present with non-neoplastic endometrium to one side. (H.E. x 6).*

glands are lined with tall columnar epithelium which shows the characteristics of malignancy. Cell nuclei are placed at irregular intervals, are hyperchromatic and of varying size. Mitotic figures are present. In their proliferation the glands may bud outwards or inwards, producing papillary processes within their own lumen. In some cases, the glands may contain many layers of cells which are irregular in shape and size, filling the gland lumen. Central degeneration may occur producing spaces. Adenocarcinoma of the endometrium is usually well differentiated and slow to invade the myometrium. Distant metastases, particularly by lymphatic spread, are unlikely if the myometrial invasion is less than 3 mm (Fig. 20.7). Invasion, a characteristic of cancer, may be absent. This should not influence the diagnosis or prognosis if other features of malignancy such as lack of differentiation are present. The grade of tumour differentiation significantly influences the 5-year survival rate (Fig. 20.8).

Clinical Features

Characteristically, endometrial carcinoma presents as abnormal perimenopausal or postmenopausal bleeding. In the premenopausal woman, it may present as intermenstrual bleeding or menorrhagia. The patient is often obese, hypertensive or diabetic, but such associations have not been definitely proven. After all, obesity is often associated with hypertension and diabetes mellitus. The association between obesity and endometrial cancer is thought to be due to a higher than menopausal level of

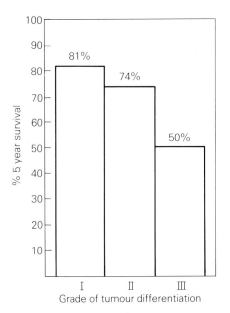

Fig. 20.8 *Survival rate for tumours of Grades I–III.*

circulating oestrogens caused by increased peripheral conversion of androstenedione to oestrone and oestradiol, and a high dietary fat intake leading to production of faecal oestrogens. A further clinically important point is the need to exclude breast tumours in these women.

Management

History

Details of the abnormal bleeding and discharge are taken, plus details of any exogenous source of

oestrogens. The history should distinguish urethral and rectal bleeding from vaginal bleeding.

Examination

Special attention is paid to the lymph nodes and breasts, and the presence or absence of hepatomegaly, para-aortic gland masses, as well as masses arising from the pelvis. Pelvic examination should determine the presence or absence of vaginal metastases, and rectal and parametrial involvement.

Special tests

Cervical cytology and cytology of the posterior fornix followed by diagnostic curettage are the principal investigations. Fractional curettage can be performed to determine involvement of the cervix (Stage II), but this can be assessed following removal of the uterus and its appendages. This is an argument against preoperative intracavitary radiotherapy which is advocated by some, as it will destroy the histopathological appearances, and features such as the depth of penetration and site of the tumour. These factors are of value in determining management beyond surgery, as they also determine lymph node involvement. Intravenous urography and pelvic ultrasound may help in assessing extrauterine spread of the disease. Lymphangiography can usefully be left until after surgery.

Once the diagnosis has been confirmed by histopathology of the uterine/endometrial curettings, the disease is staged.

To stage the lesion accurately the following special tests are performed:

EUA with measurement of uterine length;
Intravenous urogram;

Table 20.4

FIGO Staging for Endometrial Carcinoma

Stage	
0	Histology suspicious of malignancy, but not proven
1a	Confined to corpus, uterine cavity <3 cm
1b	Confined to corpus, uterine cavity >3 cm
2	Corpus and cervix involved
3	Spread outside uterus, but within pelvis
4	Spread outside pelvis or into bladder or rectum

Chest x-ray;

Ultrasound and computerised axial tomography (CAT) scans of the pelvis and abdomen if indicated;

Lymphangiography (after hysterectomy — if indicated by site, invasion and grade of tumour);

Liver scan.

The FIGO staging of endometrial carcinoma is defined in Table 20.4.

The routine investigations are the same as those detailed for cervical carcinoma.

Treatment

Stage 0

Carcinoma in situ of the endometrium may occur locally in an otherwise normal endometrium. There is no invasion, but very early lesions can metastasise, and this must be a worrying factor when counselling the young woman with a desire for future childbearing. In selected cases, progestogens may be given for three courses followed by curettage, or ovulation can be induced with clomiphene citrate followed by repeat curettage to ensure adequate endometrium. Such patients should be followed-up regularly and will eventually undergo total abdominal hysterectomy and bilateral salpingo-oophorectomy. At operation, washings should be taken from the peritoneal cavity for cytological analysis. The presence of tumour cells in the washings is thought to be associated with a higher recurrence rate.

Stage 1

About 70% of patients are Stage 1, although about 15% of these have positive peritoneal washings and 25% have deep myometrial invasion; 11% will have pelvic lymph node involvement, and 10% para-aortic node involvement. There is no significant difference between Stage 1a and 1b in terms of survival.

If only the endometrium is involved and the tumour is Grade 1 (G1), surgery alone is sufficient. Where the lesion is Grade 2 or 3 (G2 or G3), vault irradiation is added to reduce the risk of recurrence at this site.

If less than one-third of the myometrium is involved, G1 lesions are given postoperative vault irradiation. G2 and G3 lesions are given vault and external irradiation. If more than one-third of the myometrium is invaded, all grades of tumour receive vault and external irradiation following surgery.

Radiotherapy is given to all cases in which the lower one-third of the corpus is involved. If the lesion is situated in the cornu, spread can occur via the ovarian lymphatics, and therefore the para-aortic nodes are irradiated in addition to the pelvis.

Stage 2

Preoperative external pelvic irradiation (4000 cGy) and preoperative intracavitary irradiation using an intrauterine tube and vault ovoids (2000 cGy) is given. The rationale for this is that, following surgery, healing must occur before radiotherapy can be given, but surgery need not be delayed after radiotherapy, although some surgeons do prefer to wait 6 weeks before undertaking hysterectomy. Therefore, there is no delay in treating disease beyond the uterus in a situation which cannot be cured by surgery alone. At operation, para-aortic lymph node biopsies can be taken.

Stage 3

Treatment is by external pelvic irradiation (5000 cGy) plus intracavitary (2000 cGy). If there is a good response to radiotherapy, surgery is considered.

Stage 4

If disease is limited to the pelvis, external and intracavitary irradiation is given, and then, if it is considered feasible, a radical surgical procedure (exenteration) is carried out. Surgery is only performed if it is considered that it will cure the patient. Therefore, extensive preoperative investigations are required to exclude the presence of tumour outside the pelvis. At the time of operation, the surgeon should be prepared to send specimens from the lateral excision margins to confirm that the lines of excision are not passing through tumour and thus leaving tumour behind.

If there are distant metastases, radiotherapy is combined with hormonal therapy. Progestogens (medroxyprogesterone acetate 100 mg tid) are given on the basis that the tumour is oestrogen dependent. At some centres, there are facilities for assessing oestrogen receptor status which will help the clinician determine the usefulness of progestogen therapy. If there is an initial response to therapy and then subsequent recurrence, tamoxifen, an oestrogen antagonist which blocks receptor sites in target organs, can be given. Side-effects are uncommon. Increasingly, hormonal therapy is being given for earlier stages of the disease both pre- and postoperatively. Although there is evidence that this treatment alters the biochemistry and appearance of the tumour, there is, as yet, no proof that survival is prolonged.

Follow-up

Ideally this is conducted in a combined gynaecology/radiotherapy clinic, the first visit being 6 weeks postsurgery or radiotherapy. Thereafter, visits are at 3 monthly intervals for the first year, 4 monthly for the second year, 6 monthly for the third to fifth years and then annually up to 10 years.

At each visit, the woman should be asked about abnormal vaginal discharge or bleeding, micturition, bowel habit and sexual activity. She should be weighed and the breasts, abdomen, vagina and rectum examined. A vault smear is taken. A chest x-ray is performed annually, plus ultrasound scans of the pelvis, abdomen and liver as required.

CARCINOMA OF THE VULVA

Carcinoma of the vulva is a squamous carcinoma that is at present a rare disease. The origin of these tumours may be related to chronic irritation and may be preceded by the changes known as vulval dystrophies, or by vulval intraepithelial neoplasia.

Vulval Intraepithelial Neoplasia (VIN)

This condition is being seen increasingly. Its cytological and histological pattern and grading are similar to that of CIN. It occurs in the same group of women as CIN, often in association with the latter. It occurs normally on the labia minora, posterior forchette and round the clitoris. Its aetiology may be viral and it is frequently multifocal.

Small lesions may be treated expectantly and merely observed. However, larger or growing lesions require ablative treatment for which laser therapy is effective.

Vulval Dystrophies

These lesions are thought to be relatively common among women over 60 years of age. About 3% of them will progress to carcinoma. Considerable confusion has grown up because a variety of terms, often merely macroscopically descriptive, have been used. These include leukoplakia and kraurosis vulvae, neither of which gives any indication of the histological abnormality. There is a spectrum of epithelial atypia which is not as clearly defined as that for the cervix (CIN) but, nevertheless, the degree of atypical maturition is important in determining the progress and treatment for the condition.

Hyperplasia

Vulval hyperplasias range from typical to extremely atypical. Typical hyperplasia corresponds to chronic dermatitis, with hyperkeratosis and proliferation of the epithelium producing acanthosis. The maturation of the epithelium is normal and so there is no malignant potential.

Moderate degrees of atypia involve abnormal maturation of the epithelium with an increase in the numbers of immature cells and a lack of the normal layers of mature cells on the surface of the epithelium. There are increased numbers of basal and parabasal cells, and there may be some intraepithelial 'pearl' formation.

In marked atypia, there is definite pearl formation in the tips of the rete pegs and there are considerable variations in individual cells. The abnormal maturation at the tips of the rete pegs can take the place of the normal basal layer of cells. In all types, there may be subepithelial lymphocytic infiltration.

These lesions present with pruritus vulvae, and the skin will show white shiny areas that may appear thickened in mild cases, or thin and perhaps excoriated in the more abnormal cases. All cases require a vulval biopsy to make the diagnosis, and then symptomatic treatment — usually with steroid creams. With moderate to severe atypia, repeated biopsies may be necessary. All cases should be followed-up annually and a further biopsy performed if the area of abnormal skin has extended or its edges have proliferated, as these may indicate malignancy.

Lichen Sclerosis

This condition is characterised microscopically by hyperkeratosis, thinning of the epithelium, the presence of collagen and a chronic lymphocytic infiltration beneath the epithelium. The keratin layer may be quite thick, while the epithelium is thin, but contains atypical cells. The skin contains thin, grey and shiny areas. There may be excoriation with hyperplasia depending on the degree of pruritis.

These macroscopic and microscopic changes have been referred to as atrophic leukoplakia, primary senile atrophy or kraurosis. These terms should no longer be used. Lichen sclerosis is almost always a benign condition but, as occasional cases can become malignant, continued follow-up is desirable.

Treatment is symptomatic, with topical corticosteroids being the most effective. Other antipruritic preparations such as calamine lotion or topical antihistamines can be tried.

Kraurosis Vulvae

This is a descriptive term and not a histological diagnosis. It describes vulval atrophy, with loss of subcutaneous fat, labial adhesions and excoriation of atrophic skin. Microscopically, the appearances are the same as for lichen sclerosis. The cause of the vulval atrophy is lack of oestrogen action, possibly due to reduced circulating levels, but also may be due to a deficiency in oestrogen receptors in the tissues. The condition is benign and treatment is not usually effective. Pain is a prominent feature when excoriation of the skin is severe. Nerve blocks may be tried for pain relief in severe cases.

Bowen's Disease

Bowen's disease is a primary carcinoma of the epidermis, but which is restricted to the epidermis (in situ). The diagnosis is made on the malignant

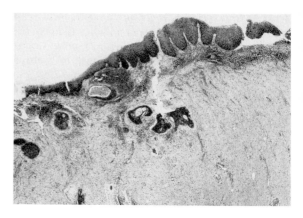

Fig. 20.9   *Carcinoma of the vulva showing epithelial thickening and small foci of invasion.*

characteristics of the cells and lack of structural maturation within the epidermis. Spread may take place laterally within the epidermis. The condition may be multifocal. Treatment is by excision with adequate (2 cm) skin margins.

Squamous Carcinoma of the Vulva

This presents either de novo or as a change in pre-existing vulval dystrophy. The presenting symptoms are those of itching, pain and possibly bleeding from a raised, indurated and ulcerated area of vulval skin. It is a slowly growing tumour, proceeding with continuing induration, ulceration and diffuse spreading margins. The lesion will probably have been present for some time before the patient seeks advice. It occurs usually in women over 60 years of age. The FIGO classification is a follows:

Stage 1: primary tumour <2 cm — no suspicious nodes.

Stage 2: primary tumour >2 cm — no suspicious nodes.

Stage 3: tumour invading urethra, vagina, perineum or anus; or tumour of any size with suspicious nodes.

Stage 4: tumour with fixed nodes and spread to bladder and/or rectum, or elsewhere.

Microscopically, the early changes include thickening of the epithelial layers and downgrowth of the interpapillary processes, which penetrates deeply invading tissue spaces, and destroys the intervening tissue (Fig. 20.9). The tumour at this stage often assumes the shape of an inverted cauliflower.

During later stages of tumour development, cells become detached and further invade tissue spaces or lymphatics. Cells in the centre of the tumour become concentrically arranged flattened and hyalinised or keratinised. These cells nests or epithelial pearls are characteristic of squamous carcinoma in general. In squamous carcinoma of the vulva, these cell nests have a keratinised centre and are relatively common. There is marked lymphocytic infiltration around the tumour. Polymorphonuclear leukocytes and foreign body giant cells may also be seen (Fig. 20.10).

Tumour spread is by direct infiltration or by lymphatics to the superficial and deep inguinal and femoral nodes.

Treatment

Treatment is by excision of the lesion and its lymph drainage — radical vulvectomy. This means removal of vulva including clitoris, mons pubis and a block dissection of the inguinal and femoral nodes. It is a major operation with problems of primary skin closure. Lymphoedema may be a chronic problem. In old women, unable to stand radical surgery, a simple vulvectomy, i.e. no node dissection, will often suffice. Radiotherapy and chemotherapy are not effective treatments for vulval carcinoma.

The vulva may be the site of other forms of malignancy such as basal cell carcinoma, melanoma, lymphoma, fibroleiomyosarcoma and rhabdomyosarcoma. These tumours are very rare and their consideration is not within the scope of this book.

CARCINOMA OF THE VAGINA

Vaginal Intraepithelial Disease (VAIN)

This has the same underlying cytological and histopathological features as cervical intraepithelial disease. It can either arise as a single vaginal focus or, along with CIN, as part of a multifocal epithelial abnormality. Aetiology of VAIN is not known, but it could be viral in origin. Treatment is by complete local ablation of the affected area defined at colposcopy, particularly if it is close to a pre-existing cervical focus. Laser treatment is effective for this. If the disease is separated from the cervix, it may either be watched regularly, on the basis that its natural history is not known, or ablated with laser therapy or 5-fluorouacil in the form of vaginal cream.

Invasive Carcinoma of the Vagina

This is a rare disease. It has been induced in some women by exposure to diethylstilboestrol before birth, when this drug was administered in high doses to their mothers as a treatment for threatened abortion during the first and early second trimesters of pregnancy. Otherwise, its aetiology is unknown, although VAIN may proceed to invasive carcinoma in due course. The incidence of carcinoma of the vagina may, therefore, increase in time. Treatment is either with radiotherapy or colpectomy or in some cases both.

OVARIAN TUMOURS OF BORDERLINE MALIGNANCY

Within the group of epithelial ovarian tumours is a substantial number which are reported by the pathologist as of 'borderline' malignancy. These tumours are neither benign nor malignant in terms of histology and biological activity. They form a grey area and often not a little disagreement between clinicians and pathologists.

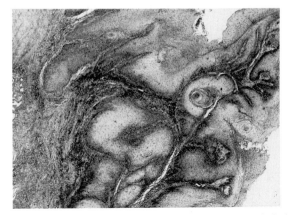

Fig. 20.10 *Carcinoma of the vulva showing epithelial pearl formation.*

The World Health Organization (WHO) has defined a borderline tumour as:

'One that has some, but not all, of the morphological features of malignancy; those present include, in varying combinations, stratification of epithelial cells, apparent detachment of cellular clusters from their sites and mitotic figures and nuclear abnormalities intermediate between those of clearly benign and unquestionably malignant tumours of a similar cell type; on the other hand, obvious invasion of the adjacent stroma is lacking.'

There are no specific clinical features to permit recognition of a borderline malignancy. Prognosis for patients with epithelial ovarian neoplasms of borderline malignancy is good, at least for 5-year survival. For serous tumours of borderline malignancy 90–95% survive 5 years, and 75–90% 10 years. For mucinous tumours of borderline malignancy the 5-year survival is 81–95% and 68–95% survive 10 years.

MALIGNANT TUMOURS OF THE OVARY

Serous cell tumours (Fig. 20.11)

Serous cystadenocarcinoma is the most commonly encountered type of ovarian carcinoma, accounting for just over half of all ovarian adenocarcinomas. They tend to be large tumours, ranging from 5 cm

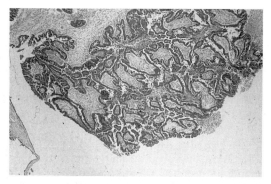

Fig. 20.11   *Serous papillary cystadenocarcinoma. Histological section through a papillary process projecting into the lumen of the cyst. The cells show characteristics of malignancy and a small element of the corrective tissue support is visible.*

to over 15 cm in diameter. The majority are cystic with both multiple papillary masses and solid nodules of adenocarcinoma obliterating the cystic cavities and invading adjacent ovarian parenchyma. The contents are usually thin and watery like its benign counterpart. About 8% are solid adenocarcinomas with virtually no cystic element. Unlike the benign form, the carcinoma is characterised by tumour growth on the capsule of the tumour which occurs in almost 50% of cases. Very rarely, the tumour is entirely exophytic. These surface papillary lesions are often difficult to detect at pelvic examination due to their small size.

Microscopically, the cells resemble those of fallopian tube epithelium. The well-differentiated tumours contain finely branched papillae with little or no connective tissue support. Stromal invasion is usually apparent. As differentiation lessens, the cells form solid sheets and surround small, irregular spaces. Cystic spaces and papillae become less frequent. The nuclei are large with prominent nucleoli, the latter increasing in number with increasing grade of malignancy. The most malignant variant is solid, containing totally undifferentiated cells which may be large and bizarre.

Psammoma bodies which are intracellular areas of calcification are frequently found in papillary cystadenocarcinomas, and especially in their accompanying peritoneal implants. The claim for a better prognosis when psammoma bodies are present probably reflects the better differentiation of the tumours which contain them.

Serous cell tumours are bilateral in 35–50% of cases. The tumour spreads rapidly and, at diagnosis, it is estimated that at most only 20% of patients have growth confined to one ovary. Intra-abdominal spread is likely to be due to the tendency of exophytic growth of the tumour and prognosis is correspondingly poor.

Mucinous cell tumours (Fig. 20.12)

Mucinous tumours account for up to 15% of primary ovarian carcinomas. Approximately 10% are bilateral. They may attain large proportions ranging from 5 cm to over 20 cm in diameter.

In contrast to serous tumours, which are relatively uniform throughout, mucinous tumours often contain benign, borderline and malignant elements within a single specimen. Careful gross examination and judicious sampling is, therefore, required to ensure accurate diagnosis.

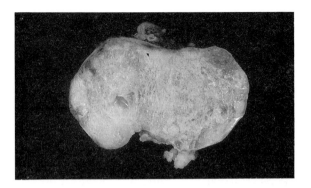

Fig. 20.12 *Mucinous cystadenocarcinoma. A predominantly solid tumour with small cystic spaces and some mucus. Small surface projections are visible.*

In general, the prognosis for mucinous adenocarcinoma is better than for its serous counterpart. This is due to a large number remaining still confined to the ovary at the time of diagnosis, and the lack of capsular involvement in the majority.

Endometrioid cell tumours

Endometrioid tumours are characterised by tubular glands lined by stratified, non-mucin-producing epithelium bearing a resemblance to proliferative endometrium. It is thought to arise from either the epithelium of existing endometriosis or from the surface epithelium of the ovary. During the last 25 years, the appreciation that such a lesion represented a primary ovarian tumour, as opposed to a metastatic deposit from an endometrial carcinoma, has led to an increasing incidence of recognition, and it is thought such lesions account for from 15 to 30% of all ovarian carcinomas.

The tumours are mainly solid with occasional cystic areas and 10–30% are bilateral. The solid portions are nodular and often dark red in colour due to haemorrhage. They range in size from 2 to 35 cm. Surface projections are rare, but intracystic papillae may be found in some.

Microscopically, most are well-differentiated adenocarcinomas with tubular glands. However, the other varieties of endometrial carcinoma may be encountered including secretory adenocarcinoma, adenoacanthoma and adenosquamous carcinoma.

Mixed epithelial and stromal tumours of endometrioid type and pure endometrial stromal tumours are included in the endometrioid category.

The highly malignant carcinosarcoma and malignant mixed mesodermal tumour, mesodermal adenosarcoma and endometrioid stromal sarcoma are rarely encountered.

Malignant gonadal stromal tumours of the ovary

Gonadal stromal tumours arise from cells derived from the sex cords or mesenchyme of the embryonic gonad. Thus granulosa cells, theca cells, Sertoli cells, Leydig cells or their precursors are found singly or in combination within these tumours, and secretion of sex steroids is common. The tumours are of low grade, malignancy usually presenting as a result of abnormal endocrine production.

Granulosa and thecal cell tumours vary in size, usually present with postmenopausal bleeding with evidence of abnormal oestrogen secretion (Fig. 20.13). Arrhenoblastomas are rare androgen secreting tumours of the ovary with malignant potential. Androblastomas include Sertoli or Leydig cell tumours. The former are very small and secrete oestrogen, while the latter are mostly androgenic, causing virilisation. A mixture of Sertoli and Leydig cell types can coexist. All these tumours are unilateral and oophorectomy is adequate treatment.

Truly malignant germ cell tumours of the ovary are very uncommon. They are solid, can be quite large, and occur in younger women. Dysgerminoma is one type which has a low malignant potential. Treatment by oophorectomy may suffice. Endodermal sinus tumour is rapidly growing with a much greater malignant potential.

One per cent of benign teratomas undergo some malignant transformation. Malignant teratomas

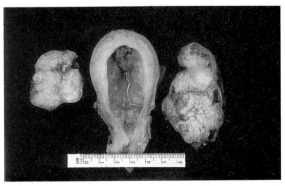

Fig. 20.13 *Granulosa cell tumour of the ovary with endometrial hyperplasia.*

are solid, fairly large tumours which present as a mass or with pain. Treatment of endodermal sinus tumours and teratomas is surgical excision and chemotherapy as appropriate.

Metastatic tumours of the ovary

Malignant neoplasms frequently metastasise to the ovary, and 10–30% of ovarian cancers are metastatic. The common primary sites are the gastrointestinal tract (Krukenberg tumours), the breast and the endometrium. Lymphomas, sarcomas, melanomas and carcinoid are also known to establish secondary growth in the ovaries. The majority of ovarian metastatic tumours are bilateral and can reach large dimensions. The histological features of the primary tumour are usually faithfully reproduced. Such metastatic spread carries a poor prognosis.

Clear cell tumours

Clear cell carcinoma accounts for 5–11% of all ovarian carcinoma. Although once firmly believed to be of mesonephric origin, and thus designated mesonephroid carcinoma, clear cell carcinoma is now regarded as being müllerian in origin, and closely related to endometrioid carcinoma and endometriosis. In fact, these tumours are more often associated with ovarian and pelvic endometriosis than any other tumour (up to 24% of cases).

The tumour is often quite large, exceeding 15 cm. The majority are both solid and cystic, with a few being mainly solid containing small cystic spaces. They are rarely bilateral.

Transitional cell tumours — Brenner

Approximately 3% of all ovarian neoplasms are composed of benign transitional cell epithelium closely resembling the epithelium of the bladder. They probably originate from the surface epithelium of the bladder, although some (about 5%) are associated with teratomas.

The vast majority of Brenner tumours are benign and are often unrecognised clinically, being an incidental finding at histological examination.

Malignant Brenner tumours are rare, and may arise from malignant transformation of the epithelium of a benign tumour or by direct malignant transformation of inclusions of surface ovarian epithelium.

Mixed epithelial tumours

These tumours are rare and contain significant quantities of two or three cell types within an epithelial tumour.

Undifferentiated and unclassified carcinomas

A small number of primary ovarian carcinomas resist categorisation, because the component cells are totally undifferentiated. They are usually very aggressive tumours with the majority at an advanced stage by the time of diagnosis, and have a correspondingly poor prognosis.

Clinical Features of Malignant Ovarian Tumours

Age

Malignant epithelial tumours of the ovary are most common between 40 and 70 years of age.

Symptoms

There are no specific symptoms of the disease, but the most common are abdominal pain and swelling with associated gastrointestinal complaints and cachexia. When the tumour is small, there are no symptoms.

Bloatedness, dyspepsia, nausea, vomiting, diarrhoea and epigastric discomfort may occur, mimicking biliary, gastric or intestinal pathology and diverting attention from the pelvis. Abnormal uterine bleeding may occur. Rarely, an ovarian carcinoma may undergo torsion, rupture or cause intra-abdominal haemorrhage.

Physical Findings

With the frequent late presentation of ovarian carcinoma, it is not surprising that from 40 to 75% of patients have a palpable abdominopelvic mass and 20–30% have ascites when first examined. Those with ascites may have coexisting pleural effusion. As few as 1–2% will have a negative clinical examination.

Malignant tumours are often solid, fixed, irregular and bilateral. Supraclavicular, axillary and inguinal lymphadenopathy may be present. Skin metastases, bilateral leg oedema, generalised weight loss and, rarely, the stigmata of abnormal hormone production may be evident.

Diagnosis

While pelvic examination may confirm suspicions of potential ovarian malignancy, often the true confirmation of the diagnosis depends on the findings at operation. The preoperative investigations are directed at the exclusion of other causes of an abdominopelvic or pelvic mass (Table 20.5).

Table 20.5

Causes of a Pelvic Mass

---

1. Distended bladder
2. Pregnancy
3. Utero leiomyomata
4. Broad ligament tumour
5. Pyosalpinx or hydrosalpinx
6. Ectopic pregnancy
7. Pelvic abscess
8. Endometriosis
9. Diverticular disease
10. Tumour of sigmoid colon or rectum
11. Pelvic kidney or gallbladder
12. Retroperitoneal tumour

Examination under anaesthetic, endocervical curettage and endometrial curettage may help in excluding other sites within the genital tract as being the seat of the disease.

A plain x-ray of the abdomen is often helpful in diagnosing dermoid cysts. Chest x-ray is routinely performed. There may be metastases within the lung parenchyma, elevation of the diaphragm due to metastatic deposits and pleural effusion.

Barium enema is warranted due to the frequency with which rectosigmoid carcinoma metastasises to the ovary. Intravenous urography demonstrates ureteric involvement by an ovarian neoplasm, excludes any ureteric anomaly and confirms their position.

Ultrasonography is commonly employed to further assess a pelvic or abdominopelvic mass. Being non-invasive, it is particularly useful and

may distinguish uterine and adnexal masses, as well as delineating cystic and solid lesions.

Computerised axial tomography (CAT) also allows assessment of both abdomen and pelvis. It is being used with increasing frequency to assess the efficacy of adjuvant chemotherapy.

Bipedal lymphangiography is also used for localising lymph node metastases. It is useful for localising suitable nodes for sampling, either by percutaneous fine needle aspiration or at laparotomy. There is a high incidence of false positives.

Staging

The stage of the disease is based on clinical and surgical findings, the final histology and the cytology of peritoneal fluid, including the cytology of peritoneal washings when ascites is absent. At laparotomy, a systematic exploration of the abdomen and pelvis is essential.

Partial or total omentectomy is commonly performed, as it is such a common metastatic site. Sampling of retroperitoneal nodes remains controversial. There is no certain clinical method for distinguishing involved nodes. Even when palpable, the nodes are not necessarily the site of metastatic disease, but should be excised for histological examination.

Accurate staging helps to decide the best treatment for an individual and also permits accurate assessment of the efficacy of treatment and allows comparison of results from one centre to another.

Treatment

Surgery

Surgery is not only important in establishing the diagnosis and staging of ovarian carcinoma, but is the primary, most effective treatment. As much as possible of the primary tumour and its metastases are removed without jeopardising the patient's life.

In the rare event of unilateral ovarian carcinoma, and when future fertility is important, salpingo-oophorectomy is performed. When fertility is not a consideration, the contralateral adnexa and the uterus are removed.

Omentectomy should be performed, as it is a

common site for metastases and it facilitates subsequent laparoscopy which is used for assessing the efficacy of adjuvant therapy.

Second-look surgery is used as a diagnostic procedure to assess patients known previously to have had widespread disease, but no clinically detectable disease after treatment for 12–18 months. Laparoscopy may detect occult persistent disease, but if negative, careful laparotomy with multiple biopsy and washings is required.

Chemotherapy

Adjuvant chemotherapy has become particularly important given the incidence of disease which is too widespread for cure by surgical methods.

Cytotoxic treatment may be administered as single agent therapy or combination therapy. The alkylating agents, melphalan, cyclophosamide, chlorambucil and dihydroxybusulphan have been used longest. Cis-platinum (dichlorodiaminoplatinum — DDP) has been increasingly used as front line chemotherapy based on its known efficacy against alkylating agent failures. The limiting factor with all drug therapy is the production of side-effects at cytotoxic doses, and the search for better, more successful, agents continues. At present cis-platinum is the most widely used cytotoxic drug for ovarian carcinoma.

Radiotherapy

Ovarian carcinomas are only moderately sensitive to radiation therapy, so it is hardly surprising that such therapy proves disappointing. Whole abdominal radiotherapy is now employed, especially when minimal tumour remains after previous surgery and/or chemotherapy.

FURTHER READING

DiSaia P.J., Creasman W.T. (1981). *Clinical Gynaecologic Oncology*. St Louis: Mosby.

Ovarian Tumour Panel of the Royal College of Obstetrics and Gynaecology (1983). Ovarian epithelial tumours of borderline malignancy: pathological features and current status. *Brit. J. Ost. Gynae*; **90**: 743–50.

Piper M.S. (1983). Ovarian malignancies: the clinical care of adults and adolescents. In *Current Reviews in Obstetrics and Gynaecology*. (Singer A. et al., eds.) Edinburgh: Churchill Livingstone.

Raz S. (1985). Gynaecological oncology. In *Clinics in Obstetrics and Gynaecology*, Vol. 12, No. 2. London: W. B. Saunders.

Singer A., ed. (1985). Cancer of the cervix, diagnosis and treatment. In *Clinics in Obstetrics and Gynaecology*, Vol. 12, No. 1. London: W. B. Saunders.

21

Female Infertility

Whether termed infertility or subfertility, the inability to reproduce is a problem which can become all-consuming for the couple concerned. Both partners *should* be seen together in the clinic throughout their management. Unfortunately, this is rarely the case, because often the man is unable to attend, but at some stage in the management it should be insisted that he be involved. The physician must be constantly aware of the psychological well-being of the couple, sensitive to the stresses and strains of the situation and sympathetic to any fear or anxieties that arise. Subfertility is an emotionally charged situation and, even before the couple enters the consulting room on their first visit, all sorts of psychological pressures, fears and other anxieties will have arisen. Most people will feel a mixture of embarrassment at their problem, and a fear and anxiety that something serious is wrong. As investigations and treatment proceed, these feelings may give way to frustration or even hopelessness at the lack of results. Emotional rapport with the physician is of extreme importance from the very start, so that fears can be allayed, the stress of the situation partly defused and confidence built up between both partners and the physician.

The rates of normal conception (Fig. 21.1) show that 10% of 'normal couples' will not conceive during the first year of attempting to get pregnant. When should investigations start? The fact that a couple seek medical help means that they perceive that there is a problem. Thus it is important to take the request for help seriously from the start, although the vigour of investigation may be modified somewhat if the duration of exposure to pregnancy has been short.

Potential areas leading to inability to reproduce will be considered under the headings of (1) defects in ovulation, (2) cervical problems preventing the entry of spermatozoa into the uterus, (3) structural problems interfering with ovum transport and (4) failure of implantation.

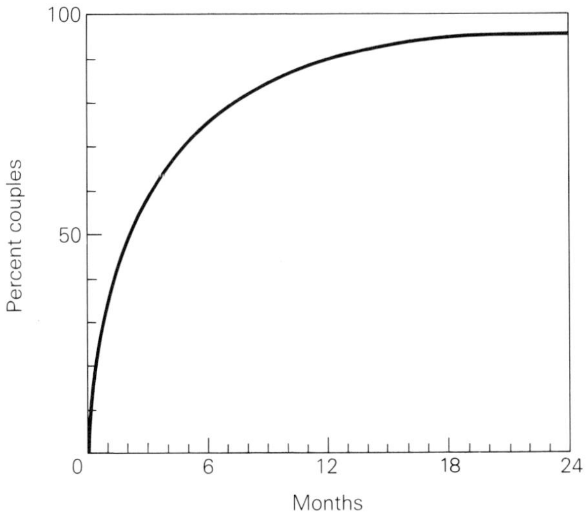

OVULATION

In the average infertility clinic, as many as 30% of couples seen will have some defect concerning maturation of the ovarian follicle. Any variation in the subtle interplay of hormonal balance, whether at hypothalamic, pituitary or ovarian level, may lead to a defect in follicular development, ovum release or maintenance of corpus luteal function. There are many signs suggestive of ovulation, but perhaps the only definite proof is pregnancy.

Menstrual History

Regular menstrual bleeding does not necessarily indicate ovulation, but scanty irregular menses is more suggestive of anovulation. Primary amenor-

Fig. 21.1 *Normal conception rates.*

rhoea, which means no spontaneous bleeding before 18 years of age, unusually presents as infertility, and the underlying cause, for instance Turner's syndrome or gynaetresia, can usually be diagnosed by an accurate clinical history and examination. Secondary amenorrhoea — cessation of menstruation after the regular occurrence of normal menstrual periods — and oligomenorrhoea, defined as scanty, irregular bleeding, may be due to many defects (Table 21.1) and treatment is by the induc-

---

Table 21.1

Causes of Secondary Amenorrhoea and Oligomenorrhoea

Hypothalamic	Weight change
	Drugs (oral contraceptives, tranquillisers)
	Psychological disturbances
Pituitary	Adenoma
Ovarian	Premature ovarian failure
	Polycystic ovarian syndrome
Uterine	Synaechiae
	Asherman's syndrome
	Cervical stenosis

---

tion of regular ovulation. Special investigations may include hysterosalpingography to exclude intrauterine pathology and measurement of follicle stimulating hormone (FSH), luteinising hormone (LH) and prolactin. If the ovary has failed prematurely (all ovaries fail at the menopause), serum FSH and, to a lesser extent, LH levels will be raised, and the diagnosis is confirmed by ovarian biopsy, when no primordial follicles will be seen. Other, less common, causes of secondary amenorrhoea are due to abnormal thyroid function (hyper or hypo) and pituitary tumours. Thyroid function tests (T4:TSH) and x-ray examination of the sella turcica of the pituitary fossa will aid diagnosis.

Cervical Mucus

Because of the high levels of circulating oestrogen, the preovulatory mucus is clear and of low viscosity allowing the free passage of spermatozoa. It has the property of forming into threads when stretched between two points (Spinnbarkeit) and, when spread on a microscope slide, it dries in the form of 'fern-like' structures (ferning). At the time of maximum mucus production, the cervical os is open to its greatest extent, but after ovulation, it closes and the mucus abruptly becomes scant, sticky, viscous and impenetrable to sperms. Women can be taught to recognise these changes in the cervical mucus both in quantity and consistency, and this is one of the most useful symptomatic markers of ovulation. Mastalgia, which is pain or tingling in the breasts, reflecting distension or fluid retention secondary to the preovulatory oestrogen rise, and Mittelschmerz, which is unilateral, midcycle pain of ovulation felt in the iliac fossa are inconstant markers.

Basal Temperature

During an ovulatory cycle, the body temperature shows a biphasic pattern with a rise of about 0.5°C following ovulation. Classically, there is a slight temperature fall (approximately 0.3°C) immediately preovulation, followed by a rise in response to the thermogenic effect of progesterone or its metabolites. The resting basal body temperature is taken daily, usually orally in the morning before getting out of bed and recorded on a temperature graph: the basal temperature chart (BTC). This biphasic chart may indicate ovulation and, occasionally, the preovulatory fall in temperature may be a useful predictor of ovulation. However, this fall immediately preovulation is often recognised only in retrospect and hence its cinical predictive value is limited. The BTC is cheap and simple to complete and hence is a popular aid in the investigation of the infertile couple. Its usefulness, however, is extended beyond that of recording basal temperature by enlarging the data recorded to include the pattern of menstruation (duration, periodicity and degree), symptoms of mastalgia and cervical mucus changes. Hence, a well completed BTC will give a comprehensive summary of all the symptomatic changes already discussed. The frequency of intercourse should also be recorded, information which is often quite revealing and important.

Endometrial Biopsy

The endometrial lining is one of the end organs of hormonal effect, and histological changes, mainly reflecting progesterone effect, are well documented. Premenstrual endometrial biopsy was widely used to demonstrate the effects of progesterone and hence indicated ovulation, but, since serum progesterone assays became available, endometrial biopsy is rarely justified except when genital tuberculosis is to be excluded. Endometrial biopsy increases the risk of uterine infection, may necessitate dilatation of the cervix with risk of damage and, if over vigorous, may lead to intrauterine adhesions and hence compound the infertility problem.

Hormones

Radioimmunoassay has enabled the measurement of most hormones involved in the ovulation mechanism. For the detection of ovulation in a menstruating woman, it is usually sufficient to measure the raised plasma progesterone levels in the potentially luteal phase of the cycle (usually Days 19–25). Values of 30 nmol/l or more are highly suggestive of ovulation and adequate luteal function. The detection of hyperprolactinaemia may also be important.

Visualisation

Perhaps the best method of detecting ovulation is actually to visualise the active ovary. This may be done by direct visualisation at time of laparotomy or conveniently at laparoscopy or by means of ultrasound scanning. The dominant preovulatory follicle measures about 25 mm in diameter and rupture and ovum release results in the formation of the characteristic punctate 'stigma'. The remaining granulosa cells then appear haemorrhagic (corpus haemorrhagica) and later have a yellow appearance (corpus luteum). These characteristic changes on the ovarian surface may be visualised directly at laparoscopy or by ultrasound. The developing fluid-filled follicles can be observed easily, especially if ovarian localisation is aided by a full bladder, and the subsequent disappearance of the dominant follicle may indicate ovum release.

In practice, a combination of these investigations and signs — usually BTC, cervical mucus observation, serum progesterone assays and possibly laparoscopy — are used to arrive at a diagnosis of anovulation or ovulation.

Treatment

First, general measures should be considered. A sudden increase in weight or, more commonly, loss of weight as seen typically in anorexia nervosa may act at the hypothalamic level to interfere with hormonal release. Simple advice on diet or perhaps psychiatric aid may be sufficient to regain hormonal balance. Other, more nebulous factors, such as stress or a great desire for pregnancy, may influence the higher centres and treatment by reassurance and the alleviation of stress may often lead to conception. Derangement of other endocrine systems, e.g. thyroid, may need to be investigated and treatment instigated. The main treatment, however, of anovulation is by ovulation induction using either:

1. Clomiphene citrate or taxomifen, or
2. Gonadotrophins, or
3. Gonadotrophin releasing hormone, or
4. Bromocriptine.

Clomiphene citrate, which is a weak oestrogen with antioestrogenic actions, is the treatment of choice for patients with anovulatory cycles and oligomenorrhoea and should always be tried first in patients with secondary amenorrhoea with normal FSH and LH and prolactin levels. Clomiphene's main action is at the hypothalamic level where, by virtue of its antioestrogenic action, it causes an increased output of pituitary gonadotrophins. It is usually prescribed for 5 consecutive days, starting at a dose of 50 mg daily and increasing to a maximum of 200 mg until ovulation as monitored by BTCs and progesterone is occurring. The mild antioestrogenic effect of clomiphene on the cervical mucus may be minimised by commencing it early in the cycle, e.g. Days 2–6. Occasionally, this effect may need to be counteracted by taking oral oestrogen in midcycle. In the absence of spontaneous menstruation, a withdrawal bleed may be stimulated by prescribing Norethisterone 5 mg twice daily for 5 days, and clomiphene is then added on the day after bleeding starts. There is about a 10% incidence of twin pregnancy following clomiphene therapy. Human chorionic gonadotrophin may sometimes be added in the middle of clomiphene stimulated cycles to enhance ovulation and improve luteal function.

Gonadotrophin therapy, a mixture of FSH and LH, acts directly on the ovaries, and hence dosage and response must be carefully monitored by oestrogen assays and ultrasound to avoid overstimulation, multiple follicle development and multiple pregnancies. Gonadotrophins should only be used in centres where good hormonal and ultrasonic monitoring of ovarian function is readily available.

Gonadotrophin releasing hormone (GnRH) has recently become available and, when given in pulsatile doses, by portable infusion pumps, is extremely effective in treating defective hypothalamic function. Its use is at present confined to specialised centres and is still being assessed.

Bromocriptine inhibits secretion of prolactin by the anterior pituitary and so is the specific treatment of anovulation due to hyperprolactinaemia. The normal dose is 2.5 mg or 5 mg daily and the response is monitored by serum prolactin assay. Hyperprolactinaemia will also be suspected if clinically galactorrhoea is demonstrated and, in this circumstance, serum prolactin assays are mandatory. Serum prolactin levels may also be raised by stress, certain drugs (e.g. phenothiazides, methyldopa, benzamines) or by a pituitary microadenoma. If hyperprolactinaemia is demonstrated, the possibility of pituitary enlargement must be investigated by x-ray, using tomograms if necessary, before treatment by bromocriptine is started. If a pituitary tumour is demonstrated, this may be treated by surgery, radiotherapy or bromocriptine. In such circumstances, the patient must be closely watched during a subsequent pregnancy for signs of pituitary enlargement by assessment of visual fields and if necessary by x-rays.

CERVICAL FACTORS

The postcoital test (PCT) involves the examination of cervical mucus on a slide under the microscope within 24 h of intercourse. This should ideally be performed when the cervical mucus is most receptive to sperm penetration, i.e. at ovulation, with maximum oestrogenisation. At the time of this examination, the following are noted: (1) whether there is evidence of oestrogenisation as seen by dilatation of the cervix; (2) the quantity and quality of the mucus (the ability to stretch being the Spinnbarkeit); (3) the numbers of sperm per high power field; (4) whether the sperm are moving in a linear direction.

Thus the presence of many motile spermatozoa in thin clear mucus should indicate that:

1. the act of coitus occurs satisfactorily;
2. good plentiful mucus is circumstantial evidence of ovulation;
3. there is no cervical barrier to the progress of healthy spermatozoa.

The most common reason for poor mucus or lack of spermatozoa is that the examination is performed at the wrong time in the cycle, or that the woman is not ovulating. Hence, a negative test must be repeated and ovulation confirmed.

If no spermatozoa are seen, this may be due to failure in coital technique, and persistently absent sperm in the presence of good mucus should raise the possibility of either a male factor, or stress and a psychological problem. The repeated finding of lack of progressive sperm movement raises the infrequent possibility of immunological factors, e.g. sperm antibodies, which have an inhibiting effect on normal sperm. This may be clarified by demonstrating cervical hostility in vitro. Cervical problems may be difficult to treat. Mucus production may be stimulated by exogenous oestrogen, e.g. ethinyl oestradiol 0.01 mg daily, and a local lesion, e.g. infection or an erosion, should be treated. However, when sperm fail to penetrate the mucus, therapy is very disappointing. Intrauterine artificial insemination with husband's sperm (AIH) may occasionally be used in these circumstances with benefit.

STRUCTURAL PROBLEMS

Interference with ovum release, its capture by the fimbrial portion of the tube (the so-called tubo-ovarian unit) and subsequent transport of the fertilised ovum into the uterine cavity caused by structural distortion accounts for perhaps 20–25% of couples attending the infertility clinic. This distortion may be major, such as complete occlusion of the fallopian tube or more subtle, such as minor peritubal adhesions interfering with the tubo-ovarian mechanism. The most common causes of such problems are infection or postoperative adhesion formation. Resolution of infection causes an inflammatory response and subsequent fibrosis, which may lead to adhesions covering the ovaries or distorting the fallopian tubes. Complete occlusion of the tube may occur and, most commonly, the most sensitive and vulnerable portions of the tube are affected, i.e. the narrow cornual isthmic portion of the tube, a cornual block, or conglutination of the fimbriae causing a hydrosalpinx. Even if tubal patency is not disturbed, the mechanism of function may be disrupted by destroying the fine sensitive cilial lining of the fallopian tube and interfering with ovum transport. Postinfective distortion is commonly symmetrically bilateral. A similar mechanism causes pelvic adhesions and distortion following any traumatic operative procedure such as ovarian cystectomy. This damage may be aggravated by postoperative infection, but postoperative adhesions may disrupt the pelvic anatomy and function.

The history may be suggestive of anatomical abnormalities contributing to the infertility problem, but confirmation of this diagnosis will be by hysterosalpingogram (HSG) and laparoscopic assessment. The x-ray demonstration by HSG allows the diagnosis of intrauterine pathology, e.g. adhesions or synaechiae and tubal occlusion (Figs. 21.2–21.5).

Introduction of a laparoscope subumbilically into a preformed pneumoperitoneum of CO_2 allows direct visualisation of the uterus, fallopian tubes, their motility and their relationship with the ovaries

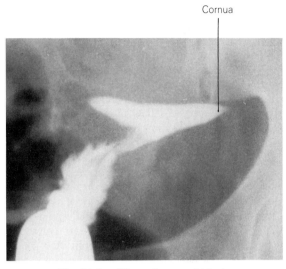

Fig. 21.3   *Bilateral cornual block.*

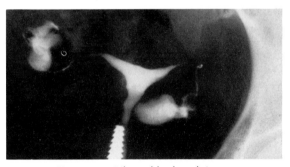

Fig. 21.4   *Bilateral hydrosalpinges.*

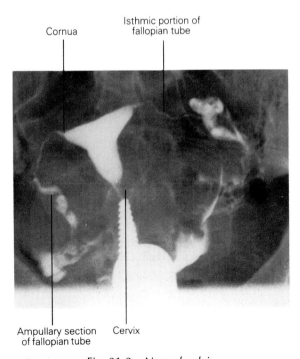

Fig. 21.2   *Normal pelvis.*

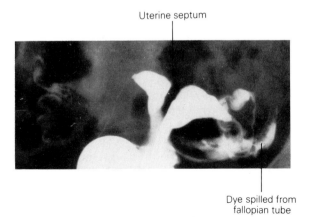

Fig. 21.5   *Septate uterus.*

as well as the ovarian surface for signs of ovulation and adhesions. Laparoscopy is a safe procedure with experience and is best performed under general anaesthesia, because manipulation of the pelvic organs necessary for adequate visualisation of the surfaces is painful. Dye may be introduced through the cervix and tubal patency demonstrated. Increased vascular markings on the external tubal serosa may indicate underlying intraluminal pathology.

Treatment of structural problems is by surgical correction, division of adhesions, and restoration of anatomy. However, even if tubal patency results, there will always be some residual scarring and damage, especially to the sensitive cilial lining of the tube. Thus results as judged by subsequent intrauterine pregnancy rates are disappointingly poor. The use of magnification allows for greater attention to detail, better conservation of healthy tissue, better restoration of anatomy and decreased postoperative adhesion formation. The correct use of the operating microscope requires special training and experience. However, its major contribution to infertility surgery has been not only to give better results, but also to teach all gynaecologists involved in fertility surgery a respect for sensitive tissues, and a better attitude towards conservation of healthy tissue, preservation of anatomy and a decrease in postoperative adhesion formation.

Endometriosis may also affect fertility by distortion of pelvic anatomy, prevention of ovum release or complete tubal blockage. The diagnosis is made by laparoscopy. Treatment may be by surgery — removing or cauterising the endometriotic deposits and restoring the pelvic anatomy — or medically. The most popular medical treatment is Danazol, a gonadotrophin inhibitor, which inhibits ovulation and causes endometrial atrophy. It is used in doses of 200–800 mg daily for 3–6 months.

Danazol is usually used in the milder forms of endometriosis, surgery being indicated when there is gross distortion. Another situation is the finding of minor endometriotic deposits on structures such as the uterosacral ligaments in infertile patients. Although not obviously interfering with the pelvic function or anatomy, it is postulated that the release of prostaglandins (mainly Pg $F_{2\alpha}$) by this ectopic endometrium interferes with tubal transport. The evidence for this is not conclusive.

Uterine leiomyomata may, by their size, cause anatomical distortion or tubal occlusion. Treatment by surgical removal, myomectomy, may be attempted but great care must be taken at the time of operation to avoid postoperative adhesion formation or haematoma in the uterus that subsequently becomes infected.

UNEXPLAINED INFERTILITY

Even with the increase in knowledge of the normal physiology of conception and also the many advances in the treatment of abnormalities which can occur, it has become apparent that there is a small group of couples who, at the end of investigation, appear 'normal' but remain infertile. These couples with 'unexplained infertility' form a difficult and demanding group for the clinician. Sometimes, on closer screening, it is apparent that the results of some of the tests are, in fact, inadequate or 'borderline', or alternatively that some areas have been overlooked, such as minor endometriosis or intrauterine pathology. Before making the diagnosis it is important to be sure that:

1. the infertility evaluation was complete in terms of most modern standards;
2. the results of studies and observations were appropriately interpreted;
3. factors, which were considered within normal limits during investigation, have not changed during the period of evaluation.

Making this diagnosis has some benefits. First, it ensures that the couple have been properly investigated and that no diagnosable abnormality has been missed. Secondly, it may allow a positive approach to counselling the couple by offering alternative treatments, for example various drugs and hormonal combinations or techniques such as in vitro fertilisation (IVF) and gamete intrafallopian transfer (GIFT). In vitro fertilisation is an expensive treatment suitable for women who have irreparable tubal disease or absent tubes, but who are otherwise fertile. The technique is described in Chapter 23. It is a stressful procedure involving detailed monitoring of the stimulated ovarian cycle, collection of eggs, preparing of fresh sperm, fertilisation and embryo culture, and finally reimplantation of the embryo should it fertilise satisfactorily. Thirty per cent of embryo replacements continue to viable pregnancies.

Gamete intrafallopian transfer is a simpler procedure than IVF. Induced ovulation and egg and sperm collection are the same. The egg and sperm are then inserted into the distal end of the fallopian tube at laparoscopy. Hopefully, fertilisation will then occur in its natural environment, namely in the ampulla of the fallopian tube. This means that a culture laboratory is not necessary but, of course, the woman must have normal tubes. The method is not suitable for those with tubal disease, but may be of some value in cases of unexplained infertility.

It is important to explain to both partners that not only has no abnormality been detected, but that there is always a possibility of spontaneous pregnancy occurring. However, it is not enough to offer open-ended psychological support, and the time usually comes when it is important for both partners and the physician to face the facts and acknowledge that, given our present state of knowledge, nothing more can be done and that persistent infertility is a definite possibility. The acceptance of this fact and the psychological adjustment required are important, if the couple are to maintain a balanced healthy attitude. At this time, it may be appropriate to raise the possibility of adoption, if this has not already been considered. Accepting the fact of probable childlessness requires social and psychological adjustment with rearrangement of emphasis on to other things such as career interests or hobbies. An open, honest, three-way discussion by the couple and their physician should set the foundation for this, often difficult, realisation.

SCHEDULE FOR INVESTIGATION

The aim is to collect as much information as quickly as possible, so that therapy can be started without delay. Each return visit should have a number of objectives, so that investigations are completed in a minimum of time and inconvenience to the woman.

First Visit

1. *History*
Take details of:

   a. duration and type of infertility;
   b. previous gynaecological and surgical history, and previous infertility history and treatment;

   c. menstrual, sexual, contraceptive and medical history.

2. *General and gynaecological examination*

3. *Investigation*
   a. *General*
      Basal temperature chart (BTC);
      Prolactin assay;
      Arrange progesterone and second prolactin assay about Day 21 of cycle (midluteal phase);
      Bring seminal analysis (SA).
   b. *Specific*
      If history indicates, arrange hysterosalpingogram (HSG) and/or laparoscopy.

Second Visit

1. Timed midcycle for postcoital test.
2. Review hormones, BTC and SA (p. 313).
3. Arrange HSG (if done too early, this may be traumatic and discourage patient) or book laparoscopy.
4. Arrange repeat of any abnormal tests.

Third Visit

1. Review all data.
2. If HSG abnormal, then arrange laparoscopy.
3. If SA x 2 abnormal, arrange examination of male.
4. If PCT abnormal, repeat and review ovulation/mucus.
5. If anovulation, commence treatment, clomiphene citrate.

Fourth Visit

Definite abnormality should by now be identified and appropriate treatment instigated. Review findings and outline subsequent management. If no abnormalities are detected, and laparoscopy has not yet been performed, it should be done at this stage.

FURTHER READING

Chamberlain G.V.P., Winston R.M.L., eds. (1981). *Tubal Infertility*. London: Blackwell Scientific Publications.

Insler V., Lunenfeld B., eds. (1986). *Infertility: Male and Female*. Edinburgh: Churchill Livingstone.

Muse K.N., Wilson E.A. (1982). How does endometriosis cause infertility? *Fertil. Steril*; **38**: 145–52.

Pepperell R. J., Hudson B., Wood C., eds. (1981). *The Infertile Couple*. Edinburgh: Churchill Livingstone.

22

Reproduction and the Male

ANATOMY

The male reproductive system consists of the testes, epididymes, vasa deferentia, seminal vesicles, prostate, the penis (including its erectile tissue), male urethra and accessory structures including the bulbo-urethral glands.

Testes

The testis lies supported in the scrotum by the scrotal tissue and spermatic cord. Its dimensions are approximately 4 x 3 x 2 cm and it is ovoid in shape. It is covered by a dense fibrous fascia, the tunica albuginea, which is invaginated posteriorly as the mediastinum. Internally, it is divided by fascial septa into some 200 lobules, these septa radiating from the mediastinum. Each lobule contains some three or more seminiferous tubules supported by stroma containing the interstitial cells of Leydig. The seminiferous tubules are lined by cells that produce spermatozoa and are of two types, the supporting cells of Sertoli and the spermatogenic cells themselves. The efferent ducts converge as the rete testes in the mediastinum, efferent ducts from the rete pass superiorly to the apex of the testis and into the head of the epididymis (Fig. 22.1).

The blood supply of the testis is from the testicular artery which arises from the abdominal aorta just below the renal arteries and courses downwards and laterally behind the peritoneum to enter the deep inguinal ring and thence the spermatic cord. This wayward course is due to the embryological origin and descent of the testis *in utero*. The venous drainage enters the pampiniform plexus in the spermatic cord and then into the testicular vein which empties into the inferior vena cava on the

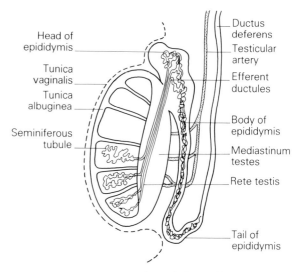

Fig. 22.1   *Cross-section through the testis.*

right and into the left renal vein on the left. Lymph drains to the lumbar lymph nodes and thence to the mediastinum.

Epididymis

The epididymis is essentially a long (6 cm) convoluted tube lined by pseudostratified columnar epithelium and is usually described as having a head, a body and tail. The head is closely apposed to the upper pole of the testis where the efferent ducts of the rete testis perforate the tunica albuginea. The body lies posterior and lateral to the testis and descends to its lower pole, where the tail is attached by dense fibrous tissue and the reflection of the tunica vaginalis. The tail drains into the ductus deferens.

Blood supply is from the testicular artery and venous drainage is similar.

Ductus Deferens (Vas Deferens)

The ductus deferens is a thick-walled muscular tube consisting of an internal mucosa and submucosa with three well-defined layers of smooth muscle: an internal longitudinal layer, which fades out proximally, and an inner circular and external longitudinal layer. It courses from the tail of the epididymis superiorly into the posterior part of the spermatic cord, through the superficial inguinal ring and along the inguinal canal to enter the pelvis, separating from the other structures in the cord to pass, initially, superiorly, anterior to the external iliac artery and then, posteriorly, into the pelvis on its lateral wall, crossing the ureter on the posterior surface of the bladder to join the duct of the seminal vesicle as the common ejaculatory duct. This duct pierces between the median and lateral lobes of the prostate to open into the prostatic urethra through the veru (verumontanum) on its posterior wall (Fig. 22.2).

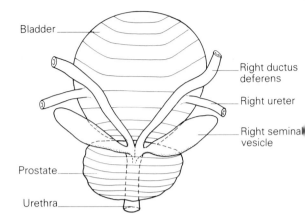

Fig. 22.3   *Posterior representation of bladder and prostate.*

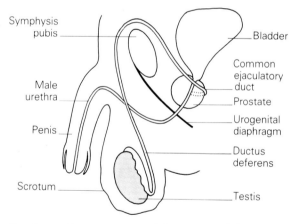

Fig. 22.2   *Representation of the course of the ductus deferens and male urethra.*

Seminal Vesicles

The left and right seminal vesicles lie attached to the posterior wall of the bladder, just superiorly and posteriorly to the prostate (Fig. 22.3). Each vesicle, approximately 6 cm long, joins the ductus deferens as the ejaculatory duct. The ureters lie somewhat

superiorly and medially to each vesicle with the ductus deferens crossing the ureter from above.

Each vesicle is lined with pseudostratified columnar epithelium with diverticulae containing goblet cells that secrete a large part of the seminal fluid. They do not form a reservoir for spermatozoa. Surrounding the mucosa is a muscular layer, thinner and less well-defined than that of the ductus, but, nevertheless, with a discernible inner circular and outer longitudinal coat. The vesicles contract during ejaculation. The blood supply comes from the inferior vesical and middle rectal arteries and the venous drainage is via the prostatic and pelvic plexuses. Lymph vessels backtrack along the arteries and nerve supply is derived from the pelvic plexuses.

Prostate

The prostate is a walnut-sized gland, weighing approximately 8 g, that has a tendency to enlarge with age. It is inferior to the bladder surrounding the prostatic part of the male urethra. It is supported, anteriorly, by the puboprostatic ligaments and, inferiorly, by the urogenital diaphragm and lies directly behind the symphysis pubis. Posteriorly, it is separated from the rectum by the rectovesical fascia of Denonvilliers (Figs. 22.2 and 22.3).

It can easily be palpated through the rectal wall and feels, to the probing finger, to have a median sulcus separating the gland into right and left lobes. Structurally, the prostate is enveloped in a thin capsule which is firmly adherent and continuous with the stroma of the gland. It contains smooth muscle fibres, which necessarily surround the urethra and can be seen to be continuous with fibres from the neck of the bladder, thus forming the involuntary sphincter of the urethra. The stroma of the gland itself consists of much elastic tissue and smooth muscle fibres, in which are embedded many epithelial glands that drain, via 25 or so ducts, into the urethra in the sulcus lateral to the verumontanum.

Blood supply comes from the inferior vesical and middle rectal arteries and some from the internal pudendal. Venous drainage is via the prostatic plexus and veins to the internal iliac veins. A rich nervous innervation of both sympathetic and parasympathetic origin is found. Lymph drains to the hypogastric, sacral, vesical and external iliac nodes.

Penis and Male Urethra

The penis is the male organ of copulation. It contains erectile tissue that brings about an increase in length and rigidity to enable vaginal penetration to occur.

It consists of two parts: the root, attached to the urogenital diaphragm, and the body, which hangs limply and is completely covered in loose fitting skin. Internally, the penis consists of three main parts: the left and right corpora cavernosa, and the median corpus spongiosum. The corpora cavernosa take origin from the base of the pubic arch and the lateral aspect of the urogenital diaphragm, here called the crura. Passing forward, these two corpora meet in the midline and continue into the body of the penis. The corpus spongiosum contains the bulb and spongy parts of the male urethra and arises in the midline from the urogenital diaphragm. Here the urethra pierces the urogenital diaphragm to enter the corpus. It continues forward into the pendulous portion and expands distally as the glans penis. It lies on the ventral aspect of the two corpora cavernosa (Fig. 22.4).

Each corpora is surrounded by a strong fibrous membrane called the tunica albuginea. The tunica of the two corpora cavernosa are fused in the midline as the septum penis. Surrounding the three corpora is a loose fitting layer of fascia (Buck's fascia) that is continuous with fascia from the anterior abdominal wall and, covering the whole, is a loose layer of skin that distally extends as a hood-

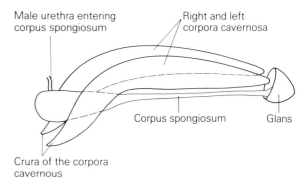

Fig. 22.4 *Diagrammatic representation of the corpora.*

Male urethra entering corpus spongiosum

Right and left corpora cavernosa

Corpus spongiosum

Glans

Crura of the corpora cavernous

like structure, the prepuce, which covers the glans penis. The body of the penis is supported by the suspensory ligament attached to the front of the pubic symphysis and blending with the tunica albuginea of the corpora cavernosa.

The blood supply is derived from the internal pudendal artery via three main branches. The bulbar artery pierces the urogenital diaphragm to enter the corpus spongiosum. Just distal to this artery, a second branch, the urethral artery, also pierces the diaphragm to follow the course of the urethra. Lastly, the penile artery divides into two branches: the deep artery, which pierces the urogenital diaphragm to supply each crura and corpus cavernosum, and the dorsal artery, which passes forward, under the arcuate ligament, into the dorsal aspect of the penis deep to the fascia. The dorsal artery sends some 5 or 6 circumflex branches around the shaft, forming a rich anastomosis, branches of which perforate the tunica albuginea and supply the corpus cavernosum as well.

Many arteriovenous anastomoses exist in the corpora and these play an important part in the mechanism of erection.

The venous drainage can be divided into three components.

1. *The superficial veins:* a rich network that merges as the superficial dorsal vein and empties commonly into the left saphenous vein, but variants are common, e.g. the right saphenous vein, the epigastric and even the femoral veins.
2. *The intermediate veins* deep to Buck's fascia that drain into the deep dorsal vein which passes under the suspensory ligament and anterior to the anterior free edge of the urogenital diaphragm into the prostatic plexus.

3. *The deep veins* which drain the corpora directly into the pudendal prostatic plexus.

Emissary veins exist that communicate between the corpora and the deep dorsal vein and, also, anastomoses exist between the superficial and deep dorsal veins.

The nerve supply of the penis comes from the pudendal nerve (root value S 2, 3, 4).

Lymph drains from the skin to the superficial inguinal nodes, from the glans to the deep inguinal and external iliac nodes, and from the urethra to the hypogastric and common iliac nodes.

Male urethra

The male urethra is divided into several parts: the prostatic part, within the prostate, 3 cm long, connects the bladder with the membranous part; the spongy urethra lies within the corpus spongiosum and terminates at the external urethral orifice. The urethra is lined with transitional epithelium throughout, except distally, where it becomes squamous in nature.

PHYSIOLOGY

Normal male potency requires all the intrinsic parts of the reproductive system to function correctly and in conjunction. The various stages involved are spermatogenesis, transport of active spermatozoa, production of semen, erection and ejaculation.

Spermatogenesis

Spermatogenesis occurs in cycles, each consisting of three stages of approximately 23 days. Successive phases of the cycle occur at consecutive intervals along the length of the tubule. In the first phase, the primitive germ cells replicate by mitotic division and produce several generations of spermatogonia. Each spermatogonium divides into two diploid primary spermatocytes, which undergo a meiotic or reduction division with the formation of two haploid spermatocytes. A second maturation division then occurs, resulting in four haploid spermatids arising from every primary spermatocyte. After a number of nuclear and cytoplasmic changes, the spermatids become spermatozoa. The mature sper-

matozoa is an actively motile cell consisting of two main parts. The head is covered in its anterior two-thirds by the acrosomal cap, and the tail provides motility and correct orientation at the time of fertilisation.

Steroidogenesis

Leydig cells of the testes produce 90% of circulating testosterone. The remainder comes from the adrenals and peripheral conversion of precursor steroids. Androgens are important for the development of the fetal genitalia and for the development and maintenance of secondary sexual characteristics and normal sexual activity. The very high intra-testicular concentration of testosterone may be necessary for germ cell maturation.

Endocrine control of spermatogenesis

The testes are affected by the gonadotrophins, luteinising hormone (LH) and follicle stimulating hormone (FSH) (Fig. 22.5). Testicular hormones

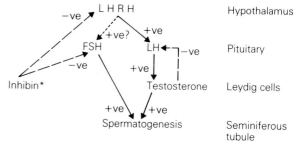

Fig. 22.5 *Hormonal control of spermatogenesis. Inhibin is a polypeptide hormone found in high levels in the seminiferous tubules. It has been shown to decrease FSH secretion. It is thus postulated that this hormone is the feedback required to control FSH secretion. It may prove to be useful as a male contraceptive.*

exert a negative feedback on LH production and, to a small extent, that of FSH. However, the failure of androgens to suppress FSH to normal levels after castration suggests an additional feedback mechanism. Inhibin, a peptide produced by the Sertoli cells, may be responsible for this. The Sertoli cells are probably the sole target for FSH within the testes. In response to both testosterone and FSH they produce a high affinity androgen binding protein which maintains the high androgen content within the seminiferous tubules. Significantly elevated levels of LH and FSH are found in infertile men with severe degrees of germ cell damage. Normal levels of reproductive hormones in males are shown in Table 22.1.

Table 22.1

Normal Levels of Reproductive Hormones in Males

Testosterone	10	– 28	nmol/l
Leuteinising hormone	4	– 14	iu/l
Follicle stimulating hormone	1.5	– 8	iu/l
Prolactin	75	– 375	mu/l

Semen

The bulk of the ejaculated fluid consists of secretions from the seminal vesicles and the prostate gland, 60% being produced from the seminal vesicles. Normal semen has a pH of 7.3–7.5 and a reasonable ejaculate volume would be 2.5–5 ml containing approximately 100×10^6 spermatozoa per ml (less than 20×10^6 normal spermatozoa per ml would render the individual subfertile).

The chemical content of semen is summarised in Table 22.2. For semen to be impregnated, a two-part mechanism occurs: erection and ejaculation.

Table 22.2

Chemical Content of Seminal Fluid

Seminal vesicle	60%	Fructose
		Phosphotidylcholine
		Vit C
		Prostaglandins
		Flavins
Prostate	35%	Spermine
		Citric acid
		Cholesterol and phospholipids
		Zinc
		Acid phosphatase
		Phosphate and bicarbonate buffers

Erection

Erection involves the lengthening and increased rigidity of the penis and is essentially a vascular phenomenon. There has been much debate in the medical literature as to the relative importance of various events that occur. It would appear, however, that there are three components to erection.

1. Increased arterial flow
2. Active relaxation of sinusoidal spaces within the corpora cavernosa
3. Active and passive venous constriction.

Stimulation of the nerve supply to the corpora cavernosa produces a three-phase response.

1. *Latent phase:* the shaft increases in length with an increase in arterial flow (both systolic and diastolic) with no change in intracorporeal pressure, suggesting decrease in resistance to flow.
2. *Tumescence:* the corpora harden and there is an increase in intracorporeal pressure and, at the same time, arterial flow remains increased.
3. *Full erection:* the intracorporal pressure reaches 5–10 mmHg below that of systolic aortic pressure and the flow decreases, but does stay higher than the prestimulation level.

Lastly, on removal of stimulus, detumescence occurs and all the parameters return to prestimulus level.

The nervous and humoral mechanisms that bring about this process are by no means clear-cut. It would appear that the flaccid state is due to an intrinsic tone in the afferent arteriolar sphincters that is under sympathetic alpha-adrenergic stimulation. By releasing this tone, either by decreasing the sympathetic drive or by active dilatation by some other, as yet, undetermined mechanism, erection will occur. One such neurotransmitter, a non-adrenergic, non-cholinergic substance (NANC), vasoactive polypeptide (VIP) has been shown to produce erection in normal subjects and can be found in nerves in the corpora cavernosa. There is no doubt that intracorporeal injection of alpha adrenergic blockers produces erection, but whether a decrease in adrenergic tone is the major event is not yet clear.

It must also be said that venous leakage does cause some cases of human erectile impotence, and it is this that suggests that active venous constriction is a required mechanism. Venous leakage can be demonstrated in these cases by such techniques as dynamic cavernosography.

Ejaculation

Ejaculation is essentially a spinal reflex, but higher centres are also intricately involved. There are three phases:

1. Seminal emission
2. Formation of a pressure chamber
3. Expulsion of fluid from the urethra.

Seminal emission is controlled via the sympathetic nervous system and noradrenaline can be found in large quantities within the vas and ejaculatory ducts. Sympathetic stimulation results in contraction of the smooth muscle within the seminal vesicles, ejaculatory duct and prostate to express secretions into the prostatic urethra. As emission occurs, pressure increases within the urethra, between the vesicle neck and the urogenital diaphragm. It is this increase in pressure that forces fluid into the bulbar urethra. An intact bladder neck is required to prevent retrograde ejaculation into the bladder. Rhythmic contractions of the bladder neck under alpha adrenergic stimulation have been demonstrated during ejaculation and, at the same time, relaxation of the external sphincter under somatic control via pudendal nerves allows semen to pass through the urogenital diaphragm into the bulbar urethra. Finally, expulsion of semen from the urethra is brought about by rhythmic contractions of the bulbospongiosus and bulbocavernosus muscles also under somatic control by the pudendal nerves.

Orgasm

Orgasm is the sensation of pleasure that normally accompanies the sequence of events already described. Part of the pleasure of orgasm is the feeling of tension and inevitability associated, temporarily, with contraction of smooth muscle in the seminal vesicles and prostate, with the development of the pressure chamber and, finally, the release of ejaculation. Whether the contraction of smooth muscle

is appreciated at a cortical level is unknown as, in other parts of the body, smooth muscle contraction is rarely associated with conscious appreciation.

The nervous pathways are obviously complicated and probably involve sensory information in both autonomic and somatic systems. Sensation, via the pudendal nerves, probably starts the sequence and a positive feedback circuit can be envisaged. As each phase of the sequence begins, further sensory afferents are stimulated and the sensations summate as orgasm on ejaculation.

Orgasm can occur without sensory stimulation of the genitalia, as seen in the phantom orgasmic imagery of paraplegics and stimulation of the septal area of the brain can lead to the experience. It would appear, therefore, that there is a cortical association area that, when stimulated, leads to orgasm, either via sensory afferents or by some other mechanism.

Orgasm can occur without emission and ejaculation in this way and, similarly, emission and ejaculation can be brought about without local stimulation (the nocturnal emissions of adolescence).

Orgasm is, as yet, a subjective phenomenon, the neurophysiology involved being complicated and ill-understood.

INFERTILITY

In the past, male dominated societies have been unable and unwilling to accept the fact that the male partner of an infertile marriage could be responsible. This is exemplified by many of the ancient gods such as Osiris of Egypt, Frey of Sweden and Priapus of the Romans being depicted with an erect or enlarged phallus (Fig. 22.6). In India, 'sterile' women would visit temples of Siva, where they would press their naked bodies against the massive phallus of the god's statue.

Between 8 and 15% of marriages are childless, though not all of these are involuntary. Male disorders are responsible in 30% of couples and contributory in a further 20%. It is now accepted that the investigation and treatment of infertility involves both partners, and most centres now run clinics where the husband and wife are seen and investigated together. In younger couples this is normally after two years of unprotected intercourse

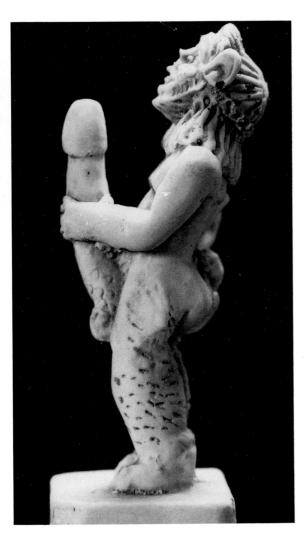

Fig. 22.6 *Statue with enlarged phallus used as a fertility symbol.*

Table 22.3
Abnormalities of Sperm Count

Azoospermia	Absence of sperm in the ejaculate
Severe oligospermia	$<5 \times 10^6$ spermatozoa/ml
Oligospermia	$<20 \times 10^6$ spermatozoa/ml
Asthenospermia	$<60\%$ motile at 3 hours

Male infertility can be classified into:
1. Pretesticular causes, which are mainly hormonal in origin;
2. Testicular causes due to damage to the germinal epithelium; or
3. Post-testicular causes due to abnormalities of the normal sperm transport pathways.

The clinical history and physical examination are aimed at determining the likely cause, so that appropriate investigations for the individual patient, rather than a full battery of tests for all, can be carried out.

History and Examination

It is essential to see both partners together and individually. A history of a previous child does not exclude either partner from further investigation.

Fertility status is often a good reflection of general fitness, particularly in relation to smoking, alcohol intake and obesity, all of which impair spermatogenesis. The frequency and timing of intercourse is important, but knowledge of the fertile period is not essential. In cases where sexual intercourse is infrequent, due to absence of one or other partner, this knowledge becomes more important.

Occupational history

Exposure to pesticides, drugs used in the treatment of nematodes, cadmium, lead, arsenic and zinc, and a variety of organic chemicals impairs spermatogenesis. Occupations which result in an increase in scrotal temperature, for example boiler workers, long-distance lorry drivers and fighter pilots, may impair fertility.

Drug history

Many drugs used in the treatment of malignancy

though, in couples where one partner is over the age of thirty, this period should be considerably less. The treatment of male problems is both controversial and very much in its infancy, and aims to provide a reliable prognosis based on probabilities derived from semen analysis, hormone levels and antibody studies. Recent research using hamster egg penetration tests, cervical mucus penetration and photographic determination of sperm motility can now provide a specific prognosis for the individual patient based on the categories of sperm count abnormalities shown in Table 22.3.

significantly affect spermatogenesis sometimes permanently. These include most alkylating agents, e.g. chlorambucil, cyclophosphamide, nitrogen mustard and melphelan. Other drugs such as sulphasalazine used in the treatment of ulcerative colitis results in oligospermia. Cimetidine and spironolactone inhibit androgen action, and ethanol, marijuana and opiates, through a variety of different mechanisms, may affect spermatogenesis (Table 22.4).

Medical history

Impaired spermatogenesis may occur in men with a history of undescended testes or previous scrotal or inguinal surgery. Many infections, including mumps, syphilis, gonorrhoea, tuberculosis and typhoid may result in an orchitis. Some congenital and chromosomal disorders also affect fertility, e.g. prune belly syndrome, cystic fibrosis, Kartagener's syndrome and Klinefelter's syndrome. Damage to the pituitary or hypothalamus may result in secondary infertility.

Physical examination

This is aimed at identifying syndromes associated with infertility and local abnormalities, which may impair sperm production or transport. The male partner should be examined in both the erect and supine positions with all clothes removed to assess build and any other general abnormalities sugges-tive of endocrine or chromosomal abnormality. In Klinefelter's syndrome (XXY), the limbs are disproportionately long in proportion to the trunk and gynaecomastia may be present. Gynaecomastia is also found in men with hyperprolactinaemia, though most men with this condition usually present with impotence or lack of libido rather than infertility. It is unusual for men with pituitary failure to present primarily with infertility.

Local examination

The penis. Meatal stenosis, phimosis, or hypospadias may result in ineffective ejaculation and require correction. If impotence is a problem, the femoral pulses should be palpated for evidence of vascular deficiency and, with a Doppler probe, the blood pressure in the penis should be measured. A difference of 40 mmHg or more between that and the brachial blood pressure suggests that an arterial perfusion defect is likely to be the cause of the impotence. Prolongation of the bulbo cavernosa reflex may suggest a neurological component to impotence.

Scrotal contents. The testes should be examined for their position, consistency and size, the latter being measured by using an orchiometer (Fig. 22.7) for a more accurate assessment of volume. The epididymes are more often affected by infection than the testes. A hard irregular epididymis is often associated with a past history of venereal disease, bacterial epididymitis or tuberculosis. A swelling in

Table 22.4
Drugs Commonly Affecting Fertility

Chemotherapeutic agents	Effect	Recovery
Mustine Vincristine Prednisolone and Procarbazine	Invariable profound oligospermia	Rare
Doxorubicin bleomycin Vinblastine docarbazine	Occasional azoospermia	Occasional
Chlorambucil	Azoospermia	Usual
Anabolic steroids	Oligospermia	Usual
Sulphasalazine	Oligospermia	Usual
Cimetidine Spironolactone	Androgen inhibition	Usual
Propanolol	Decreases motility	Usual

the head of the epididymis may be associated with an obstruction. Both vasa deferentia should be palpated, as bilateral absence accounts for up to 2% of men attending an infertility clinic. The presence of a varicocele should be sought with the patient standing, breathing quietly and also during a Valsalva manoeuvre. The use of Doppler or thermography increases the diagnostic accuracy. Ninety per cent of varicoceles occur on the left, but they can occur solely on the right, or rarely bilaterally.

Abdomen. Both groins should be examined for scars from previous herniorrhaphies or attempts to locate or bring down an undescended testis. The prostate should always be examined and the expressed prostatic secretion collected and examined for the presence of white blood cells and bacteria.

Investigations

Seminology

Seminal analysis should be carried out after 3 days' abstinence from sexual intercourse and at least two samples, 3 weeks apart, should be examined. No more than 2 h should pass from the time of ejaculation to the time of examination. The seminal fluid should be produced by masturbation and collected into a glass container with a screw cap. If coitus interruptus is used, the sperm rich first part of the ejaculate is often lost. Condoms contain spermicides and should not be used. Routine analysis (Table 22.5) will report volume, liquefaction, viscosity, motility, the presence of sperm agglutination, bacteria and leucocytes. The sperm density, i.e. numbers of sperm per ml, must always be related to the total sperm count. The percentage of abnormal forms is also reported. Unless the patient is azoospermic, it is difficult, using the above measurements, to produce an accurate prognosis for the individual patient. Three tests, mucus penetration, zona free egg penetration and photographic determination of motility, now being used more commonly, determine the capability of the best spermatozoa in the sample and give a much better prognosis for the individual patient.

Endocrine studies

It is not necessary to carry out endocrine studies in all patients. The majority of patients presenting with infertility have hormone changes secondary to seminiferous tubule damage rather than any primary endocrine abnormality. Acquired lesions of the pituitary may give rise to hypogonadotrophic hypogonadism, but this is usually associated with other pituitary defects, which require more urgent treatment. Hyperprolactinaemia is usually associated with impotence and its significance in men present-

Table 22.5

Seminal Analysis – Normal Values and Common Causes of Abnormalities

Normal range	Abnormality	Common causes
Volume 2–6 ml	Low	Inadequate collection, absent prostate and seminal vesicles, retrograde ejaculation
	High	Prolonged abstinence
Concentration > 60 x 10^6 spermatozoa/ml	Low	Chronic systemic disorders, acute febrile illness. Toxic agents or drugs, accessory gland infection, varicocele, cryptorchidism
	High	Low seminal volume
	Absent	Epidydimal obstruction, absent vasa, absent spermatogonia. Drugs, toxic agents, pituitary failure, retrograde ejaculation
Motility > 60% showing forward progressive at 3 h	Low	High scrotal temperature, occupations, varicocele
Liquefaction complete in < 20 min	Failure	Prostatic infection
Agglutination > 10%	> 10%	Infection, antibodies
Bacteria None	Present	Prostatic infection, contamination, non-sterile container
Fructose	Absent	Absent prostate and seminal vesicles

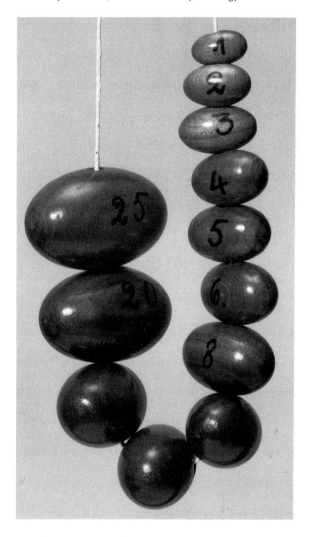

Fig. 22.7   *An orchiometer. This is used to provide an accurate assessment of testicular volume, and consists of wooden beads of varying sizes.*

ing with infertility is doubtful on present evidence. A high FSH level in the presence of small testes signifies irreversible testicular damage.

Antibody studies

Autoantibodies to certain spermatozoal antigens can exert pathological effects causing infertility. Antibodies to sperm surface antigens are usually detected by agglutination or complement mediated cytotoxic reactions. Approximately 10% of men from couples with unexplained infertility have antisperm antibodies. It is usual to examine their serum first and to test seminal plasma in all those with serum antibodies. Antibodies are more likely to be found in couples with a poor postcoital test, i.e. less than five motile sperms per high power field present in normal preovulatory cervical mucus. Antibodies are also likely to be present when there is massive agglutination of fresh semen.

A useful test for screening spermatozoa for antisperm antibodies is the mixed erythrocyte spermatozoa antiglobulin reaction (MAR) test, which can detect both IgG and IgA antibodies. Using an indirect version of the technique, serum antibodies can be determined while a direct technique determines antibodies bound to the surface of spermatozoa in the ejaculate.

The clinical significance of serum titres of antibodies is determined using the sperm cervical mucus contact test. Using fertile donor sperm and normal cervical mucus as controls with sperm and cervical mucus from the infertile couple, positive evidence as to which partner is likely to have significant antibodies can be obtained. A positive reaction is shown by a change in sperm motility when in contact with cervical mucus. The spermatozoa change from a progressive movement to a characteristic non-progressive shaking or jerking movement.

Testicular biopsy

Testicular biopsy may be indicated in the following situations:

1. Azoospermia with a mild elevation of FSH to distinguish between obstruction, germinal cell damage, maturation arrest of the developing spermatozoa or the Sertoli cell only syndrome, where the patient is born without spermatogonia.
2. Severe oligospermia with normal FSH.
3. Infertility of long duration with non-contributory tests on both husband and wife. Certain rare disorders of meiosis may be detected by meiotic analysis.
4. Where chemicals or cytotoxic agents might be implicated as a cause of infertility.

Treatment of Specific Clinical Situations

Varicocele

The mechanisms by which a varicocele affects

testicular function and how often this occurs in the male population is not known. Many patients with varicoceles have normal fertility. One suggested mechanism is the bilateral elevation of testicular temperature. Reflux of adrenal metabolites, changes in prostaglandin levels and alteration in testosterone levels have also been reported in association with a varicocele. There are many reports of improvement in semen quality and an increased rate of pregnancy after varicocele ligation. However, there are also reports questioning the efficacy of varicocelectomy in subfertile men. In one controlled study, no changes were seen in motility and motile sperm count following varicocelectomy compared with preoperative sperm counts when there were less than 10 million per ml. Treatment of varicoceles by embolisation of the testicular veins is being tried, but it is too early to assess the results. The site of choice for division and ligation of the internal spermatic vein is at the internal inguinal ring through an inguinal approach. The treatment of varicoceles is still controversial and before infertility is ascribed to the presence of a varicocele it is important to ensure that the female partner is normal.

Azoospermia

The complete absence of sperm on seminal analysis is usually due to a blockage of sperm transport or spermatogenic arrest, i.e. a failure at some stage during sperm production, in which case the plasma FSH will be normal. Other causes such as anorchism, germinal aplasia (Sertoli cell only syndrome) or previous cytotoxic therapy will usually be associated with an elevated FSH level. The presence of small testes and grossly elevated FSH levels requires counselling of the couple with regard to the hopeless prognosis and the discussion of adoption or artificial insemination using donor's sperm. If the FSH and testicular size are normal, operation should be advised. This enables the testes and epididymes to be inspected, to perform vasography, to biopsy the testicles and carry out any reconstructive procedure that may be indicated. The results of surgery for obstruction in the epididymis, however, are not good.

Antisperm antibodies

If it has been decided that antisperm antibodies are significantly interfering with fertility and that the wife has patent tubes and ovulation is occurring regularly, then treatment of the male partner should be initiated. Treatments include artificial insemination after sperm washing, prednisolone, given either as a long-term low dose regimen or in a high dose given to the male on Days 21–28 of his wife's menstrual cycle. Side-effects such as dyspepsia, haematemesis, diabetes, acne or avascular necrosis of bone may occur and the patient must be advised accordingly. The degree of response to treatment can be checked using the MAR and postcoital tests.

Erectile and ejaculatory disorders

Organic impotence due to previous trauma, operations, priapism, neuropathy or vascular insufficiency are probably best treated by implanting a penile prosthesis or by autoinjection of vasoactive drugs. The result of microsurgical revascularisation of the penile arteries have so far been disappointing. Patients with psychogenic impotence should be seen by a therapist with a particular interest in this type of disorder. Ejaculatory disorders, such as premature ejaculation or failure to ejaculate, usually require psychosexual counselling. Retrograde ejaculation is the most common cause of an absent ejaculate. The semen passes backwards through the bladder neck into the bladder. This is usually due to congenital dysfunction of the bladder neck, previous surgery to the bladder neck, or surgical injury causing damage to the sympathetic supply to the bladder neck. The most effective treatment is to ejaculate with the bladder full. Alternatively, drugs to stimulate bladder receptors such as sympathomimetic agents or antihistamines may be used. Occasionally, surgery may be required, or retrieval from the bladder of semen by postejaculatory catheterisation and artificial insemination.

Non-specific Treatments

Few controlled trials have been performed to evaluate treatment of the husband when no specific abnormality causing defective spermatogenesis has been found. In men with very abnormal seminal analysis, including poor mucus penetration, poor swim-up tests and poor zonal free egg penetration, it is unlikely that pregnancies will ensue and adoption or AID should be considered.

Possible Therapies

Clomiphene produces an increase in the secretion of pituitary gonadotrophins. A recent multicentre trial showed that no group or subgroup benefited from clomiphene when compared with vitamin C.

Androgen therapy

There are many anecdotes which report their benefit, but the appropriate subgroup has not been defined.

Bromocriptine

In a randomised study of infertile men with slightly elevated prolactin levels, and other infertile men with normal prolactin levels, there were no beneficial results in terms of improved semen analysis or pregnancies. Various vitamins, particularly vitamin C, and some metals, including zinc, have been tried, and some improvement in seminal parameters has been reported. Cold scrotal bathing and the avoidance of tight under-clothing have been reported to improve motility and improve low counts in some men.

AID and adoption

There is no evidence that artificial insemination of the husband's sperm (AIH), with defective spermatozoa, is of benefit. It may be the only form of therapy in cases of physical deformity preventing intercourse, and may have a role for those couples where antisperm antibodies interfere with sperm transport.

Despite an improvement in our knowledge of the abnormalities of the male reproductive system, many men will be unable to father a child. One of the main purposes of an infertility clinic is to identify those couples, so that they can be counselled and advised early with regard to Artificial Insemination by Donor (AID) or adoption. Despite the increase in public acceptance, and a dramatic increase in demand, AID is not yet readily available in most NHS clinics in the United Kingdom. The main indications are non-remediable azoospermia or oligospermia. The process of selection of patients should ensure that the man has a non-remedial problem, that the woman is fertile and the couple are suitably counselled and prepared to have a child by this method.

FURTHER READING

Belsey M.A., Moghiffi K.S., Eliasson R., Poulsen C.A. *et al.*, eds. (1980). Laboratory manual for the examination of human semen, and semen cervical mucus interaction. In *World Health Organisation and Special Programme of Research, Development and Research Training in Human Reproduction.* Singapore: Press Concern.

Hargreave T.B. (1983). *Male Infertility.* Berlin, Heidelberg, New York, Tokyo: Springer Verlag.

23

In Vitro Fertilisation

There are over 250 000 infertile couples in the UK and for some in vitro fertilisation (IVF) is often the only successful treatment. IVF treatment comprises several key procedures (Table 23.1). After assessment and pretreatment, if necessary, the woman is given a course of hormone therapy designed to stimulate the development of multiple follicles in her ovaries. The eggs which ripen (ideally at least three) are removed from the follicle by aspiration at laparoscopy, or non-laparoscopically using ultrasound control. They are then fertilised in a test-tube or dish using her husband's sperm or that of a donor. The embryo that develops from each egg is cultured for 1–2 days in culture medium at 37°C. Those embryos whose cells appear to divide normally are replaced into the uterus. When possible, three embryos are replaced simultaneously. This increases the chance of a pregnancy, but it is unusual for more than one baby to develop.

This chapter examines in some detail the major steps involved in a course of IVF treatment, and considers the results currently being obtained, the future developments and the political controversies which can be anticipated. Because it is a new clinical procedure, there is no general consensus on a standard treatment regimen. Specific details given here are from the protocols used in the Hammersmith Hospital IVF programme.

PROCEDURES INVOLVED IN CLINICAL IVF

Patient Selection and Pretreatment

IVF is becoming the treatment of choice for women whose fallopian tubes are absent or have been irreparably damaged due to disease or previous surgery. Those couples most likely to succeed in achieving a viable pregnancy will usually fulfil the selection criteria listed in Table 23.2. If other pathology exists, it should be resolved before IVF treatment begins. It is axiomatic that the general health and psychological condition of both partners should be adequate to undergo this as for any other form of infertility treatment.

Table 23.1

Steps Involved in IVF Treatment

Patient assessment/selection
Ovarian stimulation
Egg collection
Sperm processing
Fertilisation and embryo culture
Embryo replacement
Luteal phase support

Table 23.2

Patients Most Suited to IVF Treatment

Age	≤35 yr
Cause of infertility	Tubal
Menstrual cycles	Ovulatory (±28 d)
Endocrine status	'Normal'
Ovaries	Accessible
Uterine cavity	'Normal'
Cervix	Sounded*
Semen	'Normal'†

* Embryo transfer catheter can be passed
† Total count ≥40 x 10^6/ml
  Motility ≥40%

The Male Partner

Up to a fifth of the husbands of women whose infertility can be treated by IVF can be expected to have abnormal semen. Although IVF still might be possible, the results are unacceptably poor in most cases. Thorough assessment of the male is, therefore, needed to exclude a pathological semen profile. 'Normal' values for a semen analysis are those given on p. 313. The analysis should be repeated shortly before the IVF treatment cycle is due to begin. It should be emphasised here that semen specimens which do not fulfil all 'normal' criteria are not necessarily infertile and *vice versa*. Probably, the most meaningful parameter is the number of sperm and their motility. Viscous semen or pronounced sperm clumping can cause problems in the isolation of motile sperm for IVF.

Semen can contain many potentially pathogenic organisms, although their effect of IVF outcome is unknown. It is expedient to carry out a microbiological examination and, if pathogens are isolated, give appropriate chemotherapeutic agents before the IVF treatment starts. Prophylactic antibiotic therapy in the week leading up to semen production for IVF may also be beneficial.

Limited IVF success has been obtained for men with oligospermia (semen with low sperm concentration) and asthenospermia (low sperm motility). However, in these cases or if there is sterility due to absence of sperm (azoospermia), donor insemination can be considered.

The Female Partner

For the woman, factors which have a major impact on IVF outcome are age; the condition of her ovaries, uterus and cervix; and ovarian accessibility for egg collection. A woman is born with her full complement of about one to two million eggs; they diminish in number and age, as she grows older. The eggs which are ovulated by older women are more likely to develop abnormally if they are fertilised. Miscarriage rates and the incidence of various birth anomalies such as Down's syndrome increase with age. For these reasons, IVF is rarely offered to women over 40 years of age.

Pelvic examination

Preliminary laparoscopy is needed to determine the extent of any pelvic disease and assess the accessibility of the ovaries for oocyte collection. Active pelvic inflammatory disease, endometriosis, tubo-ovarian masses and ovarian cysts are contraindications for IVF. If the ovaries are inaccessible, it may be possible to remove adhesions and/or resite them surgically as appropriate.

Ovarian and uterine function

A history of regular approximately 28-day menstrual cycles is important evidence that ovarian function is 'normal'. Average menstrual cycle length can also be used to predict the length of the follicular phase and hence to help time egg collection in the IVF treatment cycle. Therefore, the patient should keep a daily temperature chart and/or record the first day of full menstrual flow for at least six consecutive cycles before IVF treatment begins. Progesterone measurements in blood collected during the midluteal phase of one of these cycles are a minimal requirement to determine if they are 'ovulatory'. Values of $\geqslant 30$ nmol/l suggest normal luteal development.

The best evidence that uterine function is normal is previous parity. A hysterosalpingogram is advisable. Certain abnormalities, such as fibroids or congenital malformations of the uterus, may interfere with implantation or cause early miscarriage.

Cervix

Transcervical replacement of embryos to the uterus is the climax of an IVF treatment cycle; it is essential that this step is carried out quickly and easily. This is facilitated if depth, curvature and ease of uterine sounding are checked during a pretreatment menstrual cycle.

Infections in the cervix may be carried into the uterus by the embryo replacement catheter. Microorganisms and/or the local tissue responses which they engender in the uterine cavity may interfere with implantation. Some pathogens can even infect the baby at birth. A cervical swab should be taken to exclude the presence of harmful organisms and prophylactic antibiotic therapy can be given at the time of embryo replacement.

Endocrine status

Plasma levels of luteinising hormone (LH), follicle-stimulating hormone (FSH), oestradiol, testosterone, progesterone, prolactin and thyroid-stimulating hormone (TSH) should be within the normal ranges for women with regular ovulatory menstrual cycles.

Ovarian stimulation

The number of ripe eggs which can be recovered from the ovaries is a major factor limiting the outcome of IVF. Success rates increase dramatically if multiple embryos are replaced in the uterus. Since either ovary produces only one ripe egg in a spontaneous menstrual cycle, the follicular phase before IVF must be supplemented with exogenous hormones in order to stimulate the number of eggs which develop for collection. To appreciate the underlying strategies involved in successful 'superovulation', it is necessary first to consider how preovulatory follicular development is regulated in a spontaneous ovarian cycle. This has been described in detail in Chapter 3.

When the preovulatory follicle has become fully mature and the circulating oestradiol level is at a zenith, the pituitary gland suddenly discharges increased amounts of LH. This midcycle gonadotrophin surge initiates the final stages of follicle and oocyte maturation culminating in rupture of the ripe preovulatory follicle approximately 37 h later. Among the important intrafollicular changes stimulated by the LH surge is the deposition by granulosa cells in the cumulus oophorus of a viscous mucopolysaccharide-rich matrix. The egg is embedded in this large sticky mass (up to 5 mm diameter), and the entire oocyte-cumulus complex becomes detached from the follicle wall at the time of follicle rupture. This development aids the rapid retrieval and identification of the egg for IVF.

Superovulation

To increase the number of ripe follicles available for egg collection, the ovaries must be exposed to supraphysiological gonadotrophin levels during the follicular phase of the IVF treatment cycle. The strategy is to increase the stimulus to follicular recruitment and override the process of follicular selection, whereby only one follicle would otherwise mature and ovulate. Usually, this is accomplished by giving clomiphene citrate, a mixed oestrogen antagonist/agonist, to increase pituitary secretion of endogenous LH and FSH and/or by injecting human menopausal gonadotrophin (HMG) which

is an extract of postmenopausal women's urine rich in both LH and FSH activity.

Because of the innate tendency to produce only one ripe egg in each cycle, even if multiple follicles are induced, egg maturity is usually variable at the time of follicle aspiration. Often, the eggs do not all fertilise and some of those that do give rise to embryos with variable potential for further development. This problem of follicular 'asynchrony' is presently a major barrier to consistent IVF success.

Another problem is that the uterus may be overstimulated by the high level of oestrogen secreted by multiple preovulatory follicles, so even if several embryos are produced by IVF, implantation may be impaired.

Follicular phase monitoring

To assess the ovarian response to superovulation therapy, follicular development is usually monitored by ultrasound scanning of the ovaries combined with serial measurements of oestrogen in blood or urine. Using modern ultrasound equipment, it is possible to visualise follicles within the ovaries and measure their diameters reasonably accurately when they exceed approximately 1.0 cm. At this size and beyond, preovulatory follicles begin to secrete important amounts of oestrogen; during the second half of the follicular phase, oestrogen levels correlate with the number and size of the follicles which are developing.

When the follicular phase is completed as judged by the combination of ovarian ultrasound, oestrogen measurements and predicted follicular phase length, an injection of human chorionic gonadotrophin (HCG) is given shortly before the expected onset of the LH surge. The egg collection has to be carried out within approximately 36 h after giving the HCG, since ovulation usually occurs at about 37 h. Egg collection can also be timed to the onset of the LH surge. However, this is often inconvenient since the surge can occur at any time of day and the facilities and staff required to collect eggs at the right time may not always be available.

Egg collection

Approximately 24 h after HCG injection or onset of the LH surge, cumulus expansion in preovulatory follicles starts and the oocyte-cumulus complex begins to loosen its attachment to the follicle wall and, by 36 h, it can be 'free-floating' in the follicular fluid. During this time, the egg undergoes the final stages of meiotic maturation so that, by the time of follicular rupture, it should contain only the haploid number of chromosomes, ready for fertilisation.

Egg collection is usually timed to take place 34–36 h after HCG injection shortly before the expected time of follicular rupture. Usually, it is done laparoscopically employing general anaesthesia. If the egg is not present in the first aspirate, the follicle can be refilled with culture medium and the aspiration repeated. A more recent development is to collect the eggs transvesically or transvaginally using ultrasonic visualisation and local anaesthesia. In this technique, preovulatory follices are located and the aspirating needle is usually passed along a guide attached to the ultrasound transducer into the follicles.

The cumulus-oocyte complex, easily visible with the naked eye, is picked up from the follicular fluid with a pipette and transferred into a plastic testtube containing 1.0 ml culture medium kept at physiological pH (7.4) and temperature (37°C). The egg is cultured under these conditions for at least 5 h, before it is inseminated (Fig. 23.1). This is to make sure that the egg is fully mature before fertilisation is attempted. Particularly immature eggs may need to be incubated for up to 24 h or more before insemination.

LABORATORY PROCEDURES

Culture Medium

The culture medium used for human IVF must be formulated with chemical reagents of the highest quality, which includes the water. As a 'quality-control' check, each batch of medium should be tested for its ability to sustain the development of two-cell mouse embryos to the hatching blastocyst stage. Anything with which the medium is liable to come into contact during the clinical procedure should also be checked for potential embryotoxicity using mouse embryo cultures.

Sperm Preparation

An hour or so before egg collection, the male partner produces a semen sample by masturbation

into a sterile, non-toxic plastic pot. He should refrain from ejaculation for at least three days beforehand to keep his sperm-count as high as possible. After liquefaction is complete, 0.5–1.0 ml

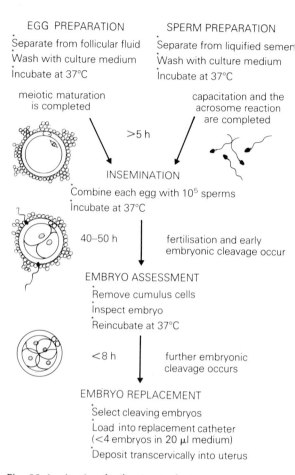

Fig. 23.1   *In vitro fertilisation technique.*

semen is carefully layered under 2.0 ml culture medium in a testtube which is then incubated at 37°C in the tissue culture incubator. During the next hour or so, the most motile spermatozoa in the semen will swim up into the culture medium above. This 'swim-up' method is a highly effective way of collecting motile sperm free from other cellular material and debris present in semen. The sperms collected in this way are diluted in fresh culture medium, pelleted by gentle centrifugation and then resuspended in more culture medium. Washed spermatozoa are then incubated for up to a further 5 h or so to ensure that capacitation and the acrosome reaction are completed before IVF is attempted.

Insemination and Embryo Culture

Each egg is cultured in a test-tube containing approximately 100 000 motile sperm per ml culture medium. After 40 h or so at 37°C, fertilisation and the first and second cleavage steps normally should have occurred, producing a 4-cell embryo. The stage of development is assessed by inspection under a stereodissecting microscope.

Embryo Replacement and Luteal Phase Support

Rapid and symmetrical cell cleavage in vitro is a sign of embryo vitality. A limited number (<4) of the most well-developed embryos should be selected for replacement to the uterus. The aim is to deposit the embryo(s) in the uterine cavity close to the fundus, avoiding contamination with blood and without traumatising the endometrium or cervix.

The catheter is loaded with a small drop of medium (about 20 µl) containing the embryos and gently passed through the cervical canal into the uterus. The embryo droplet is displaced into the fundus of the uterus with a small amount of air (<40 µl) and the catheter is withdrawn immediately.

To offset the consequences of uterine hyperstimulation by high circulating oestrogen levels caused by ovarian stimulation in the follicular phase, the women can be given a course of progesterone therapy as injections or pessaries to support corpus luteum function. This is usually started immediately after embryo replacement and continued for the remainder of the luteal phase. Blood samples for serum βHCG measurement are drawn at intervals after the replacement. If implantation occurs, serum βHCG should be raised on Days 10–12 after replacement and should approximately double every 1–2 days thereafter if a viable pregnancy develops. Clinical pregnancy should be confirmed by ultrasonic visualisation of the gestation sac approximately 4 weeks after embryo replacement.

RESULTS

Several thousand babies conceived by IVF have now been born, and almost every major city in Western Europe, Australia, Japan and the USA has at least one centre specialising in IVF and related techniques. The incidence of abnormalities in these 'test-tube' babies appears to be lower than that in the population at large.

The success of IVF as a clinical procedure can be influenced by numerous variables (*see* Table 23.1). Most internationally recognised centres are reporting overall results (pregnancy rate/embryo replacement) of around 25–30%, although this seems to vary with the type of patient treated. The best results are consistently achieved in younger women (≤35 years of age) with accessible ovaries, no endocrine dysfunction and whose male partner is free from sperm pathology. A majority of these can be expected to succeed within several successive IVF attempts.

Using current IVF methods, the most dramatic influence on pregnancy rates is the number of embryos replaced at any one time to the uterus. The success rate is less than 10% if only one embryo is replaced, but it rises to 50% when four or more are replaced. However, this benefit is offset by the increased incidence of multiple pregnancy which is approximately 15% in women receiving four embryos.

FUTURE DEVELOPMENTS

The development of IVF has advanced the treatment of human infertility. However, much further research is needed using human eggs, sperm and embryos if these techniques are to be perfected and made available to more couples.

Gamete Intra-Fallopian Tubal Transfer (GIFT) is a recent development being increasingly used by clinical departments which lack the laboratory facilities for IVF. Ovulation induction, egg collection and sperm washing are the same as for IVF. The oocytes and 100 000 sperm are then injected into the fimbrial ends of each tube at laparoscopy.

Research is also needed to be able to use these techniques to detect and prevent inherited diseases and the birth of deformed babies. For example, research with animal embryos indicates that it is possible to remove and culture cells from the preimplantation conceptus without causing it any harm. Chromosomal and molecular diagnostic tools could then be used to screen for defects while the embryo is held in storage (*see below*). In this way, only embryos free from recognisable defects (e.g. Down's sndrome or thalassaemia) need be removed from storage and replaced in the woman. This would be an immensely valuable advance, since it is estimated that genetic defects affect about 1% of babies born (about 70 000 babies per year in the UK). Moreover, over half of the 250 000 spontaneous abortions occurring every year in the UK have recognisable chromosome abnormalities. IVF-related research could also lead to the development of safer and more effective means of contraception.

Several babies have now been born from embryos which were stored in liquid nitrogen at −196°C. It would seem that the embryo can be kept for an unlimited period of time if stored frozen in this way. So far, the pregnancy rate following freezing of the embryo is as good as, and possibly better than, the success rate after immediate transfer. Since the hormone treatment used to stimulate the ovary may cause suboptimal conditions for embryo implantation, it might be better to return the embryo(s) one month later under the hormonal conditions of a normal menstrual cycle. When multiple embryos develop from one IVF attempt, repeated embryo replacements could be undertaken at monthly intervals until pregnancy occurs. This would be convenient, easy to organise, and would minimise the risk of multiple pregnancy if the number of embryos replaced on each occasion was restricted to three or less. Ethically, it might be more acceptable to store eggs and sperm separately rather than to store embryos. However, successful fertilisation and embryonic development after the freezing of a human egg in liquid nitrogen is as yet very limited.

FURTHER READING

Hillier S.G., Dawson K.J., Afnan M., Margara R.A. *et al.* (1985). Embryo culture: quality control before clinical *in vitro* fertilization. In *In Vitro Fertilization and Donor Insemination.* (Thompson W., Joyce, D.N., Newton, J.R. eds.) pp. 125–37. London: Royal College of Obstetricians and Gynaecologists.
Wood C., Trounson A., eds. (1984). *Clinical In Vitro Fertilization.* Berlin: Springer Verlag.

Index